Jesse Park Battershall

Food adulteration and its detection

Jesse Park Battershall

Food adulteration and its detection

ISBN/EAN: 9783337201005

Printed in Europe, USA, Canada, Australia, Japan

Cover: Foto ©Andreas Hilbeck / pixelio.de

More available books at **www.hansebooks.com**

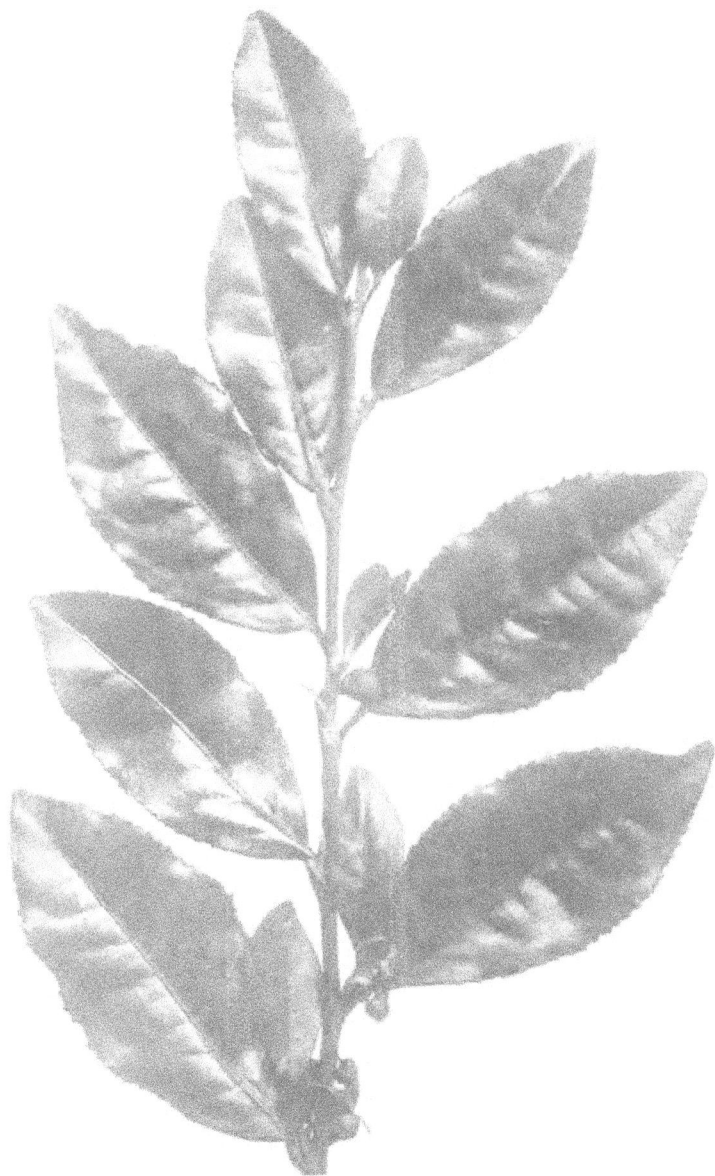

TEA PLANT.

FOOD

ADULTERATION

AND

ITS DETECTION.

WITH PHOTOMICROGRAPHIC PLATES AND
A BIBLIOGRAPHICAL APPENDIX.

BY

JESSE P. BATTERSHALL, Ph.D., F.C.S.,

CHEMIST, U.S. LABORATORY,
NEW YORK CITY.

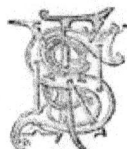

NEW YORK:
E. & F. N. SPON, 35, MURRAY STREET,
AND 125, STRAND, LONDON.
1887.

PREFACE.

To embody in a condensed form some salient features of the present status of Food Adulteration in the United States is the object of this volume. The importance of the subject, and the apparent need of a book of moderate dimensions relating thereto, must suffice as its *raison d'être*. The standard works have been freely consulted, and valuable data have been obtained from the recent reports of our State and Civic Boards of Health. The system of nomenclature accepted by the American Chemical Society has been generally adopted. It was, however, deemed advisable to retain such names as glycerine, sodium bicarbonate, etc., in place of the more modern but less well-known terms, glycerol and sodium hydrogen carbonate, even at a slight sacrifice of uniformity.

The photogravure plates, most of which represent the results of recent microscopical investigation, are considered an important feature of the book. And it is believed that the bibliographical appendix, and the collation of American Legislation on Adulteration, will supply a want for ready reference often experienced.

U. S. LABORATORY,
July 1st, 1887.

CONTENTS.

			PAGE
INTRODUCTION	..	..	1
TEA	..	..	12
COFFEE ..	..	..	29
COCOA AND CHOCOLATE		..	42
MILK	..		49
BUTTER ..	..	..	63
CHEESE ..	..		85
FLOUR, BREAD, AND STARCH			87
BAKERS' CHEMICALS ..	..		101
SUGAR ..	..	..	104
HONEY ..	..	..	121
CONFECTIONERY	..	..	129
BEER	..	..	132
WINE	..	..	157
LIQUORS ..		..	186
WATER ..		..	200
VINEGAR		..	225
PICKLES ..		..	232
OLIVE OIL		..	233
MUSTARD		..	239
PEPPER ..		..	243
SPICES ..	..	..	249
MISCELLANEOUS		..	254
BIBLIOGRAPHY ..		..	258
LAWS ..		..	268
INDEX		..	320

PLATES.

		PAGE
I.	TEA PLANT .. .. *frontispiece*	
II.	TEA LEAVES	17
III.	TEA AND OTHER LEAVES ..	18
IV.	CREAM AND COW'S MILK	61
V.	SKIMMED AND COLOSTRUM MILK ..	62
VI.	BUTTER AND OLEOMARGARINE	78
VII.	FAT CRYSTALS	79
VIII.	ARTIFICIAL DIGESTION OF BUTTER AND OLEOMARGARINE ..	82
IX.	STARCHES ..	100
X.	POLARISCOPE	112
XI.	ORGANISMS IN WATER	218
XII.	SPICES	252

FOOD ADULTERATION.

INTRODUCTION.

OF the various branches cognate to chemical research
which excite public attention, that of food adulteration
doubtless possesses the greatest interest. To the dealer in
alimentary substances, the significance of their sophistication is frequently merely one of profit or loss, and even this
comparatively unimportant consideration does not always
attach. But to the general community, the subject appeals
to interests more vital than a desire to avoid pecuniary
damage, and involving, as it necessarily does, the question
of health, it has engendered a feeling of uneasiness, accompanied by an earnest desire for trustworthy information
and data. The most usual excuses advanced by dishonest
traders, when a case of adulteration has been successfully
brought home to them—guilty knowledge being also
established—are, that they are compelled to resort to the
misdeed by the public demand for cheap commodities, that
the addition is harmless, or actually constitutes an improvement, as is asserted to be the case when chicory is added
to coffee, or that it serves as a preservative, as was formerly
alleged to be the fact when vinegar was fortified with
sulphuric acid. Pretexts of this sort are almost invariably
fallacious. The claim that manufacturers are often forced
into adulteration by the necessities of unfair trade competition possesses more weight—an honest dealer cannot as
a rule successfully compete with a dishonest one—and
has undoubtedly influenced many of the better class to

B

co-operate in attempts to prevent the practice. The general feeling of uncertainty which exists in the public mind concerning the actual extent and importance of food adulteration is probably to be ascribed to two causes. In the first place, most of the literature generally accessible relating to the subject has been limited to sensational newspaper articles, reciting some startling instance of food-poisoning, often unauthenticated and bearing upon its face evidences of exaggeration. By reason of such publications, periodical panics have been created in our large cities which, however, as a rule quickly subside, and the community relapses into the customary feeling of doubtful security, until aroused from its apathy by the next *exposé.* The fact that the only reliable results of food investigation have, until recently, been confined to purely scientific journals, and therefore not prominently brought to public notice, is another explanation of the lack of creditable information which generally prevails concerning this species of sophistication.

The adulteration of alimentary substances was practised in the civilised countries of Europe at a very remote date, and the early history of the art, mainly collated by Prof. Blyth in his valuable work on food,* is replete with interest. Bread certainly received due attention at the hands of the ancient sophisticator. Pliny makes several references to the adulteration of this food. In England, as early as the reign of King John, the sale of the commodity was controlled by the "Assize of Bread," which, although originally designed to regulate the price and size of the loaf, was subsequently amplified so as to include penalties for falsification, usually consisting of corporal punishment and exposure in the pillory. In France, in 1382, ordinances were promulgated specifying the proper mode of breadmaking, the punishment for infringement being similar in character to those inflicted in Great Britain. It is related that in the year 1525, a guilty baker "was condemned by

* 'Foods : Composition and Analysis,' pp. 1–18.

the court to be taken from the Châtelet prison to the cross
before the *Église des Carmes*, and thence to the gate of
Notre Dame and to other public places in Paris, in his shirt,
having his head and feet bare, with small loaves hung from
his neck, and holding a large wax candle, lighted, and in
each of the places enumerated he was to make *amende
honorable*, and ask mercy and pardon of God, the king, and
of justice for his fault." In Germany, during the fifteenth
century, the bread adulterator, while not subjected to a
religious penance, did not escape from a sufficiently practical rebuke, as it was the frequent custom to put him in a
basket attached to a long pole, and purge him of his mis-
deeds by repeated immersions in a pool of water.

Wine would also appear to have been exposed to
fraudulent admixture in former times. Pliny mentions
that in Rome considerable difficulty was experienced, even
by the wealthy, in securing the pure article, and in Athens
a public inspector was early appointed to prevent its adulteration. In England, during the reign of Edward the
Confessor, punishment for brewing bad beer was publicly
enforced, and, in 1529, official "ale tasters" flourished,
without whose approval the beverage was not to be sold.
In later years, Addison, referring to the manipulators of
wine of his time, writes : "These subtle philosophers are
daily employed in the transmutation of liquors, and, by
the power of magical drugs and incantations, raise under
the streets of London the choicest products of the hills and
valleys of France ; they squeeze Bordeaux out of the sloe
and draw champagne from an apple." * In the fifteenth
century, at Biebrich on the Rhine, a wine sophisticator was
forced to drink six quarts of his own stock, and it is recorded with due gravity that the test resulted fatally. Not
very many years since, a manufacturer of wine at Rheims
secured for his champagne, which was chiefly consumed in
Würtemberg, a high reputation, on account of the unusually

* *The Tatler*, 1710.

exhilarating effects following its use. Suspicion being at
length aroused, Liebig made a chemical examination of the
article, and found that it was at least unique in its gaseous
composition, being charged with one volume of carbonic acid
gas and two volumes of nitrous oxide, or "laughing gas."
These early attempts to control and punish adulteration,
while often possessing interest on account of their quaint-
ness, are chiefly important, as being the precursors of the
protective legal measures which exist in more modern times.

In 1802 the *Conseil de Salubrité* was established in Paris,
and this body has since developed into numerous health
boards, to whom the French are at present mainly indebted
for what immunity from food falsification they enjoy. A
very decided advance upon all preceding methods to regulate the public supply of food was signalised in 1874 by the
organisation in England of the Society of Public Analysts,
who formulated a legal definition of adulteration, and issued
the standards of purity which articles of general consumption should meet. This society was supported in its
valuable services by the enactment, in 1875, of the Sale of
Food and Drugs Act, which, with the amendment added
in 1879, seems to embrace all necessary safeguards against
the offences sought to be suppressed. The results of their
work are tabulated as follows :—

Year.	Samples Examined.	Samples Adulterated.	Percentage of Adulterated.
1875-6	15,989	2,895	18·10
1877	11,943	2,371	17·70
1878	15,107	2,505	16·58
1879	17,574	3,032	17·25
1880	17,919	3,132	17·47

Of the total number of samples tested, the classification
of adulterations is as below :—

Per cent.

Milk ..   ..   50·98
Butter ..   ..   5·73
Groceries ..   ..   12·90

	Per cent.
Drugs	2·52
Wine, spirits, and beer	15·18
Bread and flour	2·68
Waters (including mineral)	9·18
Sundries	0·83

More recent data concerning the falsification of food in Great Britain are as follows :—

Year.	Samples Tested.	Number Adulterated.	Per cent. of Adulterated.
1881	17,823	2,495	14·0
1882	19,439	2,916	15·0
1883	14,900	2,453	16·4

Of the samples of spirits and beer examined, about 25 per cent. were adulterated.

The results of the work done at the Paris Municipal Laboratory are the following :—

Year.	Samples Tested.	Good.	Passable.	Bad.	
				Not Injurious.	Injurious.
1881	6,258	1,565	1,523	2,608	562
1882	10,752	2,707	2,679	3,822	1,544
1883	14,686	—	—	—	—

The American characteristic of controlling their own personal affairs, and the resulting disinclination to resort to anything savouring of parental governmental interference, has probably had its effect in retarding early systematic action in the matter of adulteration. Sporadic attempts to secure legislative restrictions have, it is true, occasionally been made, but the laws passed were almost invariably of a specific nature, designed to meet some isolated case, and were destined to share the fate of most legislation of the kind—the particular adulteration being for the nonce suppressed, the law became practically a dead letter. Subse-

quent effort to obtain more comprehensive laws inclined to
the other extreme, and the enactments secured were so
general in scope, and so deficient in details, that loopholes
were inadvertently allowed to remain, through which the
crafty adulterator often managed to escape.

The present food legislation in the United States was to
some extent anticipated in 1848 by an Act of Congress to
secure the purity of imported drugs. In this enactment
these are directed to be tested by the standards established
by the various official pharmacopœias ; twenty-three are
specifically enumerated, the most important being Peruvian
bark and opium. The Act is still in force. All previous
efforts to regulate the quality of our food supply culminated
in 1877 in formal action being taken by several of the
State Boards of Health, at whose instance laws against
adulteration were formulated, and chemists commissioned
to collect and examine samples of alimentary substances,
and furnish reports on the subject. These may be found
in the publications of the same, notably in the volumes
issued by the New York, Massachusetts, Michigan, and
New Jersey Boards. The service rendered to the public
by these investigations is almost incalculable, and the
annual reports containing the results of the same are
fraught with interest. For the first time we are placed in
possession of trustworthy statistics, indicating the extent
of food sophistication in this country.

The annual report of the New York City Board of
Health for the year 1885 furnishes the following statistics :—

Milk examined	7,006 samples.
Adulterated milk destroyed	1,701 quarts.
Candy destroyed	72,700 lbs.
Cheese ,, ...	5,700 ,,
Packages of tea, ordered out of sale ..	266
Canned goods condemned	39,905 ,,
Pickles ,, ,, ...	4,000
Coffee ,. ,, ...	4,100 ,,

Pepper, spices, and baking powder .. 1,455 lbs.
Meat and fish .. .. 790,410 „
Fruit .. .. 212,000 „
Total inspections 43,665
Complaints made 5,786
Fines collected 82,070

Some of the results of the work performed by the New
York State Board of Health during the year 1882 are
tabulated below :—

Article.	Number of Samples Tested.	Number found to be Adulterated.	Per cent. of Adulterated.
Butter	40	21	52·50
Olive oil	16	9	56·25
Baking powder	84	8	9·52
Flour	117	8	6·84
Spices	180	112	62·22
Coffee (ground)	21	19	90·48
Candy (yellow)	10	7	70·00
Brandy	25	16	64·00
Sugar (brown)	67	4	5·97

In interpreting the significance of the foregoing table, it
should be borne in mind that in the vast majority of cases
the adulterations practised were not of an injurious nature,
but consisted of a fraudulent admixture of some cheaper
substance, the object being an increase of bulk or weight
resulting in augmented profit.

Much of the embarrassment experienced by health
authorities in their efforts to bring persons guilty of food
adulteration to punishment is due to the lack of explicit
detail in the law. It is far easier to substantiate the fact of
the adulteration than it is to produce the offender in court
and secure his conviction. Numerous cases are on record
illustrating the peculiar contingencies which at times arise.
Probably with the best intention, a milk vendor labelled his
wagon, "Country skimmed milk, sold as adulterated ;" an
inspector bought a sample, not noticing the label, and the

magistrate convicted the vendor, doubtless on the ground
that due attention had not been directed to the advertise-
ment.* Chief Justice Cockburn, in referring to an
analogous case, said: "If the seller chooses to sell an
article with a certain admixture, the onus lies on him to
prove that the purchaser knew what he was purchasing."
In most instances, when in ostensible compliance with the
law, a package bears a label purporting to state the actual
nature of its contents, the label is either printed in such
small type, or is placed in so inconspicuous a position, that
the buyer is in ignorance of its existence at the time the
purchase is made. A confectioner in Boston was suspected
of selling adulterated candy, and while it was proved that a
sample bought of him contained a dangerous proportion of
a poisonous pigment — chromate of lead — he escaped
conviction, on the plea that candy was not an article of
food within the meaning of the existing law, which, it seems,
has since been amended so as to embrace cases of this
kind.

In a recent action brought by the New York Board of
Health to obtain an injunction against the sale of certain
Ping Suey teas, it was held by the court, in refusing to
grant the same, that, although the teas in question had
been clearly shown to be adulterated with gypsum, Prussian
blue, sand, etc., it was likewise necessary to prove that the
effect of these admixtures was such as to constitute a
serious danger to public health.

As a result of the publicity lately given to the subject of
food adulteration, a popular impression has been produced
that any substance employed as an adulterant of, or a
substitute for another, is to be avoided *per se*. Perhaps the
common belief that for all purposes cotton-seed oil is
inferior to olive oil, and oleomargarine to butter, is the most
striking illustration of this tendency. Now, as a matter of
fact, pure cotton-seed oil, as at present found on the market,

---

* 'Analyst,' 1880, p. 225.

is less liable to become rancid than the product of the olive, and, for many culinary uses, it is at least quite as serviceable. Absolute cleanliness is a *sine qua non* in the successful manufacture of oleomargarine, and, as an economical substitute for the inferior kinds of butter often exposed for sale, its discovery cannot justly be regarded a misfortune. The sale of these products, *under their true name*, should not only be allowed, but under some circumstances even encouraged.

The benefits accruing to the community by reason of the service of our State Boards of Health are so evident and so important, that it is almost incredible that these bodies have not been put in possession of all the facilities necessary for their work. It would appear, however, that, while our legislators have been induced to enact good laws regulating adulteration, they have often signally failed to fulfil all the requirements indispensable to the efficient execution of the same. Without entering into the details of this branch of the subject, it is proper to observe that owing to the lack of necessary funds, great pecuniary embarrassment has been experienced in securing the services of a competent corps of experts, who, in addition to their inadequate remuneration, must incur the expenses of purchasing samples. The appointment of public analysts in our larger towns and cities—as has for some time been the case in Great Britain—is certainly to be urgently recommended.

All attempts to awaken public interest in the subject of food adulteration are of any real service only as they may be conducive to the adoption of more advanced and improved measures for the suppression of the practice.

In general, the adulterations to which food is subjected may be divided into those positively deleterious to health (such as the colouring of confectionery by chrome yellow), those which are only fraudulent (such as the addition of flour to mustard), and those which may be fairly considered as accidental (such as the presence of a small amount of sand in tea). It would exceed the limits of this volume to enter into a comprehensive review of the almost endless varieties of adulteration. The following list embraces the articles most exposed to falsification, together with the adulterants commonly employed :—

Article.	Common Adulterants.
Baker's chemicals	Starch, alum.
Bread and flour	Other meals, alum.
Butter	Water, colouring matter, oleomargarine, and other fats.
Canned foods	Metallic poisons.
Cheese	Lard, oleomargarine, cotton-seed oil, metallic salts (in rind).
Cocoa and chocolate	Sugar, starch, flour.
Coffee	Chicory, peas, rye, corn, colouring matters.
Confectionery	Starch-sugar, starch, artificial essences, poisonous pigments, terra alba, plaster of Paris.
Honey	Glucose-syrup, cane sugar.
Malt liquors	Artificial glucose and bitters, sodium bicarbonate, salt.
Milk	Water, and removal of cream.
Mustard	Flour, turmeric, cayenne.
Olive oil	Cotton-seed and other oils.
Pepper	Various ground meals.
Pickles	Salts of copper.
Spices	Pepper-dust, starch, flour.
Spirits	Water, fusil oil, aromatic ethers, burnt sugar.
Sugar	Starch-sugar.
Tea	Exhausted tea leaves, foreign leaves, indigo, Prussian blue, gypsum, soap-stone, sand.
Vinegar	Water, sulphuric acid.
Wine	Water, spirits, coal tar and vegetable colours, factitious imitations.

The above table includes those admixtures which have actually been detected by chemists of repute within the past few years, and omits many rather sensational forms of adulteration mentioned in the early treatises on the subject, the practice of which appears to have been discontinued.

In the following pages, some of the more important

articles of food and drink are described with especial reference to their chemical relations and the ordinary adulterations to which they are exposed. It should be added, that many of the methods of examination given are quoted in a condensed form from the more extensive works on food-analysis.

TEA.

THE early history of tea is probably contemporary with that of China, although, in that country, the first authentic mention of the plant was as late as A.D. 350; while, in European literature, its earliest notice occurs in the year 1550. The first important consignment of tea into England took place in 1657. Chinese tea made its appearance in the United States in 1711; in 1858, the importation of Japan tea began. During the season of 1883–1884, the importation of tea into this country * was—from China, 30½ millions of pounds; from Japan, 32½ millions of pounds. Recently, numerous shipments of Indian tea have been placed upon our markets, the quality of which compares very favourably with the older and better known varieties. During the past four years the consumption of tea in this country has materially decreased; whilst that of coffee has undergone an almost corresponding increase. The *per capita* consumption of tea and coffee in the United States as compared with that of Great Britain is as follows:—United States, tea, 1·16 ; coffee, 9·50 ; Great Britain, tea, 4·62 ; coffee, 0·89. In the year 1885 our importation of tea approximated 82 millions of pounds, that of coffee being nearly 455 millions of pounds.

Genuine tea is the prepared leaf of *Thea sinensis*. The growth of the tea shrub is usually restricted by artificial means to a height of from three to five feet. It is ready for picking at the end of the third year, the average life of the plant being about ten years. The first picking is made in the middle of April, the second on the 1st of May, the third in the middle of July, and occasionally a fourth during

---

* I.e. the United States.

the month of August. The first pickings, which obviously consist of the young and more tender leaves, furnish the finer grades of tea. After sorting, the natural moisture of the leaves is partially removed by pressing and rolling; they are next more thoroughly dried by gently roasting in iron pans for a few minutes. The leaves are then rolled on bamboo tables and again roasted, occasionally re-rolled and re-fired, and finally separated into the various kinds, such as twankay, hyson, young hyson, gunpowder, etc., by passing through sieves. The difference between green and black tea is mainly due to the fact that the former is dried shortly after gathering, and then rolled and carefully fired, whereas black tea is first made up into heaps, which are exposed to the air for some time before firing and allowed to undergo a species of fermentation, resulting in the conversion of its original olive-green into a black colour. The methods employed in the preparation of the tea are somewhat modified in their details in the different tea districts of China and Japan. In Japan two varieties of the leaf are used, which are termed "otoko" (male), and "ona" (female), the former being larger and coarser than the latter. After picking, the leaves are steamed by placing them in a wooden tray suspended over boiling water, in which they are allowed to remain for about half a minute. They are next thrown upon a tough paper membrane attached to the top of an oven, which is heated by burning charcoal covered with ashes, where they are constantly manipulated by the hand until the light-green colour turns to a dark olive, and the leaves have become spirally twisted. After this "firing," the tea is dried at a low temperature for from four to eight hours; it is next sorted by passing through sieves, and is then turned over to the "go-downs," or warehouses of the foreigners, where the facing process is carried on by placing the tea in large metallic bowls, heated by means of a furnace, and gradually adding the various pigments used, the mixture being continually stirred. The tea is finally again sorted by means of large fans, and is now ready for packing and shipment.

The sophistications to which tea is exposed have received the careful attention of chemists, but not to a greater extent than the importance of the subject merits; indeed, it is safe to assert that no article among alimentary substances has been, at least in past years, more subjected to adulteration. The falsifications which are practised to no inconsiderable extent may be conveniently divided into three classes.

1st. Additions made for the purpose of giving increased weight and bulk, which include foreign leaves and spent tea leaves, and also certain mineral substances, such as metallic iron, sand, brick-dust, etc.

2nd. Substances added in order to produce an artificial appearance of strength to the tea decoction, catechu and other bodies rich in tannin being mainly resorted to for this purpose.

3rd. The imparting of a bright and shining appearance to an inferior tea by means of various colouring mixtures or "facings," which operation, while sometimes practised upon black tea, is far more common with the green variety. This adulteration involves the use of soap-stone, gypsum, China clay, Prussian blue, indigo, turmeric, and graphite. The author lately received from Japan several samples of the preparations employed for facing the tea in that country, the composition of which was shown by analysis to be essentially as follows:—

1. Magnesium silicate (soap-stone).
2. Calcium sulphate (gypsum).
3. Turmeric.
4. Indigo.
5. Ferric ferrocyanide (Prussian blue).
6. Soap-stone, 47·5 per cent.; gypsum, 47·5 per cent.; Prussian blue, 5 per cent.
7. Soap-stone, 45 per cent.; gypsum, 45 per cent.; Prussian blue, 10 per cent.

8. Soap-stone, 75 per cent. ; indigo, 25 per cent.

9. Soap-stone, 60 per cent ; indigo, 40 per cent.

The "facing" or "blooming" of tea is often accomplished by simply placing it in an iron pan, heated by a fire, and rapidly incorporating with it one of the preceding mixtures (Nos. 6, 7, 8, or 9), in the proportion of about half a dram to seven or eight pounds of the tea, a brisk stirring being maintained until the desired shade of colour is produced.

Some of the above forms of sophistication usually go together ;—thus exhausted tea is restored by facing. The collection of the spent leaves takes place in China. Much of the facing was, until about three years since, done in New York city, and constituted a regular branch of business, which included among its operations such metamorphoses as the conversion of a green tea into a black, and *vice versâ*.

According to James Bell,[*] the composition of genuine tea is as follows :—

	Congou.	Young Hyson.
	per cent.	per cent.
Moisture	8·20	5·96
Theine	3·24	2·33
Albumin, insoluble..	17·20	16·83
„ soluble	0·70	0·80
Extractive, by alcohol	6·79	7·05
Dextrine, or gum	..	0·50
Pectin and pectic acid	2·60	3·22
Tannin	16·40	27·14
Chlorophyll and resin	4·60	4·20
Cellulose	34.00	25·90
Ash	6·27	6·07
	100·00	100·00

The ash of samples of uncoloured and unfaced tea, and of spent tea analysed by the author, had the following composition :—

* 'Chemistry of Foods.'

	Oolong (average of 50 samples).	Japan.	Spent Black Tea.
	per cent.	per cent.	per cent.
Total ash	6·04	5·58	2·52
Soluble in water	3·44	3·60	0·28
Per cent. soluble	57·00	64·55	11·11

Composition.

Silica	11·30	9·30	27·75
Chlorine	1·53	1·60	0·79
Potassa..	37·46	41·63	
Soda	1·40	1·12	
Ferric oxide..	1·80	1·12 }	16·00
Alumina	5·13	4·26 }	
Manganic oxide	2·10	1·30	
Lime	9·43	8·18	19·66
Magnesia	8·00	5·33	11·20
Phosphoric acid	12·27	16·62	15·80
Sulphuric acid	4·18	3·64	1·10
Carbonic acid	5·40	5·90	6·70
	100·00	100·00	99·00

"Tea dust" affords a high proportion of ash, sometimes amounting to 20 per cent., the composition of which is usually strikingly different from that of the ash of ordinary tea. It is deficient in potassa and phosphoric acid, and the amount of ash insoluble in water and acids is very excessive, as is shown by the following analysis, made by the author :—

Ash of Tea Dust.

	Per cent.
Insoluble in acids	60·30
Alumina and ferric oxide	6·60
Lime	5·10
Magnesia	7·89
Potassa	11·00
Soda	2·51
Sulphuric acid	1·23
Chlorine	0·63
Phosphoric acid	4·73
	99·99
Ash insoluble in water	80·00

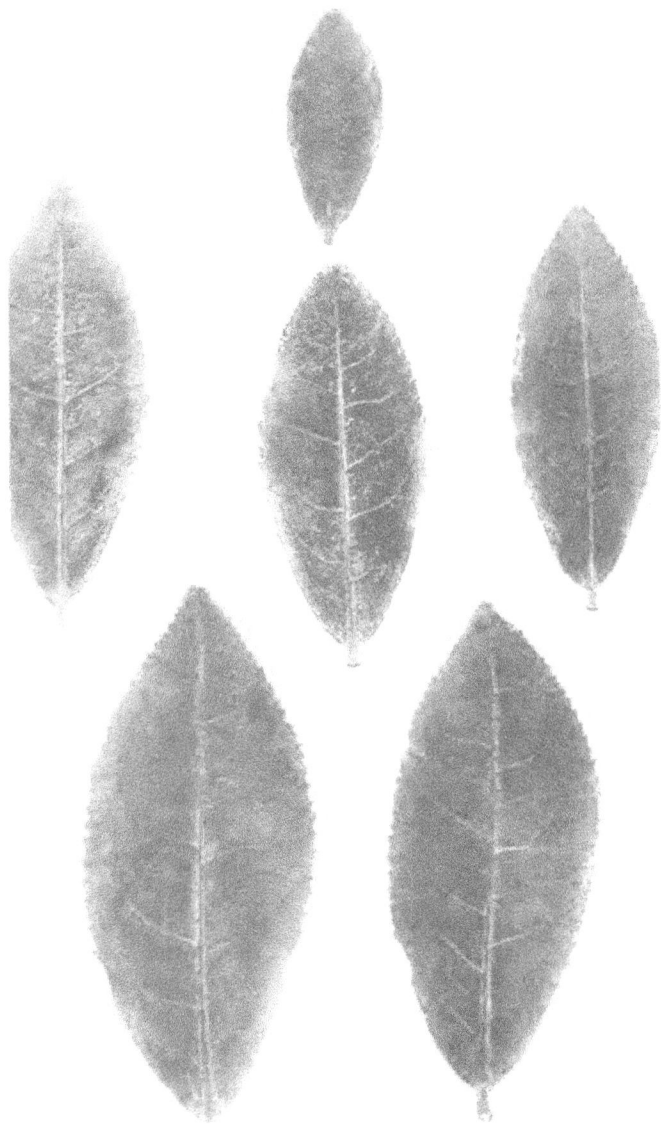

The portion of ash insoluble in acids consisted of silica, clay, and soapstone, indicating that the ash of tea dust is largely composed of the mineral substances employed for " facing" purposes.

The characteristics of the ash of unspent tea are the presence of manganic oxide, the large proportion of potassium salts present, and the solubility of the ash in water. The amount of ash in genuine tea ranges from five to six per cent. In the absence of exhausted leaves, it has been found that the finer sorts of tea afford a smaller proportion of ash than the inferior grades. It will be noticed that spent tea ash exhibits a marked increase in the proportion of insoluble compounds (silica, alumina, and ferric oxide), as well as a total absence of potassium salts.

The presence of foreign leaves, and, in some instances, of mineral adulterants in tea is best detected by means of a microscopical examination of the suspected sample. The genuine tea-leaf is characterised by its peculiar serrations and venations. Its border exhibits serrations which stop a little short of the stalk, while the venations extend from the central rib, nearly parallel to one another, but turn just before reaching the border of the leaf.

Plate I. (Frontispiece) is a photogravure of a twig of the tea plant, in possession of the author. The leaves are of natural size, but the majority are of a greater maturity than those used in the preparation of tea, which more resemble in size the few upper leaves.

Plate II. shows more distinctly the serrations and venations of the tea-leaf. The Chinese are said to occasionally employ ash, camelia, and dog-rose leaves for admixture with tea, and the product is stated to have formerly been subjected in England to the addition of sloe, willow, beech, hawthorn, oak, etc. For scenting purposes, chulan flowers, rose, jasmine, and orange leaves, have been employed. The writer has lately received from Japan specimens of

C

willow, wisteria, *te-mo-ki*, and other leaves which at one
time were used in that country as admixtures.

Plate III. exhibits some of these leaves, two genuine
Japan tea-leaves being included for purpose of comparison.
The leaves represented in this plate are : 1, beech ; 2, hawthorn ; 3, rose ; 4, Japan tea ; 5, willow ; 6, *te-mo-ki* ;
7, elm ; 8, wisteria ; 9, poplar. From very recent reports of
the American consuls in Japan and China, it would appear
that the addition of foreign leaves to tea is at present but
seldom resorted to, and this accords with the author's
experience in the testing of the teas imported into this
country.

In 1884, the Japanese Government made it a criminal
offence to adulterate tea, and instituted "tea guilds,"
which are governed by very stringent laws, and of which
most dealers of repute are members. The facing of tea
does not appear, however, to have been considered an
adulteration, its continued practice being justified by the
plea that otherwise Japan teas would not suit the taste of
American consumers.

In the microscopic examination of tea, the sample should
be moistened with hot water and spread out on a glass
plate, and then submitted to a careful inspection, especial
attention being directed to the general outline of the leaf
and its serrations and venations. The presence of exhausted tea-leaves may often be detected by their soft
texture and generally disintegrated appearance. If a
considerable quantity of the tea be placed in a long glass
cylinder and agitated with cold water, the colouring
and other abnormal substances frequently become detached, and either rise to the surface of the liquid as a sort
of scum, or fall to the bottom as a sediment. In this way
Prussian blue, indigo, soapstone, gypsum, sand, and
turmeric can often be separated, and subsequently recognised by their characteristic appearance under the microscope. The separated substances should also be subjected

PLATE III.

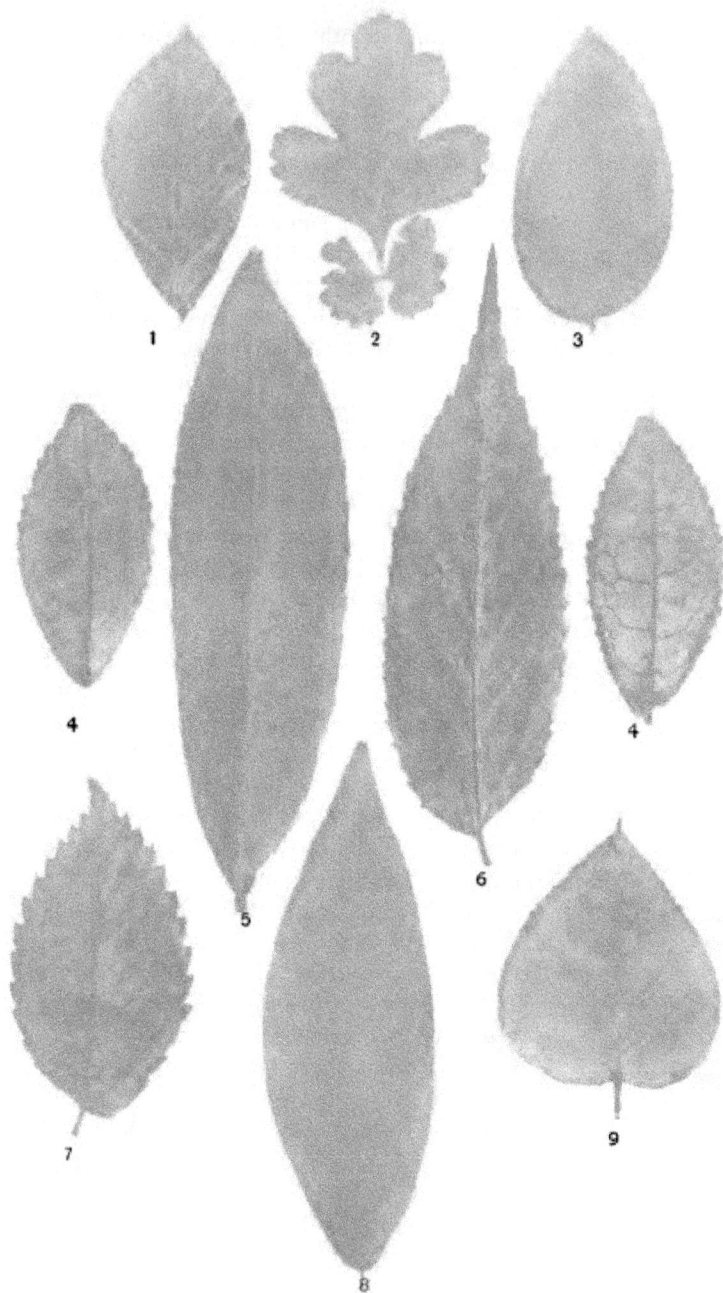

TEA AND OTHER LEAVES.

to a chemical examination. Prussian blue is detected by heating with a solution of sodium hydroxide, filtering, acidulating the filtrate with acetic acid, and then adding ferric chloride, when, in its presence, a blue colour will be produced. Indigo is best recognised by the microscopic examination. It is not decolorised by caustic alkali, but it dissolves in sulphuric acid to a blue liquid. Soapstone, gypsum, sand, and metallic iron, are identified by means of the usual chemical reactions. A compound very aptly termed "Lie-tea," is sometimes met with. It forms little pellets, consisting of tea-dust mixed with foreign leaves, sand, etc., and held together by means of gum or starch. This falls to powder if treated with boiling water. In the presence of catechu, the tea infusion usually assumes a muddy appearance upon standing. In case iron salts have been employed to deepen the colour of the infusion, they can be detected by treating the ground tea-leaves with acetic acid, and testing the filtered solution with potassium ferrocyanide. Tea should not turn black upon immersion in hydrosulphuric acid water, nor should it impart a blue colour to ammonia water. The infusion should be amber-coloured, and not become reddened by the addition of an acid.

The United States Tea Adulteration Act was passed by Congress in 1883. The enactment of this law was largely due to the exertions of prominent tea merchants, whose business interests were seriously affected by the sale (principally in trade auctions) of the debased or spurious article. It is stated in the official report of the United States Tea Examiner at New York City, that from March 1883 to December of the same year, 856,281 packages (about four millions of pounds) of tea were inspected, of which 7000 packages (325,000 pounds) were rejected as unfit for consumption. Since the enforcement in New York City of the Tea Adulteration Act, nearly 2000 samples of tea have been chemically tested under the

direction of the author. The proportion grossly adulterated
has been a little over nine per cent. But this does not
apply to the total amount imported, since only those
samples which were somewhat suspicious in appearance
were submitted for analysis. As the result of the past two
years' experience in the chemical examination of tea, the
prevailing adulterations were found to be of two kinds—
the admixture of spent tea-leaves, and the application
to the tea of a facing preparation. A natural green tea
possesses a dull hue, and is but seldom met with in the
trade ; some Moyunes and uncoloured Japans (which
latter, properly speaking, is not a green tea) being almost
the only varieties not exhibiting the bright metallic lustre
due to the facing process. The addition of foreign leaves
was detected only in a few instances ; the presence of sand
and gravel occurred far more frequently. Apropos of the
practical utility of Governmental sanitary legislation, it can
be stated that, since the enforcement of the Adulteration
Act, the tea imported into the city of New York has very
perceptibly improved in quality.

Attempts in tea culture are being made in the United
States of Columbia, S.A. A specimen of the prepared
plant received by the writer, differed greatly in appearance
from the Chinese and Japanese products. The leaves,
which had not been rolled but were quite flat, possessed
a light pea-green colour and a fine but rather faint aroma.
An examination indicated that the tea, although very
delicate in quality, was seriously deficient in body.

The analysis showed :—

	Per cent.
Moisture	6·70
Total ash	4·82
Ash soluble in water	1·62
Ash insoluble in water	3·20
Ash insoluble in acid	0·16
Extract	27·40
Tannic acid	4·31
Theine	0·66
Insoluble leaf	65·90

The following Tea Assay, while not including the determinations of all the proximate constituents of the plant, will, it is believed, in most instances suffice to indicate to the analyst the presence of spent leaves, mineral colouring matters, and other inorganic adulterations.

Theine (*Caffeine*), $C_8H_{10}N_4O_2$.—Contrary to the once general belief, there does not always exist a direct relation between the quality of tea (at least so far as this is indicated by its market price) and the proportion of theine contained, although the physiological value of the plant is doubtless due to the presence of this alkaloid.

The commercial tea-taster is almost entirely guided in his judgment in regard to the value of a sample of tea by the age of the leaf, and by the flavour or bouquet produced upon "drawing," and this latter quality is to be mainly ascribed to the volatile oil.

The following process will serve for the estimation of theine :—A weighed quantity of the tea is boiled with distilled water until the filtered infusion ceases to exhibit any colour. The filtrate is evaporated on a water bath to the consistence of a syrup; it is next mixed with calcined magnesia to alkaline reaction, and carefully evaporated to dryness.

The residue obtained is then finely powdered, digested for a day or so with ether (or chloroform) and filtered, the remaining undissolved matter being again digested with a fresh quantity of ether, so long as any further solution of theine takes place. The ether is now removed from the united filtrates by distillation, whereupon the theine will be obtained in a fairly pure condition.

Theine contains a very large proportion of nitrogen (almost 29 per cent.), and Wanklyn * has suggested the application of his ammonia process (see p. 205) to the analysis of tea. Genuine tea is stated to yield from 0·7 to 0·8 per cent of total ammonia, when tested in this manner.

* ' Tea, Coffee, and Cocoa Analysis.'

Volatile Oil.—Ten grammes of the tea are distilled with water; the distillate is filtered, saturated with calcium chloride, then well agitated with ether, and allowed to remain at rest for some time. The ethereal solution is subsequently drawn off, and spontaneously evaporated in a weighed capsule. The increase in weight gives approximately the amount of oil present. A sample of good black tea yielded by this method 0·87 per cent. of volatile oil.

Tannin.—Two grammes of the well-averaged sample are boiled with 100 c.c. of water, for about an hour, and the infusion filtered, the undissolved matter remaining upon the filter being thoroughly washed with hot water, and the washings added to the solution first obtained. If necessary, the liquid is next reduced to a volume of 100 c.c. by evaporation over a water-bath. It is then heated to boiling, and 25 c.c. of a solution of cupric acetate added. The copper solution is prepared by dissolving five grammes of the salt in 100 c.c. of water, and filtering. The precipitate formed is separated by filtration, well washed, dried, and ignited in a porcelain crucible. A little nitric acid is then added and the ignition repeated. One gramme of the cupric oxide thus obtained represents 1·305 grammes of tannin. For the estimation of spent leaves (especially in black tea), Mr. Allen suggests the following formula, in which E represents the percentage of spent tea, and T the percentage of tannin found :—

$$E = \frac{(10 - T)\ 100}{8}.$$

The Ash.—a. Total Ash.—Five grammes of the sample are placed in a platinum dish and ignited over a Bunsen burner until complete incineration is accomplished. The vessel is allowed to cool in a desiccator, and is then quickly weighed. In genuine tea the total ash should not be much below 5 per cent., nor much above 6 per cent., and it should not be magnetic. In faced teas the proportion of total ash is sometimes 10 per cent.; in "lie-tea" it may reach 30 per cent.;

while in spent tea it frequently falls below 3 per cent., the ash in this case being abnormally rich in lime salts, and poor in potassium salts.

b. Ash insoluble in water.—The total ash obtained in *a* is washed into a beaker, and boiled with water for a considerable time. It is then brought upon a filter, washed, dried, ignited, and weighed. In unadulterated tea it rarely exceeds 3 per cent. of the sample taken.

c. Ash soluble in water.—This proportion is obtained by deducting the ash insoluble in water from the total ash. Genuine tea contains from 3 per cent. to 3·5 per cent. of soluble ash, or at least 50 per cent. of the total ash, whereas in exhausted tea the amount is often but 0·5 per cent. The following formula has been proposed for the calculation of the percentage of spent tea E, where S is the percentage of soluble ash obtained :—

$$E = (6 - 2\ S)\ 20.$$

A sample prepared by averaging several good grades of black tea, was mixed with an equal quantity of exhausted tea-leaves. The proportion of soluble ash in the mixture was found to be 1·8 per cent. According to the above formula, the spent tea present would be 48 per cent., or within 2 per cent. of the actual amount.

d. Ash insoluble in acid.—The ash insoluble in water is boiled with dilute hydrochloric acid, and the residue separated by filtration, washed, ignited, and weighed. In pure tea, the remaining ash ranges between 0·3 and 0·8 per cent.; in faced tea, or in tea adulterated by the addition of sand, etc., it may reach the proportion of 2 to 5 per cent. Fragments of silica and brickdust are occasionally found in the ash insoluble in acid.

The Extract.—Two grammes of the *carefully sampled* tea are boiled with water until all soluble matter is dissolved, more water being added from time to time to prevent the solution becoming too concentrated. The operation may also be conducted in a flask connected with an ascending Liebig's condenser. In either case, the infusion obtained is poured upon a tared filter, and the remaining insoluble leaf repeatedly washed with hot water so long as the filtered liquor shows a colour. The filtrate is now diluted to a volume of 200 c.c., and of this 50 c.c, are taken and evaporated in a weighed dish until the weight of the extract remains constant. Genuine tea affords from 32 to 50 per cent. of extract, according to its age and quality ; in spent tea the proportion of extract will naturally be greatly reduced. Mr. Allen employs the formula below for determining the percentage of spent tea E in a sample, R representing the percentage of extract found.

$$E = \frac{(32 - R)\,100}{30}.$$

In order to test the practical value of this equation, a sample of black tea was mixed with 50 per cent. of spent tea-leaves, and a determination made of the extract afforded. The calculated proportion of spent tea was 44 per cent., instead of 50 per cent. It should be added, however, that the tea taken subsequently proved to be of a very superior quality, yielding an extract of 40 per cent.

Gum (Dextrine).—The proportion of gum contained in genuine tea is usually inconsiderable. Its separation is effected by treating the concentrated extract with alcohol, allowing the mixture to stand at rest for a few hours, and collecting the precipitated gum upon a tared filter, and carefully drying and weighing it. As a certain amount of mineral matter is generally present in the precipitate, this should afterwards be incinerated and a deduction made for the ash thus obtained. A more satisfactory method is to treat the separated dextrine with very dilute sulphuric acid, and estimate the amount of glucose formed by means of Fehling's solution (see p. 37) ; 100 parts of glucose are equivalent to 90 parts of dextrine.

Insoluble Leaf.—The insoluble leaf as obtained in the determination of the extract, together with the weighed filter, is placed in an air-bath, and dried for at least eight hours at a temperature of 110,°* and then weighed. In genuine tea the amount of insoluble leaf ranges from 47 to 54 per cent. ; in exhausted tea it may reach a proportion of 75 per cent. or more. It should be noted that in the foregoing estimations the tea is taken in its ordinary air-dried condition. If it be desired to reduce the results obtained to a dry basis, an allowance for the moisture present in the sample (an average of 6 to 8 per cent.), or a direct determination of the same must be made.

The following tabulation gives the constituents of genuine tea, so far as the ash, extract, and insoluble leaf are involved :—

Total ash ranges between 4·7 and 6·2 per cent.

Ash soluble in water ranges between 3 and 3·5 per cent. ; should equal 50 per cent of total ash.

Ash insoluble in water, not over 3 per cent.

Ash insoluble in acid ranges between 0·3 and 0·8 per cent.

Extract† ranges between 32 and 50 per cent.

Insoluble leaf ranges between 43 and 58 per cent.

The table below may prove useful as indicating the requirements to be exacted when the chemist is asked to give an opinion concerning the presence of facing admixtures, or of exhausted or foreign leaves in a sample of tea.

Total ash should not be under 4·5 per cent. or above 7 per cent.

Ash soluble in water should not be under 40 per cent. of total ash.

* The degrees of temperature given in the text refer to the Centigrade thermometer ; their equivalents on the Fahrenheit scale can be obtained by means of the formula $\frac{9}{5}$ C.° + 32 = F.°.

† In low grade, but unadulterated Congou tea, the extract occasionally falls so low as 25 per cent.

Ash insoluble in water should not be over 3·25 per cent.

Ash insoluble in acid should not be over 1 per cent.

Extract (excepting in poor varieties of Congou tea) should not be under 30 per cent.

Insoluble Leaf should not be over 60 per cent.

The British Society of Public Analysts adopt:—

Total ash (dry basis), not over 8 per cent. (at least 3 per cent. should be soluble in water).

Extract (tea as sold), not under 30 per cent.

Below are the proportions of total ash, ash soluble in water, and extract found in 850 samples of tea (mostly inferior and faced), examined under the direction of the author in the U.S. Laboratory :—

TOTAL ASH.

Range ..	5 to 5½ per cent.	5½ to 6 per cent.	6 to 6½ per cent.	6½ to 7 per cent.	7 to 8 per cent.	8 per cent. and over.
Number ..	21	76	102	194	421	36
Per cent. ..	2·47	8·94	12·00	21·64	49·53	4·23

ASH SOLUBLE IN WATER.

Range ..	Under 2 per cent.	2 to 3 per cent.	3 to 3½ per cent.	3½ per cent. and over.
Number ..	25	649	157	19
Per cent. ..	2·94	76·35	18·70	2·23

EXTRACT.

Range ..	20 to 25 per cent.	25 to 30 per cent.	30 to 35 per cent.	35 to 40 per cent.
Number ..	21	151	499	179
Per cent. ..	2·47	17·76	58·70	21·05

The following tabulation exhibits the results obtained by the examination of various grades of Formosa, Congou, Young Hyson, Gunpowder, and Japan tea, made, under the supervision of the writer, by Dr. J. F. Davis.

It will be noticed, if the same varieties of tea be compared, that, with some exceptions, their commercial value is directly proportional to the percentages of soluble ash, extract, tannin, and theine contained.

Variety.	Formosa Oolong, Choice, 1st Crop.	Formosa Oolong, Superior, 1st Crop.	Formosa Oolong, Choice, 3rd Crop.	Formosa Oolong, Superior, 3rd Crop.	Congou, Choicest.	Congou, Medium.	Congou, Common.	First Young Hyson, Regular Moyune.	First Young Hyson, Plain Draw.	Second Young Hyson, Moyune.	Third Young Hyson, Plain Draw.
Price per lb. (wholesale).	c. 70	c. 28	c. 55	c. 24	c. 65 to 70	c. 24	c. 14	c. 28 to 30	c. 25	c. 17 to 18	c. 14
Total ash ..	p. c. 6·50	p. c. 5·96	p. c. 5·80	p. c. 6·34	p. c. 6·22	p. c. 6·36	p. c. 6·58	p. c. 6·26	p. c. 5·86	p. c. 5·84	p. c. 6·20
Ash soluble in water.	3·60	2·86	3·12	3·60	3·56	3·00	2·88	3·60	3·28	3·36	3·34
Ash insoluble in water.	2·90	3·10	2·68	2·74	2·66	3·36	3·70	2·66	2·58	2·48	2·86
Ash insoluble in acids.	0·86	0·94	0·56	0·66	0·56	0·66	1·06	0·64	0·58	0·50	0·52
Extract ..	42·00	37·40	43·20	40·60	34·60	29·60	26·20	40·60	41·00	39·80	30·40
Insoluble leaf	54·90	59·55	52·70	56·55	60·75	64·80	68·75	55·50	57·70	57·15	61·95
Tannin ..	18·66	16·31	18·00	16·05	14·87	13·70	12·26	18·00	19·96	18·53	16·99
Theine ..	3·46	2·20	2·26	1·39	3·29	2·23	2·35	2·26	2·30	1·16	1·08

Variety.	Choice Gunpowder.	Third Gunpowder.	Uncoloured Japan, Choicest, First Picking.	Coloured Japan, Good Medium, First Picking.	Coloured Japan, Good Medium, Third Picking.	Japan Dust.	
						Coloured, Fine.	Uncoloured, Common.
Price per lb. (wholesale).	c. 35	c. 23	c. 30	c. 22	c. 19	c. 9	c. 6
Total ash ..	p. c. 5·76	p. c. 5·50	p. c. 5·44	p. c. 6·06	p. c. 6·50	p. c. 9·74	p. c. 6·66
Ash soluble in water.	3·26	3·14	3·46	2·84	2·90	1·48	2·78
Ash insoluble in water.	2·50	2·36	1·98	3·22	3·60	8·26	3·88
Ash insoluble in acids.	0·54	0·52	0·46	0·78	0·96	3·90	1·46
Extract ..	39·60	36·00	39·20	36·40	33·40	31·80	32·80
Insoluble leaf	56·70	57·90	56·85	57·10	59·90	61·45	60·05
Tannin ..	20·09	17·87	21·92	18·27	17·35	15·66	17·74
Theine.. ..	1·78	1·42	1·54	1·66	0·74	0·82	2·43

The following analyses of several kinds of spurious tea, received from the U.S. Consuls at Canton and Nagasaki (Japan), have been made by the author :—

	1.	2.	3.	4.
	per cent.	per cent.	per cent.	per cent.
Total ash	8·62	8·90	7·95	12·58
Ash insoluble in water ..	7·98	6·04	4·95	8·74
Ash soluble in water ..	0·64	1·86	3·00	3·84
Ash insoluble in acid ..	3·92	3·18	1·88	6·60
Extract	7·73	14·00	12·76	22·10
Gum	10·67	7·30	11·00	11·40
Insoluble leaf	70·60	70·55	67·00	60·10
Tannin	3·13	8·01	14·50	15·64
Theine	0·58	nil	0·16	0·12

1. Partially exhausted and refired tea-leaves, known as "*Ching Suey*" (clear water), which name doubtless has reference to the weakness of a beverage prepared from this article.

2. "Lie tea," made from Wampan leaves.

3. A mixture of 10 per cent. green tea and 90 per cent. "lie tea." It is sometimes sold as "Imperial" or "Gunpowder" tea, and is stated to be extensively consumed in France and Spain.

4. "Scented caper tea," consisting of tea-dust made up into little shot-like pellets by means of "Congou paste" (*i. e.* boiled rice), and said to be chiefly used in the English coal-mining districts.

The following are the results of the analysis by American chemists of samples representing 2414 packages of Indian tea.

	Per cent.	Average per cent.
Moisture	5·830 to 6·325 ..	5·938
Extract	37·800 „ 40·350 ..	38·841
Total ash	5·050 „ 6·024 ..	5·613
Ash soluble in water ..	3·122 „ 4·280 ..	3·516
Ash insoluble in water	1·890 „ 2·255 ..	2·092
Ash insoluble in acid ..	0·120 „ 0·296 ..	0·177
Insoluble leaf	47·120 „ 55·870 ..	51·910
Tannin	13·040 „ 18·868 ..	15·323
Theine	1·880 „ 3·24 ..	2·736

COFFEE.

COFFEE is the seed of the *Caffea Arabica*, indigenous to Abyssinia and southern Arabia, and since naturalised in the West Indies, Ceylon, Brazil, and other tropical countries. Its importance as an almost universal beverage is only equalled by that of tea. The ancient history of coffee is shrouded in great obscurity. It was unknown to the Romans and Greeks, but its use is said to have been prevalent in Abyssinia from the remotest time, and in Arabia it formed an article of general consumption during the fifteenth century. From its introduction, in 1575, into Constantinople by the Turks, it gradually made its way into all civilised countries. In 1690 it was carried by the Dutch from Mocha to Java, whence specimens of the tree were taken to Holland and France. Coffee houses were opened in London about the middle of the seventeenth century, and in 1809 the first cargo of coffee was shipped to the United States. As with many other articles of diet, the adulteration of coffee has kept well apace with its increased consumption. The bean is deprived of its external fleshy coatings before exportation, and is met with in commerce in a raw, roasted, or ground condition. Bell * gives the following analyses of two samples of coffee, both in the raw and roasted state :—

* Op. cit.

	Mocha.		East Indian.	
	Raw.	Roasted.	Raw.	Roasted.
	per cent.	per cent.	per cent.	per cent.
Caffeine	1·08	0·82	1·11	1·05
Saccharine matter	9·55	0·43	8·90	0·41
Caffeic acids	8·46	4·74	9·58	4·52
Alcohol extract (containing nitrogen and colouring matter).	6·90	14·14	4·31	12·67
Fat and oil	12·60	13·59	11·81	13·41
Legumin or Albumin ..	9·87	11·23	11·23	13·13
Dextrine	0·87	1·24	0·84	1·38
Cellulose (and insoluble colouring matter).	37·95	48·62	38·60	47·42
Ash	3·74	4·56	3·98	4·88
Moisture	8·98	0·63	9·64	1·13
	100·00	100·00	100·00	100·00

Other authorities have obtained the following results :—

	König.		Payen. Raw.	Smethan. (Average of 7 Varieties.) Roasted.
	Raw.	Roasted.		
	per cent.	per cent.	per cent.	per cent.
Substances soluble in water	27·44	27·45	..	..
Nitrogen	1·87	2·31	..	2·26
Nitrogenous substances	11·43	12·05	11 to 13	..
Caffeine	1·18	1·38	0·8	..
Caffetannic acid	..	..	3·5 to 5	..
Fat	13·23	15·03	10 to 13	10·99
Ethereal oil	..	..	0·013	..
Sugar	3·25	1·32	..	..
Sugar and Dextrine ..	..	..	15·5	..
Other non-nitrogenous substances.	31·52	38·41	..	..
Cellulose	27·72	24·27	34·0	29·28
Ash	3·48	3·75	6·7	4·19
Soluble ash	..	..	..	3·37
Moisture	11·19	3·19	12·0	2·87

It will be noticed from these analyses that the amount of sugar is greatly diminished by the process of roasting. According to some analysts, the proportion of fat experiences an increase, but it is more probable that this constituent is simply rendered more susceptible to the action of solvents by a mechanical alteration of the structure of the berry. Recent determinations of the ash in coffee place its average proportion at 4 per cent. ; 3·24 being soluble in water, and 0·74 per cent. insoluble. The soluble extract in roasted coffee usually amounts to about 30 per cent.

An analysis made by Beckurts and Kauder * gives the general composition of roasted chicory, dried at 107°, as follows :—

	Per cent.
Substances soluble in water	57·40
„ insoluble „	41·90
Ash	7·66
Fat	0·73
Nitrogenous substances	7·12
Grape sugar	4·35
Cane sugar and dextrine	5·33
Starch	2·45
Other non-nitrogenous substances	49 13
Woody fibre	26·23

The most common adulterations to which coffee is liable consist in the addition of chicory, caramel, and numerous roasted grains, such as corn, wheat, and rye, as well as such roots and seeds as dandelion, mangold wurzel, turnips, beans, peas, etc. The roasted and ground article is naturally most exposed to falsification, although letters patent have been issued for the fictitious manufacture of a pressed "coffee bean," containing absolutely no coffee. The addition of chicory is by far the most prevalent adulteration of coffee. Of thirty-four samples examined by Hassall, thirty-one (91 per cent.) contained this root. In regard to the moral aspects of its use, it can safely be asserted that, while the addition of chicory to coffee is largely sanctioned, and indeed demanded by the existing tastes of many coffee-

* Pharm. Centralbl., 1885, p. 346.

drinkers, its use constitutes a true adulteration, and should be condemned, unless its presence is prominently stated on the label of the package. In chicory the active principles of coffee, which exert valuable physiological effects on the system (viz. caffeine, the essential oil, etc.), are totally absent ; moreover, its comparative cheapness is a constant temptation to employ a proportion largely in excess of the amount requisite to produce any alleged improvement in the flavour of the resulting admixture.

The sophistications of coffee may be detected, in a general way, by physical tests, by chemical analysis, and by microscopic examination, in which processes great aid is derived from the characteristic properties exhibited by the pure roasted and ground berry which distinguish it from its more usual adulterants.

(a) *Physical Examination.*—The following tests, while not always decisive in their results, are often of service.

A small portion of the suspected sample is gently placed upon the surface of a beaker filled with cold water, and allowed to remain at rest for about fifteen minutes. If pure, the sample does not imbibe the water, but floats upon the surface without communicating much colour to it ; if chicory or caramel be present, these substances rapidly absorb moisture and sink, producing brownish-red streaks in their descent, which, by diffusion, impart a very decided tint to the entire liquid. A similar coloration is caused by many other roasted roots and berries, but not so quickly or to so great an extent. The test may be somewhat modified by shaking the sample with cold water, and then allowing the vessel to stand aside for a short time. Pure coffee rises to the surface, little or no colour being imparted to the water ; chicory, etc., fall to the bottom as a sediment, and give a brownish colour to the liquid.

If a small quantity of the sample is placed upon a clean plate of glass, and moistened with a few drops of water, the pure coffee berries remain hard, and offer resistance when tested with a needle ; most grains employed for their adulteration become softened in their texture.

A considerable portion of the mixture is treated with boiling water and allowed to settle. Genuine coffee affords a clear and limpid infusion ; many foreign grains yield a thick gummy liquor, resulting from the starchy and saccharine matters contained. An infusion of pure coffee, if treated with solution of cupric acetate and filtered, will show a greenish-yellow colour ; if chicory be present, the filtrate will be reddish-brown. As a rule, samples of ground coffee which are much adulterated, pack together when subjected to a moderate pressure.

Owing to the low density of a coffee infusion (due to its almost entire freedom from sugar), as compared with that of the infusions of most roots and grains, it has been suggested by Messrs. Graham, Stenhouse and Campbell, to apply the specific gravity determination of the infusion obtained from the suspected sample as a means for detecting adulteration. The results afforded are fairly approximate. The solution is prepared by boiling one part of the sample with ten parts of water and filtering. The following table gives the densities, at $15°·5$, of various infusions made in this manner :—

Acorns	1·0073
Peas	1·0073
Mocha coffee	1·0080
Beans	1·0084
Java coffee	1·0087
Jamaica coffee	1·0087
Costa Rica coffee	1·0090
Ceylon coffee	1·0090
Brown malt	1·0109
Parsnips	1·0143
Carrots	1·0171
Yorkshire chicory	1·0191
Black malt	1·0212
Turnips	1·0214
Rye meal	1·0216

D

English chicory	.. ..	1·0217
Dandelion root	.. ..	1·0219
Red beet ..	.. ..	1·0221
Foreign chicory	.. ..	1·0226
Mangold wurzel	.. ..	1·0235
Maize	.. ..	1·0253
Bread raspings	.. ..	1·0263

Assuming the gravity of the pure coffee infusion to be 1·0086, and that of chicory to be 1·0206, the approximate percentage of coffee, C, in a mixture, can be obtained by means of the following equation, in which D represents the density of the infusion:—

$$C = \frac{1·00 \, (1·020 - D)}{12} \, .$$

This was tested by mixing equal parts of coffee and chicory, and taking the specific gravity of the infusion; it was 1·01408, indicating the presence of 49 per cent. of coffee. Some idea of the amount of foreign admixture (especially chicory) in ground roasted coffee may be formed from the tinctorial power of the sample. It has already been mentioned that coffee imparts much less colour to water than do most roasted grains and roots. The table below shows the weights of various roasted substances which must be dissolved in 2·000 parts of water in order to produce an equal degree of colour: [*]—

Caramel	.. ..	1·00
Mangold wurtzel	.. ..	1·66
Black malt	.. ..	1·82
White turnips ..	.. ..	2·00
Carrots	.. ..	2·00
Chicory (darkest Yorkshire) ..	.. .. ..	2·22
Parsnips	.. ..	2·50
Maize	.. ..	2·86
Rye	.. ..	2·86
Dandelion root ..	.. ..	3·33
Red beet	.. ..	3·33

[*] Graham, Stenhouse and Campbell.

Bread raspings	.. ..	3·36
Acorns	.. ..	5·00
Over-roasted coffee	.. ..	5·46
Highly-roasted coffee	.. ..	5·77
Medium-roasted coffee	.. ..	6·95
Peas	.. ..	13·33
Beans	.. ..	13·33
Spent tan	.. ..	33·00
Brown malt	.. ..	40·00

The comparative colour test may also be applied as follows :*—One gramme each of the sample under examination, and of a sample prepared by mixing equal parts of pure coffee and chicory, are completely exhausted with water, and the infusions made up to 100 c.c. or more ; 50 c.c. of the filtered extract from the suspected sample are then placed in a Nessler cylinder, and it is determined by trial how many c.c. of the extract from the standard mixture, together with enough distilled water to make up the 50 c.c., will produce the same colour. In calculating the chicory present, it is assumed that this substance possesses three times the tinctorial power of coffee.

(b) *Chemical Examination.*—Some of the chemical properties of roasted coffee afford fairly reliable means for the detection of an admixture of chicory. Coffee ash dissolves in water to the extent of about 80 per cent. ; of the ash of roasted chicory only about 35 per cent. is soluble. Coffee ash is almost free from silica and sand, which substances form a notable proportion of the constituents of the ash of chicory.

The following (see p. 36) are the results obtained by the writer from the analysis of the ash of coffee and chicory.

It will be observed from these analyses, that the most distinctive features presented by coffee ash are the absence of soda, and the small amounts of chlorine, ferric oxide and silica present. In these respects, it is very different from the ash of chicory. The proportion of phosphoric acid

* Leebody, Chemical News,' xxx. p. 243.

D 2

	Java Coffee.	Chicory Root.
	per cent.	per cent.
Percentage of ash	3·93	4·41
Potassa	53·37	23·00
Soda	..	13·13
Lime	5·84	9·40
Magnesia	9·09	5·88
Alumina	0·43	..
Ferric oxide	0·53	5·00
Sulphuric acid	3·19	9·75
Chlorine	0·78	4·93
Carbonic acid	15·26	4·01
Phosphoric acid	11·26	8·44
Silica and sand	0·25	16·46
	100·00	100·00

found in the latter is in excess of that given by some
authorities. Several analyses of chicory ash have been made
by the author, and, in every instance, the amount of phosphoric acid was over 8 per cent. ; in one sample of the ash
of commercial chicory it approximated 13 per cent.

Blyth gives the annexed table, showing the characteristic
differences between coffee and chicory ash : *—

	Coffee Ash.	Chicory Ash.
	per cent.	per cent.
Silica and sand	none	10·69 to 35·88
Carbonic acid	14·92	1·78 „ 3·19
Ferric oxide	0·44 to 0·98	3·13 „ 5·32
Chlorine	0·26 „ 1·11	3·28 „ 4·93
Phosphoric acid	10·00 „ 11·00	5·00 „ 6·00
Total soluble ash	75·00 „ 85·00	21·00 „ 35·00

The following formula has been suggested for determining the percentage of pure coffee, in mixtures :—

$$C = 2 \frac{(100\ S - 174)}{3}$$

where S represents the percentage of soluble ash.

Another noteworthy difference between roasted coffee
and chicory, is the amount of sugar contained. As a rule,
in roasted coffee, it ranges from 0·0 to 1·2 per cent. ; in

* 'Foods : Composition and Analysis.'

roasted chicory, it varies from 12· to 18· per cent. The quantity of sugar in a sample can be determined by Fehling's method as follows:—

A standard solution of pure cupric sulphate is first prepared by dissolving 34·64 grammes of the crystals (previously ground and dried by pressing between bibulous paper) in about 200 c.c. of distilled water; 173 grammes of pure Rochelle salt are separately dissolved in 480 c.c. of a solution of sodium hydroxide of sp. gr. 1·14. The solutions are then mixed and diluted with distilled water to one litre. Each c.c. of the above solution represents 0·05 gramme of grape sugar. The test is applied by taking 10 c.c. of the copper solution, adding about four times its volume of water, and bringing it to the boiling point. The coffee infusion is then gradually added from a burette, until the copper salt is completely reduced to the red sub-oxide, which point is recognised by the disappearance of its blue colour, and can be more accurately determined by acidulating the filtered fluid with acetic acid and testing it (while still hot) for any remaining trace of copper with potassium ferrocyanide. In preparing the coffee solution for the foregoing test, it is advisable to exhaust a weighed quantity of the sample with hot water. The infusion is treated with basic plumbic acetate so long as a precipitate forms; it is then filtered, the precipitate being well washed, and the lead contained is removed by conducting sulphuretted hydrogen gas through the fluid which is subsequently again filtered and boiled until the dissolved gas is expelled. The sugar determination is now made. Wanklyn employs the following equation to estimate the amount of chicory in an adulterated sample :—

$$E = \frac{(S-1)\ 100}{14},$$

where E is the percentage of chicory, and S the percentage of sugar.

According to the analysis of König, the proportions of
sugar and other constituents in some of the adulterants of
coffee, are as follows :—

	Chicory.	Figs.	Acorns.	Rye.
	per cent.	per cent.	per cent.	per cent.
Water	12·16	18·98	12·85	15·22
Nitrogenous substances	6·09	4·25	6·13	11·84
Fat	2·05	2·83	4·61	3·46
Sugar	15·87	34·19	8·05	3·92
Other non-nitrogenous substances.	46·71	29·15	62·	55·37
Cellulose	11·0	7·16	4·98	5·35
Ash	6·12	3·44	2·12	4·81
Substances soluble in water	63·05	73·81	..	45·11

Estimations of the amount of sugar obtained upon boiling the suspected coffee with water containing a little
sulphuric acid (see p. 37), and the proportion of the
sample which is soluble in hot water should be made.
The presence of chicory is shown by a decided increase
in the amount of soluble substances ; that of rye, by the
notable quantity of sugar produced by the inversion with
acid, due to the starch contained in the grain.

In this connection, the following determinations of
Krausch are of interest :—

	Substances Soluble in Water.	Ready-formed Sugar.	Sugar after Inversion.
	per cent.	per cent.	per cent.
Roasted coffee	23·81	0·20	24·59
„ chicory	65·42	23·40	22·14
„ rye	31·92	..	75·37
„ coffee + 10 per cent. chicory	30·63	2·30	23·15
„ coffee + 10 per cent. rye ..	25·98	0·19	29·60

The presence of roasted rye, corn, and other grains in
coffee, may be qualitatively recognised by testing the cold
infusion of the sample with iodine solution for starch, which

COFFEE.

is not contained in a ready formed state in coffee. Caffeine is absent in chicory and the other usual adulterants of coffee, and the estimation of this alkaloid is of decided service (see p. 21). Roasted coffee contains about 1 per cent. of caffeine.

A popular brand of ground coffee received by the author for examination, and labelled "Prepared Java Coffee," had the following approximate composition :—Coffee, 38 ; peas, 52 ; rye, 2 ; and chicory, 7 per cent.

A sample of "acorn" coffee, analysed by König, gave the following results :—

	Per cent.
Water	12·85
Nitrogenous substances	6·13
Fat	4·01
Sugar	8·01
Other non-nitrogenous substances	62·00
Cellulose	4·98
Ash	2·02

The non-nitrogenous constituents contained from 20 to 30 per cent. of starch, and from 6 to 8 per cent. of tannic acid.

The composition of the well-known German coffee-substitutes, prepared by Behr Bros., is stated to be as follows :—

"Rye Coffee-substitutes."

	Per cent.
Substances soluble in water	61·33
Substances insoluble in water	36·45
Cellulose	9·78
Starch	8·34
Dextrine	49·51
Nitrogenous substances	11·87
Other non-nitrogenous substances	9·83
Fat	3·91
Ash	4·54
Moisture	2·22

" Malt Coffee-substitute."

		Per cent.
Soluble in hot water	Albuminoid substances	4·22
	Dextrine	50·19
	Alcoholic extract	7·57
	Inorganic matter, containing phosphoric acid, 0·54	2·27
Insoluble in hot water		35·00
Moisture		0·35

The raw coffee bean is sometimes subjected to a process termed "sweating," which consists in treating it with moist steam, the object being to artificially reproduce the conditions present in the holds of vessels, by means of which the bean is increased in size, and also somewhat improved in colour and flavour. Another form of manipulation, analogous to the facing of tea, is to moisten the raw bean with water containing a little gum, and agitate it with various pigments, such as indigo, Prussian blue, Persian berries, turmeric, alkanet, Venetian red, soap-stone, chrome-yellow, and iron ochre. Mexican coffees are sometimes made to resemble the more expensive Java in appearance. The chemist of the New York City Board of Health has found in the quantity of such treated coffee commonly taken to make a cup of the beverage 0·0014 gramme of cupric arsenite. Indigo may be detected in the artificially coloured product by treating a considerable portion of the sample with dilute nitric acid, filtering and saturating the filtrate with sulphuretted hydrogen. If indigo be present, it can now be extracted upon agitating the solution with chloroform. Alkanet root and Prussian blue are separated by warming the coffee with solution of potassium carbonate, from which these pigments are precipitated upon addition of hydrochloric acid.

(c) *Microscopic Examination.*—Great aid to the chemical investigation is afforded by the microscopic examination of ground coffee. It is necessary to first become familiar with the appearance of the genuine article—low magnifying powers being employed—and then make comparative examinations of the adulterant suspected to be present.

The coffee bean mainly consists of irregular cells inclosed in very thick walls which are distinguished by uneven projections. The cells contain globules of oil. Most of the roots added to coffee exhibit a conglomeration of cells (provided with thin walls) and groups of jointed tubes, often quite similar to one another in structure. The microscopic appearance of some of the starch granules, occasionally met with in coffee mixtures, is represented on p. 100.

Of 151 samples of ground coffee recently purchased at random and tested by various American chemists, 69 (45·7 per cent.) were found to be adulterated.

COCOA AND CHOCOLATE.

Cocoa is prepared from the roasted seeds of the tree *Theobroma cacao*, of the order *Byttneriaceæ*. It sometimes appears in commerce as "cocoa-nibs" (*i. e.* partially ground), but it is more frequently sold in the powdered state, either pure or mixed with sugar and starch, and also often deprived of about one-half of its fat. Chocolate usually consists of cocoa-paste and sugar flavoured with vanilla, cinnamon, or cloves, and commonly mixed with flour or starch. According to Wanklyn, the average composition of cocoa is as follows :—

	Per cent.
Cocoa butter	50·00
Theobromine	1·50
Starch	10·00
Albumin, fibrine and gluten	18·00
Gum	8·00
Colouring matter	2·60
Water	6·00
Ash	3·60
Loss, etc.	0·30

R. Benzeman * has furnished the following averages of the results obtained by the analysis of cocoa and chocolate. The air-dried cocoa berries gave—husks, 13·00 per cent. ; nibs, 87·00 per cent. :—

* Jahresberichte, 1883, p. 1002.

	Cocoa Nibs.	Chocolate made from Cocoa and Sugar.
	per cent.	per cent.
Moisture at 100°	6·41	1·65
Fat	51·47	22·57
Starch	11·75	4·58
Other organic substances, insoluble in water.	18·03	8·58
Organic substances, soluble in water	8·54	60·63
Mineral Ash	3·80	1·99
	100·00	100·00
Ash of insoluble substances	0·89	0·30

Recent analysis of shelled cocoa-beans, made by Boussingault, gave the following results :—

	Fresh.	Dry.
	per cent.	per cent.
Fat	49·9	54·0
Starch and starch-sugar	2·4	2·5
Theobromine	3·3	3·6
Asparagine	traces	..
Albumin	10·9	11·8
„ gum	2·4	2·5
Tartaric acid	3·4	3·7
Tannin	0·2	0·2
Soluble cellulose	10·6	11·5
Ash	4·0	4·4
Water	7·6	..
Undetermined	5·3	5·8

Dr. Weigman [*] obtained the following results from an examination of several varieties of the shelled beans :—

	Water.	Fat.	Ash.	Nitrogen.
	per cent.	per cent.	per cent.	per cent.
Machala	4·97	47·80	3·88	2·25
Arriba	6·57	47·44	3·52	2·31
Caracas	6·00	46·39	4·19	2·23
Puerto Cabello	5·71	48·74	3·94	2·13
Surinam	5·01	46·26	2·99	2·20
Trinidad	6·07	45·74	2·04	2·04
Port au Prince	4·73	48·58	3·89	2·33

[*] Agrikulturchemische Versuchstation, in Münster.

The most important constituents of cocoa are the fat (cocoa-butter), and the alkaloid (theobromine).

Cocoa butter forms a whitish solid of 0·970 specific gravity, fusing at 30°, and soluble in ether and in alcohol.

Theobromine ($C_7H_8N_4O_2$) crystallises in minute rhombic prisms, which are insoluble in benzol, but dissolve readily in boiling water and alcohol. It sublimes at 170°. Theobromine is exceedingly rich in nitrogen, containing over 20 per cent. of the element. In this and many other respects it bears a great resemblance to theine.

The proportion of mineral ash in cocoa varies from 3·06 to 4·5 per cent.

James Bell[*] gives the following composition of the ash of Grenada cocoa nibs :—

	Per cent.
Sodium chloride	0·57
Soda	0·57
Potassa	27·64
Magnesia	19·81
Lime	4·53
Alumina	0·08
Ferric oxide	0·15
Carbonic acid	2·92
Sulphuric acid	4·53
Phosphoric acid	39·20
	100·00

The most characteristic features of the ash of genuine cocoa are its great solubility, the small amounts of chlorine, carbonates, and soda, and the constancy of the proportion of phosphoric acid contained. Bell has also analysed several samples of commercial cocoa. The following will serve to illustrate their general composition :—

	Per cent.
Moisture	4·95
Fat	24·94
Starch (added)	19·19
Sugar (added)	23·03
Non-fatty cocoa	27·89
	100·00

[*] Op. cit.

	Per cent.
Nitrogen	2·24
Ash	1·52
Cocoa, soluble in cold water..	31·66
Ash in portion soluble in cold water	1·17

The comparatively low percentage of ash contained in prepared cocoas and chocolate, is of use in indicating the amount of real cocoa present in such mixtures. A large proportion of the mineral constituents of cocoa are dissolved by directly treating it with cold water. Wanklyn obtained in this way from genuine cocoa-nibs 6·76 per cent. organic matter, and 2·16 per cent. ash, the latter chiefly consisting of phosphates ; a commercial cocoa gave, extract, 46·04 per cent. ; ash, 1·04 per cent. The most common admixtures of cocoa and chocolate, are sugar and the various starches. The addition of foreign fats, chicory, and iron ochres, is also sometimes practised. Since prepared cocoas are generally understood to contain the first-named diluents, their presence can hardly be considered an adulteration, if the fact is mentioned upon the packages. Many varieties of the cocoas of commerce will be found to be deficient in cocoa-butter, a considerable proportion of which has been removed in the process of manufacture. This practice is also claimed to be justifiable, the object being to produce an article unobjectionable to invalids, which is not always the case with pure cocoa. In the analysis of cocoa the following estimations are usually made:—

Theobromine.—10 grammes of the sample are first repeatedly exhausted with petroleum - naphtha. The insoluble residue is mixed with a small quantity of paste, prepared by triturating calcined magnesia with a little water, and the mixture evaporated to dryness at a gentle heat. The second residue is boiled with alcohol and the alcoholic solution of theobromine filtered and evaporated to dryness in a tared capsule. It is then purified by washing with petroleum-naphtha and weighed. Bell has

verified the existence in cocoa of a second alkaloid, distinct
from theobromine, which crystallises in silky needles very
similar to theine.

Fat.—The proportion of fat is readily determined by
evaporating to dryness the petroleum-naphtha used in the
preceding estimation.   As already stated, it is generally
present in a proportion of 50 per cent. in pure cocoa ; the
amount contained in prepared soluble cocoas being often
less than 25 per cent.   The English minimum standard is
20 per cent.

Ash.—The ash is determined by the incineration of a
weighed portion of the sample in a platinum dish.   In
prepared cocoas and chocolates, the proportion of ash is
considerably lower than in pure cocoa.   It is of importance
to ascertain the amount of ash soluble in water (the proportion in genuine cocoa is about 50 per cent.), and
especially the quantity of phosphoric acid contained.
Assuming that prepared cocoa contains 1·5 per cent. of
ash, of which 0·6 per cent. consists of phosphoric acid, and
allowing that pure cocoa contains 0·9 per cent. of phosphoric acid, Blyth adopts the following formula for calculating the proportion of cocoa present in the article :—

$$\frac{\cdot 6 \times 100}{\cdot 9} = 66 \cdot 66 \text{ per cent.}$$

Starch.—A convenient method for estimating the starch
is to first remove the fatty matter of the cocoa by exhaustion with petroleum-naphtha, and then boil the residue with alcohol.   The remaining insoluble matter is
dried, and afterwards boiled until the starch becomes
soluble.   It is next again boiled for several hours with
a little dilute sulphuric acid, after which the solution
is purified by addition of basic plumbic acetate.   The
liquid is then treated with sulphuretted hydrogen, in
order to remove the lead, and the sugar contained in
the filtered solution is determined by means of Fehling's

solution, and calculated to terms of starch. The proportion of starch normally present in cocoa is to be deducted from the results thus afforded. The variety of starch contained in cocoa differs in its microscopic appearance from the starches most frequently added.

Sugar.—The sugar may be determined by evaporating the alcoholic solution obtained in the preceding process, and then subjecting the residue to the same method of procedure.

The proportion of woody fibre in cocoa can be approximately estimated by the method of Henneberg and Stohman,* which consists in extracting the fat with benzole, boiling the remaining substances for half an hour, first with 1·25 per cent. sulphuric acid, then with 1·25 per cent. solution of potassium hydroxide. The residue is washed with alcohol and with ether, and its weight determined. Unwashed cocoa-berries, when treated in this manner, gave from 2 to 3 per cent. of cellulose, while cocoa husks furnished from 10 to 16 per cent. The presence of chicory in soluble cocoa and chocolate is easily recognised by the dark colour of the extract obtained, upon digesting the suspected sample with cold water ; ochres and other colouring matters are detected by the reddish colour of the ash as well as by its abnormal composition. The addition of foreign fats to chocolates is stated to be occasionally resorted to.

The melting point of pure cocoa-butter varies from 30° to 33°. The identification of foreign fats can sometimes be accomplished by means of their higher melting point, and by an examination of the separated fat, according to Koettstorfer's method (see p. 71). The table following gives the melting points of various fats, and the number of milligrammes of K(OH) required for the saponification of one gramme of the same.

* Repert. f. Analyt. Chemie, 1884, p. 345.

Fat.	Melting point.	m.g. K(OH) to saponify one gramme.
	° °	
Cocoa-butter	30 to 33	198 to 203
Arachidis oil	..	191·3
Sesamé oil	..	190·0
Cotton-seed and olive oil	..	191·7
Almond oil	..	194·5
Palm oil	35 to 36	202·5
Lard	32 „ 33	195·5
Mutton tallow (fresh)	42·5 „ 45	..
Mutton tallow (old)	43·5	196·5
Bone fat	21 to 22	190·0
Beeswax	63	..

Other tests have also been suggested for the detection of foreign fats in cocoa-butter :—

(a) Treat the fat with two parts of cold ether ; pure cocoa-butter dissolves, forming a clear solution, whereas in presence of tallow or wax a cloudy mixture is obtained.

(b) Dissolve 10 grammes of the suspected fat in benzole, and expose the solution to a temperature of 0°. By this treatment a separation of pure cocoa-butter in minute grains is produced. The liquid is now heated to 14°·4, when the cocoa-fat will re-dissolve to a transparent solution, while the presence of tallow will be recognised by the turbid appearance of the liquid.

MILK.

OWING to the very important sanitary relations of milk as a model food, the subject of its sophistication has during the past ten years received particular notice at the hands of the food-chemist. The investigations of our public sanitary authorities have shown that milk adulteration is exceedingly common. It is stated upon good authority that until quite recently (1883) the 120 millions of quarts of milk annually brought into New York city were intentionally diluted with 40 millions of quarts of water, the resulting product rivalling in richness the famous compound once lauded by the philanthropic Squeers.

The results of the examination of milk instituted by the New York State Board of Health are given below, in which, however, the specimens of skimmed milk are not included:—

Year.	Number of Samples tested.	Number showing addition of Water.	Per cent. of Adulterated.
1880	1514	167	11·0
1881	1110	51	4·6
1882	1775	120	6·7

From October 1883 to March 1884, of 241 samples of milk examined by the Public Analyst of Eastern Massachusetts, 21·37 per cent. were watered; of 1190 samples tested during the year 1884, 790 were watered.* Over 73 per cent. of the milk supplied to the city of Buffalo in 1885 was found to be adulterated. A very marked improve-

* In 1885, out of 2024 samples tested, 880 fell below the standard of 13 per cent. total solids.

E

ment in the quality of the milk received in New York city
has taken place since the appointment of a State Dairy
Commissioner (1884). Under the direction of this official
the metropolitan milk supply has been subjected to a most
rigid inspection, and with very satisfactory results. During
the years 1884 and 1885 nearly 45,000 samples of milk
were examined.

A very common sophistication practised upon milk consists in the partial or complete removal of its cream. This
process of skimming is conducted at establishments called
"creameries," of which sixty-three were formerly known to
send their impoverished product to New York city. The
State Dairy Commissioner has likewise accomplished
much towards stopping this form of adulteration.

Milk is the secretion of the mammary glands of female
mammalia. It is an opaque liquid, possessing a white,
bluish-white, or yellowish-white colour, little or no odour,
and a somewhat sweetish taste. At times it exhibits an
amphigenic reaction, *i. e.* it turns red litmus blue and blue
litmus red. From the examination of nearly one thousand
cows in the States of New York, New Jersey, and Connecticut, the *minimum* specific gravity of milk was found to be
1·0290, the *maximum* being 1·0394. The opacity of milk
is only apparent, and is due to the presence of fatty
globules held in suspension ; these under the microscope
are seen to be surrounded by a transparent liquid. Upon
allowing milk to remain at rest for some time it experiences
two changes. At first, a yellowish-white stratum of cream
rises to the surface, the lower portion becoming bluish-
white in colour and increasing in density. If this latter is
freed from the cream and again set aside, it undergoes a
further separation into a solid body (*curd*), and a liquid
(*whey*). This coagulation of the curd (*caseine*) is immediately produced by the addition of rennet, and of many
acids and metallic salts.

The essential ingredients of milk are water, fat, caseine,
sugar (lactose), and inorganic salts. The following table,

collated by Mr. Edward W. Martin,* exhibits the results
obtained by numerous authorities from the analysis of pure
cow's milk :—

Authority or Analyst.	Number of cows.	Water.	Total solids.	Fat.	Solids not fat.	Sugar.	Caseine.	Salts.
		per cent.	per cent.	per cent.	per cent.	per cent.	per cent.	per cent.
James Bell ..	216	87·17	12·83	3·83	9·00	..	..	0·71
James Bell ..	24 dairies	86·78	13·22	4·12	9·10	..	..	0·72
C. Estecourt	22 ,,	87·26	12·74	3·37	9·37	..	..	
J. Carter Bell	183	86·40	13·60	3·70	9·90	..	..	0·76
J. Cameron..	42	86·53	13·47	4·00	9·47	..	..	..
C. Cameron	40	87·00	13·00	4·00	9·00	4·28	4·10	0·62
C. Cameron	100	86·75	13·85	4·60	9·25	..	..	..
Fleischmann and Veith ..	120	87·78	12·22	3·20	9·02	..	..	..
Veith	60	87·20	12·80	3·10	9·70	..	..	..
Veith	9120	86·97	13·03	3·52	9·51	..	..	..
Wanklyn ..	Average	87·50	12·50	3·20	9·30	..	..	..
A. Wynter Blyth	,,	86·87	13·13	3·50	9·63	..	..	
Marchand ..	,,	87·15	12·85	3·55	9·30	..	..	..
Henry and Chevalier ..	,,	87·02	12·98	3·13	9·85	4·77	4·48	0·60
Vernois Bec-querel ..	,,	86·40	13·60	3·60	10·00	..	..	..
Payen	,,	86·60	13·40	3·50	9·90	..	..	..
O. C. Wiggin	58	85·92	14·08	4·01	10·07	4·29	4·99	0·79
E. Calder ..	27	87·23	12·77	3·32	9·45	..	..	..
Sharpless ..	34	85·85	14·15	4·62	9·53	4·82	4·06	0·65
Haidlen ..	Average	87·30	12·70	3·00	9·70	..	..	..
Letherby ..	,,	86·00	14·00	3·90	10·10	5·20	4·10	0·80
J. König ..	,,	87·30	12·70	3·00	9·70	5·00	4·00	0·70
Boussingault	,,	87·40	12·60	4·10	8·50	5·10	3·20	0·70
Muspratt ..	..	86·43	13·57	4·43	9·14	4·73	3·74	0·67
Dieulafait ..	,,	87·64	12·36	3·11	9·25	4·22	4·18	0·85
Gorup-Bezanez ..	,,	85·70	14·30	4·31	9·99	4·04	5·40	0·55
Brinton ..	,,	86·00	14·00	4·50	9·50	3·50	5·50	0·70
Chandler ..	1700 qts.	87·45	12·55	3·83	8·72	..	..	..
Newton ..	Average	87·50	12·50	3·50	9·00	..	..	..
Bartley ..	,,	87·50	12·50	3·50	9·00	..	..	..
White	,,	87·50	12·50	3·50	9·00	..	..	..
Waller.. ..	,,	87·50	12·50	3·20	9·30	..	..	..
Babcock ..	,,	85·53	14·47	5·09	9·39	5·15	3·57	0·67
Church ..	,,	86·30	13·70	3·70	10·00	5·10	4·10	0·80
Edward Smith	,,	86·40	13·60	3·61	9·90	3·80	5·52	0·66
Martin.. ..	,,	86·50	12·50	3·20	9·30	..	..	0·67

Mr. Martin obtained the following results from the

* Second Annual Report of the New York State Dairy Commissioner, 1886.

examination of cream separated by centrifugal force, and of skimmed milk :—

	Cream.	Skimmed Milk.
	per cent.	per cent.
Water	52·21	90·34
Fat	41·16	0·15
Sugar	3·11	3·98
Caseine	3·40	4·80
Salts	0·12	0·78

The proportion of mineral constituents in milk usually ranges between 0·7 and 0·8 per cent. The average composition of milk ash is as follows : *—

Per cent.

Potassa	24·5
Soda	11·0
Lime	22·5
Magnesia	2·6
Ferric oxide	0·3
Phosphoric anhydride	26·0
Sulphuric anhydride	1·0
Chlorine	15·6
	103·5 †

The tabulation below gives the composition of human milk and the milk of various animals :—

	Specific Gravity.	Water.	Milk Solids.	Fat.	Caseine.	Milk Sugar.	Inorganic Salts.
		per cent.	per cent.	per cent.	per cent.	per cent.	per cent.
White woman	0315	87·806	12·194	4·021	3·523	4·265	0·28
Coloured woman	..	86·34	13·66	4·03	3·32	5·71	0·61
Mare	1·031	91·310	9·690	1·055	1·953	6·285	0·397
Goat	1·032	86·36	13·64	4·36	4·70	4·00	0·62
Ewe	1·038	82·94	17·00	6·97	5·40	3·63	0·97
Sow	1·044	81·80	18·20	6·00	5·30	6·07	0·83
Canine	1·036	77·26	22·74	10·64	9·21	2·49	0·44
Ass	1·033	91·95	8·05	0·11	1·82	6·08	0·34
Camel	..	86·94	13·06	2·90	3·67	5·78	0·66
Hippopotamus ..	..	90·43	9·57	4·51	4·40		0·11
Elephant	..	66·697	33·303	22·070	3·212	7·392	0·629
Porpoise	..	41·11	58·89	45·80	11·19	1·33	0·57
Cat	..	81·62	18·38	3·33	9·55	4·91	0·58
Llama	..	89·55	10·45	3·15	0·90	5·60	0·80

* Dammer's ' Lexikon der Verfälschungen,' 1887, p. 592.
† 3·50 per cent. should be deducted for chlorine and oxygen.

Several varieties of preserved and condensed milk have, for a number of years, been placed upon the market. The composition of the best-known brands of these preparations is as follows :—

PRESERVED MILK.

Brand.	Water.	Fat.	Cane and Milk Sugar.	Caseine.	Salts.
	per cent.	per cent.	per cent.	per cent.	per cent.
Alderney	30·05	10·08	46·01	12·04	1·82
Anglo-Swiss (American)	29·46	8·11	50·41	10·22	1·80
„ „ (English) ..	27·80	8·24	51·07	10·80	2·09
„ „ (Swiss) ..	25·51	8·51	53·27	10·71	2·00
Eagle	27·30	6·60	44·47	10·77	1·86
Crown	29·44	9·27	49·26	10·11	1·92

CONDENSED MILK.

Brand.	Water.	Fat.	Cane and Milk Sugar.	Caseine.	Salts.
	per cent.	per cent.	per cent.	per cent.	per cent.
American	52·07	15·06	16·97	14·26	2·80
New York	56·71	14·13	13·98	13·18	2·00
Granulated Milk Co. ..	55·43	13·16	14·84	14·04	2·53
Eagle	56·01	14·02	14·06	13·90	2·01

ANALYSIS.

The principal adulterations of milk (watering and skimming), are detected by taking its specific gravity, and making quantitative determinations of the total milk solids, the fat, and the milk solids not fat. Of these criteria, the last-mentioned is the most constant and reliable.

Physical Examination.

a. *Specific Gravity.*—The instrument employed by the New York health inspectors for testing milk is a variety of the hydrometer, termed the lactometer, and its use, which is based upon the fact that under ordinary conditions

watered milk possesses a decreased density, is certainly of
great value as a preliminary test. The Board of Health
lactometer indicates specific gravities between 1·000 (the
density of water) and 1·0348. On its scale 100° represents the specific gravity of 1·029 (taken as the
minimum density of genuine milk), and 0 represents the
density of water; the graduations are extended to 120°,
equivalent to a specific gravity of 1·0348. In taking an
observation with the lactometer, the standard temperature
of 15° should be obtained, *and the colour and consistency of
the milk noted.* If these latter properties indicate a dilution
of the sample, and the instrument sinks below the 100°
mark, it is safe to assume that the milk has been watered.
The scale is so constructed that the extent of the dilution
is directly shown by the reading, *e. g.* if the lactometer sinks
to 70° the sample contains 70 per cent. of pure milk and
30 per cent. of water. As the standard of specific gravity
(1·029) selected for the 100° mark of the lactometer is the
minimum density of unwatered milk, it is evident that the
readings of the instrument will almost invariably indicate
an addition of water less than has actually taken place. It
would therefore appear that, under normal circumstances,
the standard adopted by the New York Board of Health
errs on the side of too much leniency toward the milk
dealer. Cream being lighter than water, a sample of
skimmed milk will possess a greater specific gravity than
the pure article, and it is possible to add from 10 to 20 per
cent. of water to it and still have the resulting admixture
stand at 100° when tested by the lactometer. Vehement
attempts have been made in court and elsewhere to impeach
the accuracy of the indications afforded by the lactometer.
These have been mainly founded upon the fact that a
sample of milk unusually rich in cream will have a lower
density than a poorer grade, so that it is quite possible that
milk of very superior quality may show a gravity identical
with that of a watered specimen. Great stress has been

laid upon this by the opponents of the measures to control milk adulteration adopted by the public sanitary authorities. They have contended that a chemical analysis should be made. Recourse to this method would, however, involve a greater amount of time than it is usually practicable to devote to the examination of the numerous samples daily inspected; moreover, the process is resorted to whenever the indications of the lactometer leave the inspector in doubt. With the exercise of ordinary intelligence this contingency seldom arises, as the proportion of cream required to reduce the specific gravity to that of a watered sample would be more than sufficient to obviate any danger of mistaking the cause of the decreased density. In this connection it should be stated, that the average lactometric standing of about 20,000 samples of milk, examined by the New York State Dairy Commissioner in the year 1884, was 110°, equivalent to a specific gravity of 1·0319.

The following table shows the value of lactometer degrees in specific gravity :—

VALUE OF LACTOMETER DEGREES IN SPECIFIC GRAVITY.

Lactometer.	Gravity.	Lactometer.	Gravity.	Lactometer.	Gravity.
0	1·00000	18	1·00522	36	1·01044
1	1·00029	19	1·00551	37	1·01073
2	1·00058	20	1·00580	38	1·01102
3	1·00087	21	1·00609	39	1·01131
4	1·00116	22	1·00638	40	1·01160
5	1·00145	23	1·00667	41	1·01189
6	1·00174	24	1·00696	42	1·01210
7	1·00203	25	1·00725	43	1·01247
8	1·00232	26	1·00754	44	1·01276
9	1·00261	27	1·00783	45	1·01305
10	1·00290	28	1·00812	46	1·01334
11	1·00319	29	1·00841	47	1·01363
12	1·00348	30	1·00870	48	1·01392
13	1·00377	31	1·00899	49	1·01421
14	1·00406	32	1·00928	50	1·01450
15	1·00435	33	1·00957	51	1·01479
16	1·00464	34	1·00986	52	1·01508
17	1·00493	35	1·01015	53	1·01537

VALUE OF LACTOMETER DEGREES IN SPECIFIC GRAVITY
(*continued*).

Lactometer.	Gravity.	Lactometer.	Gravity.	Lactometer.	Gravity.
54	1·01566	77	1·02233	100	1·02900
55	1·01595	78	1·02262	101	1·02929
56	1·01624	79	1·02291	102	1·02958
57	1·01653	80	1·02320	103	1·02987
58	1·01682	81	1·02349	104	1·03016
59	1·01711	82	1·02378	105	1·03045
60	1·01740	83	1·02407	106	1·03074
61	1·01769	84	1·02436	107	1·03103
62	1·01798	85	1·02465	108	1·03132
63	1·01827	86	1·02494	109	1·03161
64	1·01856	87	1·02523	110	1·03190
65	1·01885	88	1·02552	111	1·03219
66	1·01914	89	1·02581	112	1·03248
67	1·01943	90	1·02619	113	1·03277
68	1·01972	91	1·02639	114	1·03306
69	1·02001	92	1·02668	115	1·03335
70	1·02030	93	1·02697	116	1·03364
71	1·02059	94	1·02726	117	1·03393
72	1·02088	95	1·02755	118	1·03422
73	1·02117	96	1·02784	119	1·03451
74	1·02146	97	1·02813	120	1·03480
75	1·02175	98	1·02842		
76	1·02204	99	1·02871		

Chemical Examination.

b. Water, Total Solids, and Ash.—Five grammes of the fresh milk are weighed in a tared platinum dish, having a flat bottom, which is placed on a water-bath, where it is allowed to remain for about three hours. It is then transferred to a water-oven, and the dish is subsequently weighed, from time to time, until the weight becomes constant. The loss in weight is the *water* present; the difference between the weight of the platinum capsule and its weight with the remaining contents gives the amount of *total solids*, which, in milk of good quality, should not be under 12 per cent. The inorganic salts (ash) can now be determined by carefully incinerating the residual contents of the capsule. Too high a temperature is to be avoided in this process, in order to prevent the fusion of the ash, which should, however, be ignited until it shows a greyish-white colour. The amount of ash in genuine milk ranges from 0·70 to 0·80 per cent. The addition of water naturally decreases this proportion as well as that of the total milk-solids.

c. Fat, Milk Solids not Fat, Caseine, and Milk Sugar.—An approximate estimation of the fat in milk was formerly made by the use of the *creamometer.* This instrument consists simply of a long glass tube, provided at its upper end with a scale. The milk under examination is introduced into the tube and allowed to remain at rest for about 24 hours, or until the stratum of cream has completely collected upon its surface ; the quantity is then read off by means of the attached scale. The results afforded by the creamometer are, however, far from reliable. Cream is really milk rich in fat, caseine, etc., and the quantitative relation it bears to the true amount of fat present is not always a direct one. A recent form of *lactoscope*, devised by Feser, is less objectionable, and is in very general use for the rapid estimation of fat in milk. It consists essentially of a glass cylinder, provided with two scales, one being graduated into c.c., the other, into percentages of fat. In the lower end of the instrument is a contraction, in which is placed a cylindrical piece of white glass, graduated with well-defined black lines. In using the lactoscope, 4 c.c. of the milk are introduced into the instrument by means of a pipette, and water is gradually added, with shaking, until the black marks on the small white cylinder become just visible. Upon now referring to the c.c. scale, the quantity of water used to effect the necessary dilution is ascertained, and the corresponding percentage of fat in the sample is indicated by the percentage scale.*

In the gravimetric determination of the fat (butter), 10 grammes of the milk are put into a tared platinum dish, containing a weighed amount of dry sand. The milk is evaporated as previously directed, the mixture being con-

* For description of the " Lactocrete," see 'Analyst,' Jan. 1887.

stantly stirred with a small platinum spatula. The residue is repeatedly treated with warm ether or petroleum naphtha of 70° B., and the solutions poured upon a small filter. The several filtrates are collected in a tared beaker, and cautiously evaporated, until constant weight is obtained. This will give the amount of *fat*. The undissolved residue remaining in the platinum capsule, or the difference between the quantity of fat and that of the total milk-solids, affords the proportion of *milk solids not fat* contained, which, in unadulterated milk, should amount to 9 per cent. It has been determined by experiment, that every percentage of milk-solids not fat, increases the specific gravity of milk 0·00375, whereas each percentage of fat decreases the gravity 0·0010, and the proportion of solids not fat can be calculated from the data afforded by the lactometer and Feser's lactoscope by means of the formula :—

$$\frac{S - A}{0 \cdot 00375},$$

where S is the specific gravity of the milk, as shown by the lactometer, and A is the remainder obtained upon multiplying the percentage of fat indicated by the lactoscope by 0·001 and subtracting the residue from 1·0000.

The residue remaining after the extraction of the fat is treated with warm water containing a few drops of acetic acid, or with dilute (80 per cent.) alcohol, in order to remove the sugar. The residue is dried until it ceases to decrease in weight, and is then weighed. The difference between the original weight of the sand and the weight of the sand and residue combined represents approximately the amount of *caseine* (albuminoids) present. As this contains a certain proportion of ash it is to be subsequently ignited, and the ash obtained deducted from the first weight. The alcoholic sugar solution is evaporated to dryness and weighed. The residue is then incinerated and the weight of ash is subtracted. The difference is the amount of *milk sugar* contained. The sugar may likewise be determined by means of Fehling's solution (see pp. 37, 111). About 50 c.c. of the milk is warmed with a small quantity of acetic acid to precipitate the caseine, which is removed by filtration, and the filtrate diluted to 500 c.c.; the test is then applied. 10 c.c. of the copper solution represents 0·067 gramme of milk sugar.

The sugar in milk can also be estimated by the polariscope (see under Sugar, p. 112). In case the Ventzke-Scheibler instrument is used, 65·36 grammes of the sample are weighed out and introduced into a 100 cc. flask; about 5 cc. of plumbic basic acetate solution is added, and the liquid is well shaken, and then allowed to stand at rest for a few minutes. It is next filtered, its volume made up to the 100 cc. mark, and the 20 cm. tube filled and the reading made; this divided by 2 gives the percentage of sugar in the milk.

Mr. A. Adams * has recently proposed a method of milk analysis which consists in first placing 5 cc. of the sample in a tared beaker, and then introducing a weighed paper coil made of blotting paper from which all fatty matter has previously been removed by washing with ether. As soon as the milk is completely absorbed, the paper coil is removed and dried at 100°. The increase of weight gives the amount of *total solids*. The *fat* is next extracted by petroleum naphtha or ether, and its weight determined. The proportion of *solids not fat* is ascertained by again drying and weighing the exhausted coil.

The standards adopted by the English Society of Public Analysts for pure milk, are :—

	Per cent.
Specific gravity	1·030
Ash	0·70
Solids not fat	9·00
Fat	2·50
Total solids	11·50
Water	88·50

* 'Analyst,' x. pp. 46–54.

In the State of New York, the legal standards for
milk are that it shall not contain more than 88 per cent. of
water, nor less than 12 per cent. of milk solids, and 3 per
cent. of fat.

In Massachusetts the law fixing a chemical standard of
purity for milk reads: "In all cases of prosecution, if the
milk shall be shown upon analysis to contain more than
87 per cent. of water, or to contain less than 13 per cent. of
milk solids, it shall be deemed, for the purpose of this Act,
to be adulterated."

The Board of Health of New Jersey fixes the minimum
amount of total solids at 12 per cent. and the maximum
amount of water at 88 per cent. In Paris, the minimum
limits *for condemnation* are the following :—

Fat, 2·70; milk-sugar, 4·50; caseine, albumen, and
ash, 4·30; total solids, 11·50.

The following proportion can be employed in the calculation of the amount of pure milk (x) contained in a
suspected sample :—

From the total solids :—

$$12·5 : \text{total solids found} = 100 : x.$$

From the solids not fat :—

$$9·30 : \text{solids not fat} = 100 : x.$$

From the sugar :—

$$4·40 : \text{sugar found} = 100 : x.$$

From the specific gravity :—

$$1·030 : \text{sp. gr.} = 100 : x.$$

In most cases the determination of the total milk-solids
and the fat (the difference being the solids not fat) furnishes
all the data required for determining the amount of watering which a sample of milk has undergone. The Society
of Public Analysts use 9 as the average percentage of solids

PLATE IV.

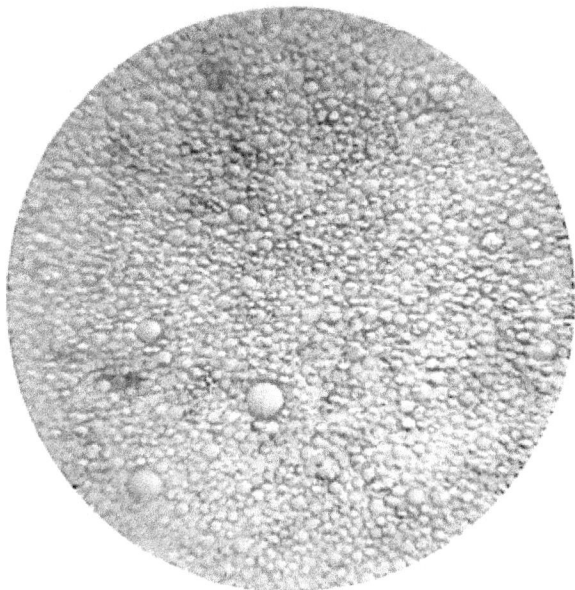

Cream × 420.

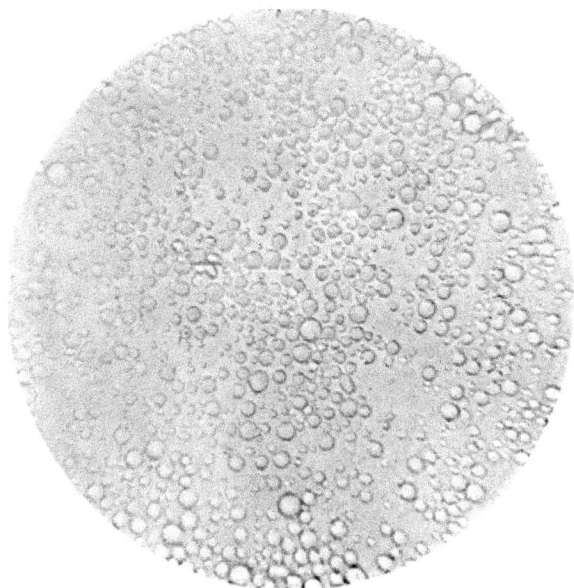

Cows Milk × 420.

not fat in pure milk (which is generally considered as too low) and adopt the formula :—

$$\frac{100}{9} S = x,$$

in which x represents the percentage of genuine milk, and S the solids not fat.

In skimmed milk the percentage of fat removed (x) can be ascertained by the formula :—

$$\frac{2 \cdot 5}{9 \cdot 0} S - f = x,$$

in which S = solids not fat, and f = the fat found. In case the sample has been subjected to both skimming and watering, the water added (x) can be calculated from the formula* :—

$$100 - \frac{100 + 2 \cdot 5}{9} S - f = x.$$

The addition of mineral salts to milk is detected by the increased proportion of ash found; the presence of an abnormal amount of common salt by the high proportion of chlorine present in the ash, which in pure milk should never exceed $0 \cdot 14$ per cent. The use of sodium bicarbonate, borax, etc., is also detected by the analysis of the ash. Glycerine, salicylic acid, flour, and starch, if added, can be extracted from the milk-solids and their identity established by the usual characteristic reactions.

The microscope is of great service in the determination of the quality of milk, and especially in the detection of the presence of abnormal bodies, such as pus, colostrum cells, and blood. In pure cow's milk the globules are in constant motion; their usual size is $\frac{1}{3000}$ of an inch, but this depends upon the nature of the food used. Plates IV. and V., which represent cream, pure milk, skimmed milk, and milk containing colostrum cells, were taken from photo-micrographic negatives furnished through the kindness of Mr. Martin.

* Blyth.

Numerous cases of severe illness have from time to time been developed by the use of milk which was apparently free from any of the usual adulterants. In a recent issue of the 'Philadelphia Medical News' (Sept. 1886) an instance of wholesale milk poisoning at Long Branch is described, and the results reached by a careful study of the epidemic are given. It was demonstrated that warm milk, fresh from the cow, if placed in closed cans under conditions which retarded the dissipation of its heat, may suffer fermentation resulting within a few hours in the genesis of a sufficient quantity of a poisonous ptomaine (termed *tyrotoxicon*) to produce dangerous toxic effects in those drinking it.

Tyrotoxicon was isolated from the milk, and obtained in needle-shaped crystals, which reduced iodic acid and gave a blue coloration when treated with potassium ferricyanide or ferric chloride. Prof. Victor C. Vaughan * discovered the same alkaloid in poisonous cheese, and has also detected its presence in ice-cream that had been the cause of sickness. In this connection it is of importance to note that the addition of gelatine to ice-cream is occasionally practised : in case this substance is used while in a state of incipient decomposition, the danger of the bacteria and other organisms present subsequently resuming activity is considerable. It has been repeatedly and conclusively demonstrated that milk from cows affected with tuberculosis and other complaints, is capable of propagating the seeds of disease, especially in children. The presence of impure water in milk constitutes another source of danger. A test based upon the fact that water which has received sewage contamination often contains nitrites, is applied by first coagulating the suspected milk with acetic acid, then filtering and adding to the filtrate a few cc. of an equal mixture of sulphanilic acid and naphthylamine sulphate, when, in presence of nitrites, a rose-red colour will be produced.

* " Ein Ptomain aus giftigem Käse," Zeit. f. Phys. Chem., x. p. 2, 1886.

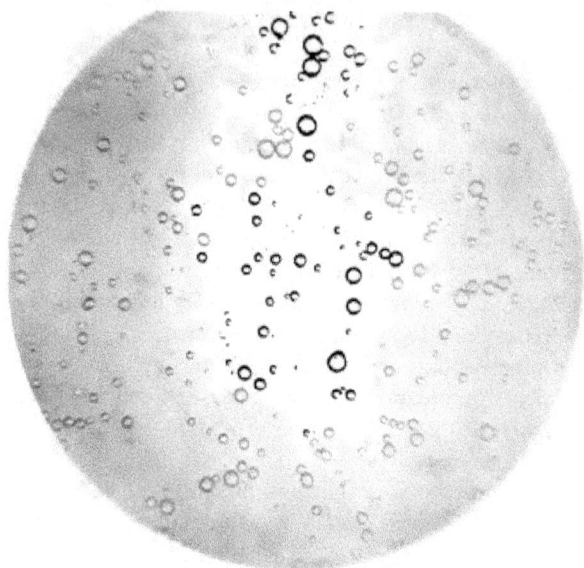

Skimmed Cows Milk × 420.

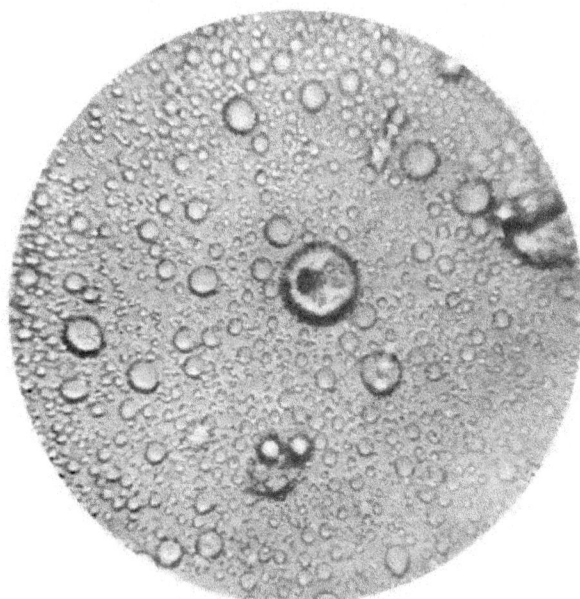

Colostrum in Cows Milk × 420.

BUTTER.

BUTTER is the fat of milk, containing small proportions of caseine, water, and salt (the latter mostly added), and possessing a somewhat granular structure. In its preparation the fat-globules of cream are made to coalesce by the process of churning, and are removed from the residual buttermilk. Its colour, due to lactochrome, varies from white to yellow, according to the breed and food of the cow. The fatty constituents of butter are butyric, caproic, caprylic, capric, myristic, palmitic, stearic, and oleic acids, which are combined with glycerine as ethers ; the first four are soluble in hot water, the remainder insoluble. It is very probable that butter fat is composed of complex glycerides, *i.e.* tri-acid (presumably oleic, palmitic, and butyric) ethers, of the following character :—

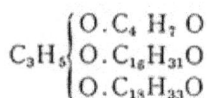

$$C_3H_5 \begin{cases} O . C_4 H_7 O \\ O . C_{16} H_{31} O \\ O . C_{18} H_{33} O \end{cases}$$

The table on p. 64 exhibits a summary of the results obtained by various chemists by the analysis of numerous specimens of genuine butter.

Dr. Elwyn Waller found the following variations in the constituents of pure butter :—Fat, from 83 to 85 ; water, from 8 to 10 ; curd, from 1 to 3 ; salts, from 3 to 5 per cent.

Butter fat fuses at 28° to 37°, and at 37°·7 its specific gravity ranges from 0·91200 to 0·91400. The

Analyst	No. of Samples	Water Maximum	Water Minimum	Water Average	Fats Maximum	Fats Minimum	Fats Average	Curd Maximum	Curd Minimum	Curd Average	Salts Maximum	Salts Minimum	Salts Average
	per cent.	per cent.	per cent.	per cent.	per cent.	per cent.	per cent.	per cent.	per cent.	per cent.	per cent.	per cent.	per cent.
König	123	35·12	5·50	14·49	85·25	76·37	83·27	4·77	0·25	1·29	5·65	0·08	0·95
Bell	117	20·75	4·15	14·2	::	::	::	4·02	::	1·2	15·08	0·5	::
Hassall	48	15·43	4·18	::	96·93	67·72	::	::	::	::	2·91	0·3	::
Hassall	48	28·6	8·48	::	96·93	67·72	::	::	::	::	8·24	1·53	::
Angell and Hehner	30	16·0	6·4	::	90·2	76·4	::	5·1	::	::	8·5	0·4	::
Wanklyn..	50	24·9	8·6	::	::	::	::	::	1·1	::	10·7	0·1	::
Caldwell	26	30·75	10·45	::	::	::	::	::	::	::	::	::	::
Ellis..	12	10·5	4·9	::	89·7	80·8	::	4·9	1·1	::	6·2	0·1	::
Larue	12	16·5	8·0	::	86·9	79·14	::	5·5	1·5	::	3·60	0·4	::
Fleischmann {fresh	::	::	::	18·0	::	::	80·0	::	::	::	::	::	2·0
Fleischmann {salt	::	::	::	12·0	::	::	83·5	::	::	2·5	::	::	6·5
Blyth	5	12·984	8·58	::	87·223	82·643	85·45	5·137	2·054	::	3·151	0·424	::
Schacht	8	9·00	1·25	::	98·00	87·00	::	0·5	::	::	6·0	0·57	::

most common adulterations of butter consist in the addition of water, salt, colouring matters, and various foreign fats (notably oleomargarine). The first two admixtures are easily recognised by the proximate analysis; the detection of the last sophistication involves a somewhat elaborate examination of the fatty constituents of the butter.

Proximate Analysis.

About five grammes of the well-averaged sample are weighed out in a tared platinum capsule, and dried for three hours (or until constant weight is obtained) over a water-bath (or over a low flame, constantly stirring with a thermometer), and the decrease in weight (water) ascertained. As a rule, the proportion of water in genuine butter varies from 8 to 16 per cent. The residue in the capsule is then melted at a gentle heat, and the liquid fat cautiously poured off from the remaining caseine and salt, these latter being afterwards more completely exhausted by washing with ether. Upon now drying the residue, the loss in weight will give the amount of fat present. The caseine is next determined by the loss in weight obtained upon incinerating the matters left undissolved by the ether, the remaining inorganic matter being the salt contained.

The proportion of fat present in genuine butter ranges from 82 to 90 per cent.; it should never be below 80 per cent. The average amount of caseine is 2·5 per cent.; greater proportions, frequently occurring in unadulterated butter, render it more liable to become rancid. The ash should consist of sodium chloride, with some calcium phosphate; the amount of salt is quite variable, but it usually ranges from 2 to 7 per cent. The proportion of ingredients, not fat, in butter may be conveniently determined by melting 10 grammes of the sample in a graduated tube, provided with a scale at its lower end, which is narrowed, adding 30 c.c. of petroleum naphtha,

F

and shaking the mixture. After standing a few hours, the non-fatty matters collect in the lower portion of the tube, and their volume is read off. Genuine butter is said to yield from 12 to 14 per cent. (assuming each c.c. to equal one gramme), while adulterated specimens may show 20 per cent. of matters not fat.

Examination of the Butter-fat.

The most common and important sophistication of butter consists in the addition of foreign fats, embracing both animal fats (oleomargarine and lard) and vegetable oils (cotton-seed, olive, rape-seed, cocoa-nut, almond, palm, etc.). Of these, oleomargarine is doubtless the most often employed. Oleomargarine is the more fusible portion of beef fat, and is prepared by straining the melted fat, allowing the oil thus obtained to stand for some time at a temperature of about 24°, when most of the stearine and palmitine will separate out, and cooling the remaining oil until it solidifies. This is next churned with milk, a little colouring matter (annato) being added, and the product is then chilled by mixing it with ice ; salt is now added, and the mass is finally worked up into lumps.

It is stated that fifteen establishments in the United States are engaged in the manufacture of oleomargarine, the annual production in the State of New York alone being about 20,000,000 pounds. The rapid increase in the manufacture of oleomargarine is shown by the following statistics :—In 1880 this country exported 39.236,655 pounds of butter and 20,000,000 pounds of oleomargarine, while in 1885 the exportation of butter declined to 21,638,128 pounds, and the exportation of oleomargarine reached nearly 38,000,000 pounds. The present production is said to approximate 50,000,000 pounds per annum. The most characteristic difference in the composition of genuine butter and oleomargarine consists in the greater proportion of soluble fats contained in the former. This is illustrated

by the following comparative analysis of the two products
(Mége Mouriès) :—

	Genuine Butter.	Oleomargarine.
	per cent.	per cent.
Water	11·968	11·203
Solids..	88·032	88·797
	100·000	100,000
Solids:		
Insoluble fats	75·256	81·191
Soluble fats	7·432	1·823
Caseine	0·182	0·621
Salt	5·162	5·162
	88·032	88·797

Lard is likewise occasionally used in the United States
as an admixture to butter, the product, "lardine," being
sold either as oleomargarine-butter, or as the genuine
article. Dr. Munsell mentions a factory in New York city
where the weekly output of larded butter is 5000 pounds.
As a result of the efforts of the New York State Dairy
Commission, it has been estimated that the sale of imitation butter in this State in 1885 suffered a decrease of
about 60 per cent., although the quantity manufactured in
the United States showed an increase of 50 per cent.

The specific gravity and melting point of butter have
been suggested as criteria for its purity; in most cases,
however, these determinations possess a rather limited
value; as already stated, butter fat, at the temperature of
$37°·7$, has a density ranging from $0·91200$ to $0·91400$.

The relation between the specific gravity of a fat and the
proportion of insoluble acids contained was first noticed by
Bell. This is shown in the following table which refers
to pure butter fat.

Specific Gravity at 37°·7.	Per cent. Insoluble Acids	Specific Gravity at 37°·7.	Per cent. Insoluble Acids.
0·91382	87·47	0·91286	88·52
0·91346	87·89	0·91276	88·62
0·91337	87·98	0·91258	88·80
0·91290	88·48	0·91246	89·00

The following results have been obtained by the analysis of samples of various animal fats, and oleomargarine butter.

	Specific Gravity at 37°·5.	Per cent, Fixed Fatty Acids.
Mutton suet	0·90283	95·56
Beef suet	0·90372	95·91
Fine lard	0·90384	96·20
Dripping (commercial)	0·90456	94·67
Mutton dripping (genuine)..	0·90397	95·48
Oleomargarine butter	0·90384	94·34
,, ,, ...	0·90234	94·83
,, ,, ...	0·90315	95·04
,, ,, ...	0·90379	96·29
,, ,, ...	0·90136	95·60

It will be noticed that the fats mostly used to adulterate butter are of a lower density. Blyth regards a gravity below 0·911 (at 37°·5) as clearly pointing to the presence of foreign fatty admixture.

The specific gravity determination is made by means of the areometer, or by the gravity bottle ; numerous indirect methods have also been proposed. P. Casamajor * suggests a process for distinguishing genuine butter from oleomargarine which is based upon the fact that the density of a liquid in which a body remains in equilibrium is the density of the body itself. As the result of his investigations it was found that pure butter at 15° would be held in equilibrium by alcohol of 53·7 per cent. (sp. gr. = 0·926), and that oleomargarine would remain in equilibrium, at the same temperature, in alcohol of 59·2 per cent. (sp. gr. = 0·905). If equal volumes of alcohol of 53·7 per cent. and 59·2 per cent. (i. e. an alcohol of 56·5 per cent.) are taken, and a drop of melted butter and of oleomargarine are delivered upon its surface, the former will sink to the bottom and the latter will remain at the top, so long as the

* Journ. Amer. Chem. Soc., iii. p. 53.

two globules are warm and liquid. In case the temperature of the alcohol is about 30°, the butter will solidify and also rise to the top, whereas the oleomargarine may remain liquid. On now keeping the alcohol for a short time at a temperature of 15°, the oleomargarine becomes opaque, but remains at the top, while the solidified butter will sink to the bottom. If alcohol of 59·2 per cent. is employed, oleomargarine will remain at the surface and genuine butter fall to the bottom at all temperatures above 15°, and at this temperature oleomargarine will be in equilibrium. Since not over 33 per cent. of butter is usually added to oleomargarine, it is proposed to use alcohol of 55 per cent., and consider as oleomargarine any sample which does not sink at 15°.

The foregoing method can be applied quantitatively by determining the strength of the alcohol which will keep in equilibrium a drop of the fat under examination. Since the difference between 59·2 and 53·7 is 5·5, the difference between the strength of the alcohol used and 53·7, divided by 5·5 (or multiplied by 0·18), will give the proportion of oleomargarine present. For example, if the globule is held in equilibrium at 15° in 57 per cent. alcohol, the sample contains about 60 per cent. of oleomargarine, for $(57 - 53·7) \times 0·18 = 3·3 \times 0·18 = 0·594$ or, say, $\frac{6}{10}$.

The melting-point of butter is below that of most of its fatty adulterants; as previously stated, it varies from 28° to 37°. The determination is made either in the ordinary manner by means of a fine tube, or a little of the chilled sample is attached to a looped platinum wire, placed near the thermometer-bulb, in water which is gradually heated until fusion takes place. Blyth gives the following table of the melting-points of various fats :—

	°
Butterine	31·3
Cocoa butter	34·9
Butter (average)	35·8
Beef dripping	43·8

Veal dripping	..	..	..	..	..	..	47.7
Mixed	..	..	..	..	..	..	42.6
Lard, from	..	..	..	..	..	..	42 to 45
Ox fat, from about		..	..	..	..	..	48 ,, 53
Mutton fat, from about		..	..	..	..	50 ,, 51
Tallow ..	..	..	..	..	..	..	53.3

Numerous qualitative tests have been proposed by various authorities for the detection of foreign fats in butter, of which the following are perhaps sometimes of use. It should be added that the value of these tests, when applied to mixtures, is limited and very uncertain.

1. A little of the sample is heated in a test-tube : pure butter froths and acquires a brownish colour; with foreign fats there is but little foaming, and, although the casein present darkens, the liquid itself remains comparatively clear.

2. If a sample containing oleomargarine is melted and the oil burned in an ordinary lamp-wick, a decided odour of burning tallow will be produced upon extinguishing the flame. Specimens of real butter, however, have been found to also emit a tallow-like odour.

3. The melted sample is filtered and treated with boiling ether; pure butter fat dissolves much more readily than do lard and tallow. Upon adding methylic alcohol to the solution the latter fats are precipitated, whereas pure butter will remain in solution.

4. If the filtered fat is distilled with a mixture of alcohol and sulphuric acid, the distillate will possess the odour of butyric ether *in a very marked degree*, in case it consists of butter.*

5. The strained fat is treated with a solution of carbolic acid (1 part acid and 10 parts water) : genuine butter dissolves to a clear solution; beef, mutton, and swine fat

* The proportion of butyrine present in commercial oleomargarine is often sufficient in quantity to cause the characteristic odour of butyric ether to a noticeable degree.

form two layers, the upper one becoming turbid upon cooling.

6. If the sample consists of butter or oleomargarine, and is mixed with about ten parts of glycerine and the emulsion digested with a mixture of equal parts of ether and alcohol, two layers of solution will be produced, without any deposit of solid matter between them; if, however, lard, suet, or starch is present it will become deposited between the layers.

It has already been mentioned that butter differs from some of its fatty adulterants in containing a considerable proportion of fatty acids which are soluble in hot water, the acids present in most foreign fats being, on the other hand, almost entirely insoluble. The estimation of the relative amounts of soluble and insoluble acids contained in a fat possesses therefore much importance ; indeed, more significance attaches to this determination than to any other. The processes most frequently employed in the quantitative examination of butter fat are those of Koettstorfer, Hehner, and Reichert.

Koettstorfer's method * is based upon the fact that, as butter fat contains the fatty acids, having a smaller molecular weight than those present in other fats, it must contain more molecules of acid, and will therefore require a greater amount of an alkali to effect saponication. The process is executed as follows :—One or two grammes of the filtered fat are weighed out in a narrow beaker and heated over a water-bath with about 25 c.c. of one-half normal alcoholic solution of potassium hydroxide. The saponification of the fat is assisted by repeated stirring ; when it is completed the beaker is removed from the bath, a few drops of alcoholic phenol-phthaleine added for an indicator, and the excess of potash used titrated back with one-half normal hydrochloric acid. It has been found that pure butter fat requires from 221·4 to 232·4 milligrammes of potassium

* Fresenius' ‘Zeitschrift,’ 1879, p. 197.

hydroxide for saponification. The following are the number of milligrammes of alkali necessary for the saponification of one gramme of various other fats :—

								mgr.
Olive oil	..	..	..	..	..	..	..	191·8
Rape-seed oil	..	..	..	..	..	..	178·7
Oleomargarine..	..	..	..	..	..	..	195·5
Beef tallow	..	..	..	..	..	..	196·5
Lard ..	..	..	..	..	..	..	195·5
Mutton suet	..	..	..	..	..	..	197·0
Dripping	..	..	..	..	..	..	197·0

Taking 227 milligrammes as the average amount of potassium hydroxide required to saponify one gramme of pure butter fat, the following formula has been suggested for the estimation of the proportion of admixture in a suspected sample :—

$$(227 - n) \times 3·17 = x,$$

in which n represents the number of milligrammes of potassium hydroxide used, and x the percentage of foreign fat added. In the Paris Municipal Laboratory, 221 milligrammes of K(OH) are regarded as a standard for the saponification of one gramme of genuine butter.

Cocoa-nut oil, unfortunately, requires a figure (250 mgr.) considerably above that of butter, and it is quite possible to prepare a mixture of this oil and oleomargarine, that by the foregoing test would show a result almost identical with that afforded by pure butter. Hehner's process,* which is often employed for the determination of the insoluble fatty acids, is as follows :—About 4 grammes of the melted and strained sample are dissolved in 50 c.c. of alcohol, containing two grammes of potassium hydroxide in solution, and the mixture is heated until complete saponification takes place. The alcohol is removed by evaporation, the residue dissolved in 200 c.c. of water, and the fatty acids precipitated by adding dilute sulphuric acid to distinct acid reaction. The fatty acids are next melted by heating the liquid and are then allowed to cool, after

* ' Zeitschrift für Analytische Chemie,' 1877, p. 145.

which the insoluble acids are poured upon a tared filter
and repeatedly washed with hot water until the washings
cease to show acidity. The filter and contents are finally
cautiously dried and weighed. In genuine butter the proportion of insoluble fatty acids ranges between 86·5 and
87·5 per cent.; it should not be above 88 per cent.* Oleomargarine, lard, mutton, beef, and poppy, palm, olive, and
almond oils contain about 95·5 per cent. of insoluble acids.†

The preceding process is also imperfect in not effecting
the detection of cocoa-nut oil, which affords only about
86 per cent. of insoluble fatty acids, and although the
presence of any considerable proportion of this oil in
butter would probably be indicated by the decreased melting point of the admixture, an estimation of the soluble
fatty acids is by far the most reliable means for its detection. For this determination Reichert's method‡ is
eminently adapted. In this process advantage is taken of
the facts that the amount of soluble acids in a mixture of
fat bears a direct relation to the proportion of genuine
butter present, and that, if the aqueous solution of a
saponified fat is decomposed by an acid and heated to
boiling, the greater portion of the soluble acids escape
with the watery vapours and can be collected and determined in the distillate. The details of this method are
essentially as follows:—2½ grammes of the filtered sample
are introduced into an Erlenmayer flask together with
1 gramme of potassium hydroxide and 20 c.c. of dilute
(80 per cent.) alcohol, and the mixture is heated over the
water-bath until complete saponification is effected, and the
alcohol *entirely* removed. The soap thus formed is dissolved in 50 c.c. of water, and decomposed by adding 20 c.c.
of dilute sulphuric acid (1 : 10). The flask is next connected

* The French standard is 87·50 per cent.
† The percentage of foreign fat (F) in a sample can be calculated by
the formula $F = (I - 88) \times 13\cdot3$, in which I = the insoluble fatty acids.
‡ Fresenius' Zeitschrift, 1879, p. 68.

with a Liebig's condenser and the contents carefully distilled until 50 c.c. have passed over. The distillate is now freed from any insoluble acids possibly present by filtration; it is then titrated with decinormal soda solution, a few drops of litmus solution being employed as an indicator. As the result of numerous tests, it has been found that genuine butter, when examined by the above method, requires from 13 to 15 c.c. of the decinormal solution. The following are the number of c.c. required by various other fats:—

Lard	..	..	..	..	..	..	..	..	0·2
Rape oil	..	..	..	..	..	..	..	..	0·25
Kidney fat	..	..	..	..	..	..	..	..	0·25
Olive oil	..	..	..	..	..	..	..	..	0·3
Sesamé oil	..	..	..	..	..	..	..	..	0·35
Oleomargarine	..	..	..	..	..	..	..	0·7 to 1·3
Cocoa-nut oil	..	..	..	..	..	..	..	3·70

Dr. Elwyn Waller [*] modifies the foregoing method of procedure by adding 50 c.c. of water to the contents of the flask remaining after the first distillation, and again distilling off 50 c.c., the process being repeated until the final distillate neutralises only 0·1 c.c. of the decinormal alkali. With butter fat, it was found that the first distillate contained about 79 per cent. of the total volatile acids present. By means of this modification, a distinction between the rate of distillation of the volatile fatty acids of different fats is possible. The non-volatile acids left in the flask are washed several times with water, in order to remove the glycerine and potassium sulphate present, and are then dried and weighed.

For estimating the percentage of pure butter fat in a sample of mixed fat, Reichert employed the formula: $B = 7·3 \ (m - 0·3)$, in which m is the number of c.c. of soda solution used in the titration.

Baron Hübl [†] has recently suggested a method for butter testing, which is founded upon the fact that the three series

* Journ. Amer. Chem. Soc., viii. p. 6.
† Dingl. Polyt. Journ., ccliii., p. 281.

of fats (acetic, acrylic, and tetrolic), unite in different proportions with the halogens (iodine, bromine, and chlorine),
to form addition products. Iodine has been found especially
well adapted to the examination of fats. The standard
solution employed is prepared by dissolving 25 grammes
of iodine in 500 c.c. of 95 per cent. alcohol, and adding to
the solution a solution of 30 grammes of mercuric chloride
in 500 c.c. of alcohol. The reagent is then standardised by
means of a solution of 24 grammes of sodium hyposulphite in 1 litre of water. The test is applied as
follows :—1 gramme of the sample under examination is
introduced into a flask and dissolved in 10 c.c. of pure
chloroform. The iodine reagent is then gradually added
from a burette, the mixture being well shaken, until the
coloration produced indicates that an excess is present, even
after standing for about two hours ; 15 c.c. of a 10 per cent.
potassium iodide solution and 150 c.c. of water are then
added and the excess of iodine present determined by means
of the sodium hyposulphite solution, and deducted from
the total quantity used. The amount of iodine (in grammes)
absorbed is calculated to 100 grammes of the fat ; this is
termed the iodine number. The examination of numerous
samples of genuine butter and oleomargarine, and other
fats, made at the laboratory of the New York State Dairy
Commissioner, furnished the following results :*—

						Iodine Number.
Genuine butter	..	..	..	from	30·5 to 43·0
Oleomargarine	..	..	..	„	50·9 „ 54·9
Cocoa-nut oil	..	..	..	..	..	6·8
Lard	..	..	..			55·0
Mutton fat	..	..	..	..	..	57·3
Oleine	..	..	..	..	..	82·3
Olive oil	..	..	..	..	..	83·0
Pea-nut oil	..	..				96·0
Sweet-almond oil	..	..	..	..	..	102·0
Cotton-seed oil	..	..	..	..	..	108·0
Poppy oil	..	..	..	..	..	134·0

* R. W. Moore notes that a certain mixture of lard and cocoa-nut
oil would give an iodine number identical with that of butter fat.—
('Analyst,' x. p. 224.)

It has been proposed to differentiate between butter and oleomargarine by a determination of the proportion of glycerine contained. Liebschütz * employs the following process for this estimation: 10 grammes of the sample are saponified by heating with 20 grammes of barium hydroxide, until the water of crystallisation has been almost entirely expelled. Alcohol is then added with constant stirring ; saponification quickly takes place, and is completed by evaporating the mass nearly to dryness. The glycerine is extracted with boiling water, the solution filtered, and the barium contained removed by means of sulphuric acid. The filtrate from the barium sulphate is then concentrated by evaporation, and the excess of sulphuric acid present neutralised by adding a little barium carbonate. The filtered liquid is now again evaporated to a small volume, and most of the salts present precipitated by addition of absolute alcohol. After filtration the alcoholic solution is evaporated over the water-bath, then dried at 100° until constant weight is obtained. It is finally ignited and the proportion of glycerine contained estimated by the loss in weight sustained. This process is certainly far from being exact, owing principally to the volatilisation of glycerine that occurs in the evaporation of its aqueous and even alcoholic solutions. The following results were obtained upon treating genuine butter and oleomargarine according to the above method :—

	Per cent. Glycerine.
Butter	3·75
Oleomargarine	7·00

Gelatine is said to have lately been used as an adulterant of butter, more especially of artificial butter. Its detection is a matter of some difficulty. The following method has been suggested. A considerable quantity of the suspected butter is boiled with water, the solution strained, a drop of acetic acid and a little potassium ferrocyanide added, and

* Journ. Amer. Chem. Soc., vii. p. 134.

the liquid boiled until the precipitate formed becomes bluish in colour. The solution is then filtered hot and the filtrate examined for gelatine by adding tannic acid to, or conducting chlorine gas through it.

A sample lately imported under the name of "butter preservative" was found by the author to consist of a dilute solution of phosphoric acid. The use of this agent does not, however, appear to be prevalent to any great extent.*

Artificial Colouring.—The list of colouring matters said to be added to butter includes the vegetable dyes, annato, carotin, fustic, turmeric, marigold, and saffron ; the coal-tar colour, Victoria yellow (potassium dinitrocresylate), and Martius yellow (potassium dinitronaphthalate), and the mineral pigment chrome yellow (plumbic chromate). Of the foregoing, annato and carrot colour appear to be most commonly employed. Mr. Edward W. Martin† has proposed a method for the isolation of the former which consists in dissolving the butter in carbon disulphide, and shaking the solution with a *dilute* solution of potassium hydroxide, in which the colouring matter dissolves ; it is subsequently identified by further tests. According to Mr. R. W. Moore,‡ the presence of carotin in butter may be detected by first agitating the carbon disulphide solution of the fat with alcohol, which fails to extract this colour. Upon now adding to the mixture a drop of dilute ferric chloride solution, again shaking the liquid and then putting it aside for a short time, the alcoholic solution dissolves the carrot colour, and if no other colouring matter is contained in the butter, leaves the carbon disulphide colourless.

The artificially coloured butter may be dissolved in alcohol and tested with the following reagents :—

(*a*) Nitric acid : greenish coloration, *saffron*.

(*b*) Sugar solution and hydrochloric acid : red coloration, *saffron*.

---

* Samples invoiced as "butter flavouring," and consisting of butyric acid, have also been imported.

† 'Analyst,' x. p. 163. ‡ Ibid., xi. p. 163.

(*c*) Ammonia : brownish coloration, *turmeric.*

(*d*) Silver nitrate : blackish coloration, *marigold.*

(*e*) Evaporate the alcoholic solution to dryness and add concentrated sulphuric acid : greenish-blue coloration, *annato ;* blue coloration, *saffron.*

(*f*) Hydrochloric acid : decolorisation, with formation of yellow crystalline precipitate, *Victoria or Martius yellow.*

(*g*) Separation of a heavy and insoluble yellow powder, *chrome yellow* (see p. 130).

Microscopic Examination. — The microscopic examination of butter has lately received considerable attention as a means for the detection of the presence of foreign fats. Genuine butter generally exhibits under the microscope a crowded mass of globules of fat, fatty crystals being commonly absent. In oleomargarine a more crystalline structure is observed, with pear-shaped masses of fat and but few globules. While the presence of crystals in a sample may justly be regarded as suspicious, it is by no means a positive evidence of adulteration, since, under certain circumstances, pure butter may present the same indications. In applying the microscopic test, a small portion of the fat is made into a thin layer on the slide, and then protected with a glass cover, applied with rather gentle pressure.

Plate VI.* represents the microscopic appearance of genuine butter and oleomargarine. It will be observed that in butter (Fig. 1) numerous globules but no crystals of fat are presented, the crystals present being those of salt. In oleomargarine (Fig. 2) the distinctive pear-shaped masses of fat, accompanied by only a small number of fatty globules, are to be seen. Dr. Thomas Taylor (of the U.S. Department of Agriculture), has made an elaborate investigation of the microscopic appearance of various fats

* The author is indebted to Mr. Edward W. Martin for the negatives used in the preparation of these and other photomicrographs of fats.

PLATE VI.

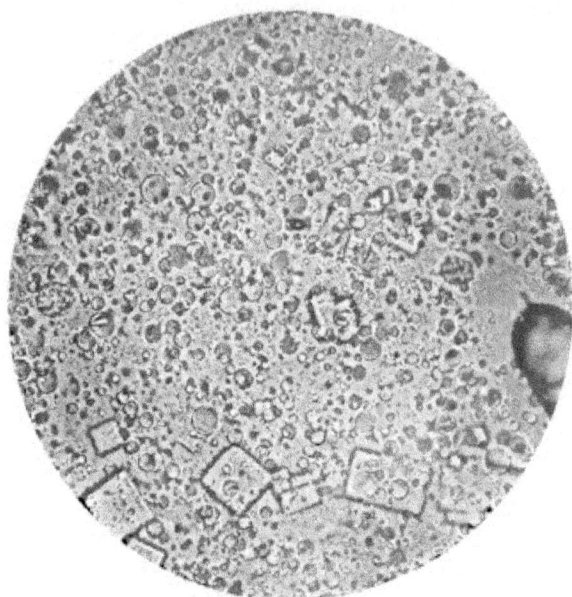

Fig. 1. Butter × 400.

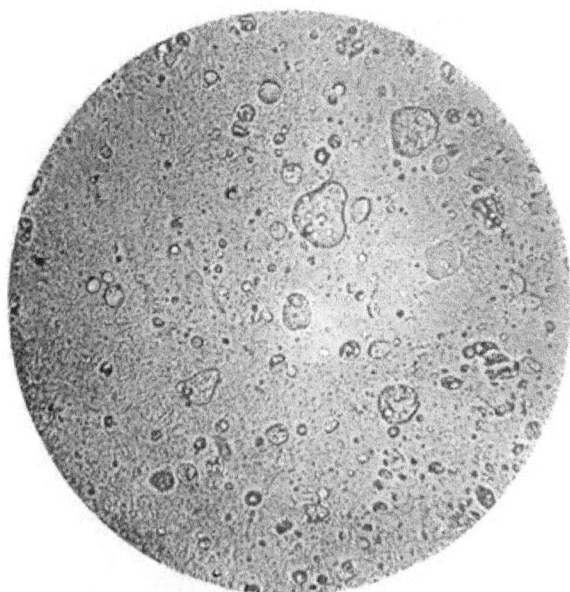

Fig. 2. Oleomargarine ×40.)

PLATE VII

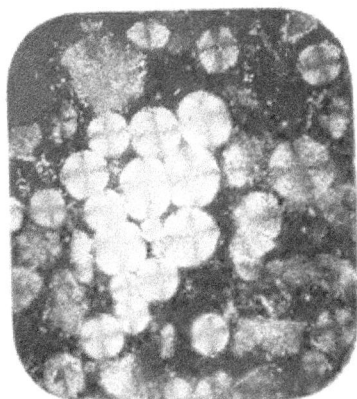

Butter × 40.

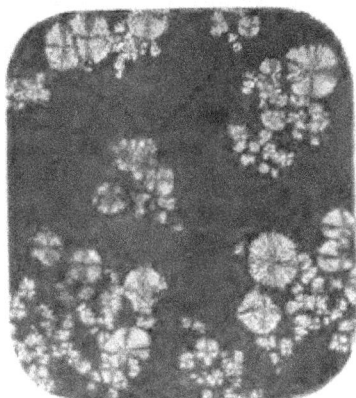

Butter × 40.

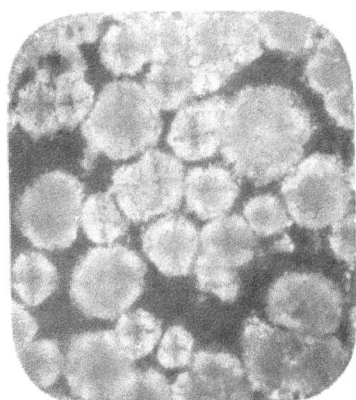

Beef × 40.

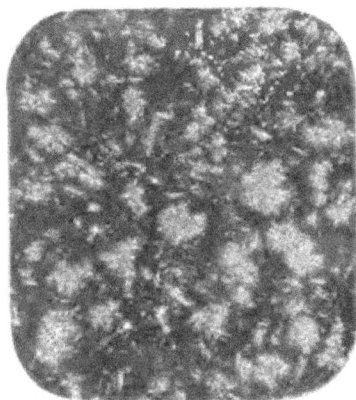

Lard × 160.

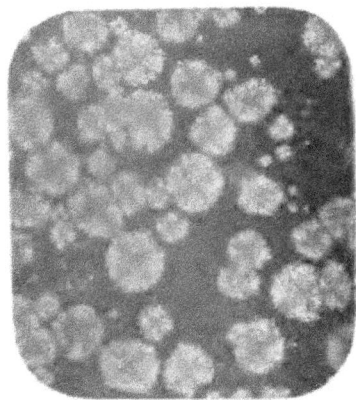

Butterine × 40.

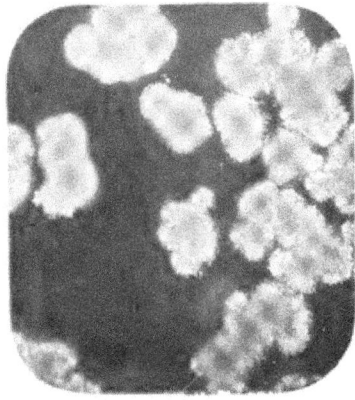

Oleomargarine × 40.

FAT CRYSTALS.

when viewed by polarised light. He regards the presence of peculiar globular crystals and the black cross commonly termed St. Andrew's cross as characteristic of genuine butter.* Lard, beef, and other fats are said to exhibit different and, to some extent, distinctive crystalline forms. Prof. Weber,† however, affirms that mixtures of lard and tallow fat, under certain conditions, cannot be distinguished from butter by means of this method of examination. More recently, Dr. Taylor states that the distinguishing difference between butter and other fats under the microscope is that the former, when observed by polarised light through a selenite, exhibits a uniform tint, whereas the latter shows prismatic colours. Although the results of these investigations cannot as yet be considered as perfectly satisfactory or conclusive, they certainly are entitled to rank as a highly valuable and important step in advance of the optical processes hitherto employed.

Plate VII. exhibits the appearance of butter, oleomargarine, beef, and some other fats, when viewed by the microscope and polarised light. It will be noticed that, while a discrimination between lard and butter is readily made, oleomargarine presents the St. Andrew's cross, stated to be characteristic of genuine butter. These photomicrographs represent the results of investigations made in the Chemical Division of the U.S. Department of Agriculture.

The question of the sanitary effects of oleomargarine and other substitutes for butter, has been studied by many scientists, and with very discordant results. Doubtless the great divergence of opinion which at present exists, is largely due to the fact that the artificial products examined have been made according to different processes, and with varying regard to the quality of the fats used in their

* *Vide* 'Proceedings of the American Microscopical Society,' May 1885.

† 'Bulletin of the Ohio Agricultural Experiment Station,' March 1st, 1886.

manufacture, and to the degree of care and cleanliness
observed. The attention of the American public has very
lately been directed to the oleomargarine question, by the
recent enactment of a national law imposing a tax upon
the manufacture of the article.

Without entering to any great extent into the subject of
the wholesomeness of artificial butter as it is generally
met with in commerce, it will be of interest to refer to the
conclusions reached by two or three sanitarians who have
devoted particular attention to this aspect of the question.
Prof. W. O. Atwater* summarises the results of his
investigation of oleomargarine as follows :—

" 1. The common kinds of imitation butter, oleomargarine, butterine, etc., when properly made, agree very
closely in chemical composition, digestibility, and nutritive
value with butter from cow's milk.

" 2. In fulfilling one of the most important functions of
food, namely, that of supplying the body with heat and
muscular energy, they, with butter, excell in efficiency all,
or nearly all, our other common food materials.

" 3. Considering the low cost at which they can be produced, as well as their palatability and nutritive value, they
form a food product of very great economical importance,
and one which is calculated to greatly benefit a large class
of our population whose limited incomes make good dairy
butter a luxury.

" 4. Imitation butter, like many other manufactured food
materials, is liable (but in actual commerce has been found
not to be so) to be rendered unwholesome by improper
materials and methods of manufacture. It is also open
to the especial objection that it is largely sold as genuine
butter. The interests of the public, therefore, demand
that it should be subjected to competent official inspection, and that it should be sold for what it is, and not
as genuine butter."

* Bradstreet's, June 19, 1886.

Dr. S. B. Sharples * states: "When well made, it (oleomargarine) is a very fair imitation of genuine butter; being inferior to the best butter, but much superior to the low grades of butter too commonly found in the market. So far as its influence on health is concerned, I can see no objection to its use. Its sale as genuine butter is a commercial fraud, and as such, very properly condemned by the law. As to its prohibition by law, the same law which prohibited it should also prohibit the sale of lard and tallow, and more especially all low-grade butters, which are far more injurious to health than a good sweet article of oleomargarine. A good deal has been said in regard to the poor grade of fats from which the oleomargarine is made. Any one making such assertions in regard to the fats is simply ignorant of the whole subject. When a fat has become in the least tainted, it can no longer be used for this purpose, as it is impossible to remove the odour from the fat after it has once acquired it."

Per contra, Dr. R. B. Clark, in an exhaustive report on butter,† affirms with great decision, that artificial butter is not a wholesome article of food, for the following reasons :—

" 1. On account of its indigestibility.

" 2. On account of its insolubility when made from animal fats.

" 3. On account of its liability to carry germs of disease into the human system.

" 4. On account of the probability of its containing, when made under certain patents, unhealthy ingredients."

The two last grounds for condemning oleomargarine are evidently affected by, and, in fact, dependent upon the character of the fat and the exercise of care employed in its manufacture. In regard to the relative digestibility of butter and its imitations, actual experiments have been

---

* Fourth Annual Report (1883) Mass. State Board of Health, p. 30.
† Second Annual Report of the New York State Dairy Commissioner, pp. 291–392.

made by several chemists. A. Mayer,* from the results of
feeding human beings for three days on butter and on
oleomargarine, found that 1·6 per cent. less of the latter
was absorbed by the system than of the former, and
inclines to the opinion, that with healthy persons this proportion is so inconsiderable, that it is of little or no importance. Dr. Clark considers these experiments of too
limited duration to be regarded as conclusive, although, so
far as they went, the results reached coincided with those
obtained by him by a more exhaustive investigation. Dr.
Clark has made an examination of the artificial digestion
of butter as compared with oleomargarine and other fats,
including beef and mutton suet, and lard, cotton-seed,
sesamé, and cod-liver oils. The method of examination
pursued was as follows :—About 2 grammes of the melted
fat was added to a digestive fluid consisting of 0·33 gramme
of "extractum pancreatis," and 0·33 gramme of sodium
bicarbonate, dissolved in 10 c.c. of distilled water. This
mixture was introduced into a test-tube, well shaken, and
then exposed to a temperature of 40°. The contents of
the test-tube were microscopically examined at the lapse
of intervals of one, four, and twelve hours. It was found
from these tests that cod-liver oil exhibited the most perfect
state of emulsion, after which came genuine butter, next
lard oil, and then commercial "oleo." Plate VIII. represents the results obtained from the experiments made with
butter and commercial oleomargarine, as presented at the
end of one, four, and twelve hours. The globules of
butter-fat, it will be observed, are smaller in size and more
uniform in appearance. Dr. Clark likewise instituted experiments which tended to demonstrate the relative insolubility of the fats used in the preparation of artificial
butter.

* 'Landwirthschaftliche Versuchsstation,' ii. p. 215.

PLATE VIII.

Butter 1 hour × 250.

Oleomargarine 1 hour × 250.

Butter 4 hours × 250.

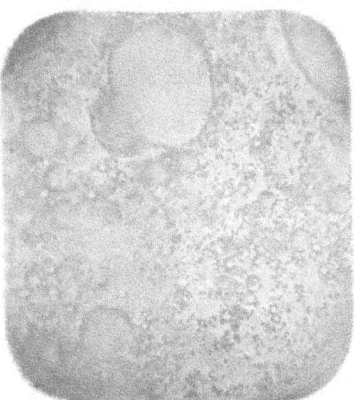

Oleomargarine 4 hours × 250.

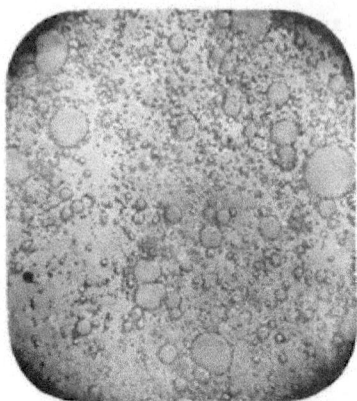

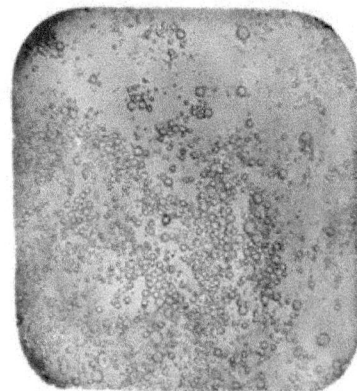

Butter 12 hours × 250.

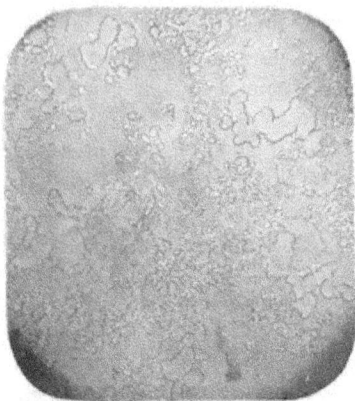

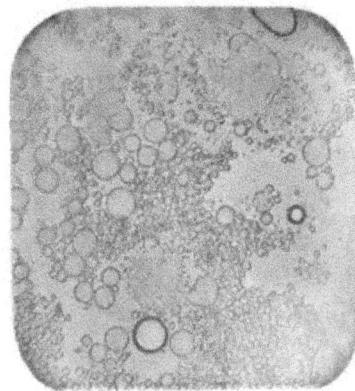

Oleomargarine 12 hours × 250.

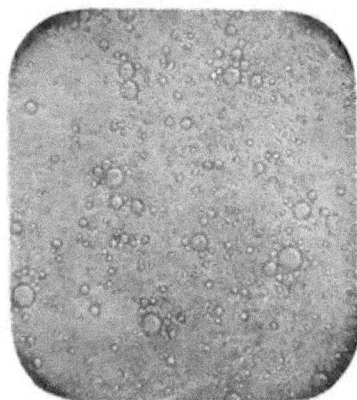

ARTIFICIAL DIGESTION OF FATS.

CHEESE.

CHEESE consists essentially of the cas: and albumen of milk, together with water, fat, lactic acid, and mineral salts. It is prepared by the coagulation of milk by means of rennet, and is usually obtained from cow's milk (either fresh, skimmed, or sour), although the milk of the goat, ewe, and other animals is occasionally used. Its colour is very often due to the addition of annato. The following table exhibits the composition of the best-known varieties of cheese, according to the analysis of various chemists :—

Variety.	Water.	Fat.	Caseine or Nitrogenous Matter.	Milk Sugar.	Free Acid, as Lactic.	Ash.	Composition of Fat.	
							Soluble Acids.	Insoluble Acids.
	per cent.	per cent.	per cent.	per cent.	per cent.	per cent.	per cent.	per cent.
American (pale)	31·55	35·93	28·83	..	0·27	3·42	4·81	88·49
American (red)	28·63	38·24	29·64	..	..	3·49	4·26	89·06
Cheddar	35·60	31·57	28·16	..	0·45	4·22	4·55	88·75
Stilton	23·57	39·13	32·55	..	1·24	3·51	4·42	88·76
Gloucester ..	35·75	28·35	31·10	..	0·31	4·49	6·68	86·89
Dutch	41·30	22·78	28·25	..	0·57	7·10	5·84	87·58
Roquefort ..	32·26	34·38	27·16	..	1·32	4·88	4·91	88·70
Brie	51·87	24·83	19·00	..	..	5·00	..	..
Cheshire	37·11	30·68	26·93	..	0·86	4·42	5·55	87·76
Gruyère	33·66	30·69	30·67	..	0·27	4·71	4·41	88·97
Gorgonzola ..	31·85	34·34	27·88	..	1·35	4·58	4·40	89·18
Neufchatel ..	37·87	41·30	17·43			3·40	..	..
Camembert ..	51·30	..	19·00	3·50		4·70	..	..
Parmesan	27·56	15·95	44·08	6·69		5·72	..	..

Dr. Muter has published the following analyses of cheese :—*

Variety.	Insoluble Acids.	Soluble Acids.	Milligrammes K(OH) to saponify 1 gr.	Water.	Fat.	Lactic Acid.	Insoluble Ash.	Soluble Ash.	Salt.
Double Gloucester ..	87·00	6·28	229·3	37·20	22·80	1·80	2·56	2·00	1·64
Stilton	86·20	7·02	231·7	28·60	30·70	1·08	1·80	2·22	0·75
English cream ..	90·01	3·26	220·0	63·64	15·14	0·90	0·72	0·20	0·12
Dutch	87·20	6·09	228·7	42·72	16·30	1·35	2·26	9·10	4·02
Gruyère	87·32	5·98	228·0	33·20	27·26	1·35	3·12	1·58	1·05
Rochefort ..	87·00	6·27	229·3	21·56	35·96	0·72	1·70	8·54	3·42
Camembert	87·15	6·09	229·0	48·78	21·35	0·36	0·16	8·64	3·46
Bondon	7·834	5·95	228·0	55·20	20·80	0·90	0·52	6·46	3·16
American Cheddar ..	89·08	3·30	220·2	29·70	30·70	0·90	2·16	1·54	1·20
Cheddar	87·66	5·00	227·5	33·40	26·60	1·53	2·30	2·00	1·52

According to this chemist, one gramme of genuine cheese should require not less than 220 milligrammes K(OH) for saponification, as executed in Koettstorfer's process (see p. 71).

The following results were obtained by Griffiths † from the analysis of American cheese, and by Gerber ‡ from the analysis of artificial American cheese :—

	American Cheese.	Lard Cheese.	Oleomargarine Cheese.
	per cent.	per cent.	per cent.
Water	26·55	38·26	37·99
Fat	35·58	21·07	23·70
Caseine, etc.	33·85	35·55	34·65
Ash	3·90	5·12	3·66

The constituents of cheese are very similar to those of milk; the relations between the soluble and insoluble fatty

* 'Analyst,' Jan. 1885, p. 3.
† Chem. News, pp. 47, 85.
‡ Dingl., vol. i. pp. 247, 474.

acids is much the same as in butter. In cheese, however, the milk-sugar is largely decomposed into lactic acid, alcohol, and carbonic acid, during the process of ripening or curing employed in its manufacture.

Another essential change effected by the curing of cheese is the partial decomposition of the caseine into ammonia, which combines with the unaltered caseine, forming soluble ammonium caseates. Other products of the ripening process, also due to the decomposition of the caseine, are tyrosine and leucine ($C_6H_{13}NO_2$). The butter-fats are likewise transformed into the corresponding fatty acids, which give rise to the formation of either the ammonia salts, acid albuminates, or amines, such as butylamine or amylamine.

The characteristic odour of many varieties of cheese is chiefly owing to the genesis of these latter compounds.

As with butter, the most important adulteration of cheese consists in the addition of foreign fats. Doubtless, the most frequent sophistication is the admixture of lard. Lard cheese (which is usually sold as " Neufchatel ") is made by first preparing an emulsion of lard and skimmed milk (in the proportion of one part of the former to two parts of the latter). This is subsequently incorporated with skimmed milk and butter-milk, the coagulation of the fat being then effected in the usual manner. In regard to the production of this species of cheese, it is stated that in the 23 factories in the State of New York, the product of six months' working (ending November, 1881), was about 800,000 pounds, of which the greater proportion was exported. The recent (1885) adoption of a New York State brand for " pure cream cheese " has had a very good effect, and accomplished much in the restriction of the manufacture and sale of the spurious article. Another variety of imitation cheese, know as " anti-huff cheese," is prepared from skimmed milk without the addition of foreign fat, but with the aid of various chemical preparations, such as caustic or carbonated soda, saltpetre, and borax. The rind of cheese is occasionally contaminated with poisonous metallic salts, including those of lead, mercury, antimony, arsenic, copper and zinc, which are added either for colouring purposes or to prevent the attacks of flies and other insects. This form of adulteration is doubtless of rare occurrence. The methods used in cheese analysis are much the same as those employed in the examination of butter. The fat is determined by exhaustion with ether (or preferably, petroleum naphtha), and evaporation, the remaining solids not fat being likewise dried and weighed. The difference between the combined weight of the fat and the solids not fat, and the amount of the sample taken, represents the proportion of water present. Lactic acid, while insoluble in petroleum naphtha, is also dissolved by ether, and can be estimated by digesting another portion of the sample with water, and titrating the filtered liquid with decinormal soda solution. Its weight is then to be deducted from the amount of fat previously obtained, in case ether was employed in this determination. The relative proportions of the soluble and insoluble fatty acids contained in cheese possess the same significance in indicating the presence of oleomargarine and other foreign fats as with butter ; and they are determined by the same methods.

The examination of the colouring matter of cheese can be made by first neutralising the free lactic acid, separating the fat by agitation with water, filtering and drying ; the fat is then tested with carbon disulphide and potassium hydroxide (see p. 77).

FLOUR AND BREAD.

WHEAT (*Triticum vulgare*) forms the principal bread-stuff of civilised nations, and is by far the most important of all cereal grasses. It has one or more slender, erect and smooth stalks, which, owing to the large proportion of siliceous matter present, possesses the strength necessary for the support of the ears. The grain is imbricated in four rows. The following are the averages of the results obtained by the analyses of 260 samples of American wheat, made by the United States Department of Agriculture, in 1883:—

	Per cent.
Water	10·27
Ash	1·84
Oil	2·16
Carbohydrates	71·98
Fibrin	1·80
Albuminoids	11·95
Nitrogen	1·91

Analyses of the ash of wheat made by the same Department, furnished the following results :—

	Dakota.	Foreign.	
		Winter.	Spring.
	Per cent.	Per cent.	Per cent.
Insoluble	1·44	2·11	1·64
Phosphoric acid	47·31	46·98	48·63
Potassa	30·63	31·16	29·99
Magnesia	16·09	11·97	12·09
Lime	3·36	3·34	2·93
Soda	1·17	2·25	1·93
Sulphuric acid	trace	0·37	0·48
Chlorine	,,	0·22	0·51
Ferric oxide	,,	1·31	0·28
Undetermined	..	0·29	1·52
	100·00	100·00	100·00
Total ash ..	1·88	1·97	2·14

FLOUR.

The name flour is usually given to the product obtained
by grinding wheat and removing the bran, or woody portion of the grain, by sifting or bolting. Its constituents are
starch, dextrine, cellulose, and sugar (carbohydrates), the
nitrogenous compounds albumen, gliadin, mucin, fibrin,
and cerealin, and fat, mineral substances and water. Upon
kneading flour with water, and removing the starch and
soluble matters by repeated washing, an adhesive body
termed *gluten* remains behind. This is chiefly composed of
gliadin, mucin, and fibrin.

According to Wanklyn,[*] the general composition of
flour is :—

	Per cent.
Water	16·5
Fat	1·5
Gluten	12·0
Modified starch	3·5
Vegetable albumen	1·0
Starch granules	64·8
Ash	0·7

The average of numerous analyses of American flour
examined by the Department of Agriculture gave :—

	Per cent.
Water	11·67
Fat	1·25
Sugar	1·91
Dextrine	1·79
Starch	71·72
Soluble albuminoids	2·80
Insoluble „	7·90
Total „	10·70
Ash	0·54

The composition of the ash of flour from Minnesota
wheat (1883), is as follows :—

	Per cent.
Insoluble	0·98
Phosphoric acid	49·63
Potassa	31·54
Magnesia	9·05
Lime	5·87
Soda	2·93

* 'Bread Analysis.'

ANALYSIS OF FLOUR.

The following are the determinations generally required in the proximate analysis of flour :—

Water.—Two or three grammes of the sample are weighed in a tared platinum dish, and heated in an air bath, until constant weight is obtained. The proportion of water should not exceed 17 per cent.

Starch.—A small amount of the flour is placed in a flask, connected with an ascending Liebig's condenser, and boiled for several hours with water slightly acidulated with sulphuric acid. Any remaining excess of acid is then neutralised with sodium hydroxide ; the solution is considerably diluted, and the glucose formed, estimated by means of Fehling's solution (see p. 111). 100 parts of glucose represent 90 parts of starch.

Fat.—The inconsiderable proportion of fat in flour is best determined by exhausting the dried sample with ether and evaporating the solution.

Gluten (albuminoids).—As previously stated, gluten is separated by kneading the flour and repeated washing with water. After the removal of the amylaceous and soluble ingredients, the residue is carefully dried and weighed. A far more accurate method is to make a combustion of a small portion of the flour with cupric oxide, and determine the quantity of nitrogen obtained, the percentage of which, multiplied by 6·33, gives the percentage of gluten.* The proportion of gluten in flour ranges from about 8 to 18 per cent. From 10 to 12 per cent. is deemed necessary in order to make good bread, and, in England,

* Wanklyn applies his ammonia process (see p. 205), to the estimation of albuminoids in vegetable substances. In this manner he obtained the following percentages of ammonia from various flours :— Rice, 0·62 ; maize and malt, 1·03 ; wheat and barley, 1·10 ; rye, 1·45 ; pea, 2·30.

any deficiency in this constituent is remedied by the
addition of bean or other flour, but in the United States
this practice is seldom required.

Substances soluble in cold water.—About five grammes
of the flour are digested with 250 c.c. of cold water, and the
solution filtered, and evaporated to dryness. Good flour
is stated to yield 4·7 per cent. of extract when treated in
this manner, the soluble matters consisting of sugar, gum,
dextrine, vegetable albumen, and potassium phosphate.
The latter salt, which constitutes about 0·4 per cent. of
the extract, should form the only mineral matter present.

The Ash.—The ash of flour is determined in the usual
manner, by ignition in a platinum dish. It varies in
amount from 0·3 to 0·8 per cent., and should never exceed
a proportion of 1·5 per cent.

When of good quality, wheaten flour is perfectly white,
or has only a faint tinge of yellow. It should be free from
bran, and must not show red, grey, or black specks, nor
possess a disagreeable odour. It should also exhibit a
neutral reaction and a decided cohesiveness, acquiring a
peculiar soft and cushion-like condition when slightly com-
pressed. Formerly, wheaten flour was mixed with various
foreign meals, such as rye, corn, barley, peas, beans, rice,
linseed, buckwheat, and potato starch ; but at present this
form of adulteration is probably but rarely resorted to, at
least in the United States. The presence of mildew,
darnel, ergot, and other parasites of the grain, constitutes
an occasional contamination of flour. The most frequent
admixture consists, however, in the addition of alum, which,
although more extensively used in bread, is also employed
in order to disguise the presence of damaged flour in
mixtures, or to improve the appearance of an inferior
grade ; its addition to a damaged article serves to arrest
the decomposition of the gluten, thereby preventing the
flour from acquiring a dark colour, and disagreeable taste
and odour.

It has recently been stated that in flour which has been kept for a long time in sacks, a transformation of the gluten sometimes occurs, resulting in the production of a poisonous alkaloid. This body may be separated by evaporating the ethereal extract of the flour to dryness, and treating the residue with water. The presence of the alkaloid in the filtered aqueous solution is recognised by means of potassium ferrocyanide. The presence of an excessive proportion of moisture is doubtless instrumental in the formation of toxic alkaloids or fungi in old flour and bread.

Pure wheaten flour is coloured yellow when treated with ammonium hydroxide, whereas corn meal assumes a pale brown colour, and the meals prepared from peas, beans, etc., become dark brown in colour when tested in this way. Nitric acid imparts an orange-yellow colour to wheaten flour, but fails to change the colour of potato-starch, with which it forms a stiff and tenacious paste.

Potato-starch is readily detected by examining a thin layer of the sample on a slide under the microscope, and adding a dilute solution of potassium hydroxide, which, while not affecting the wheaten starch, causes the potato-starch granules to swell up very considerably. Leguminous starches, such as peas, etc., contain approximately $2\cdot5$ per cent. of mineral matter; in pure flour, the average proportion of ash is only about $0\cdot7$ per cent., and this difference is sometimes useful in the detection of an admixture of the former.

The external envelope of the granules of potato-starch offers far less resistance when triturated in a mortar than that of wheat, and upon this fact a simple test for their detection is founded. It is executed by rubbing up a mixture consisting of equal parts of the sample and sand with water, diluting and filtering the paste formed, and then adding to it a solution of 1 part of iodine in 20 parts of water. In the absence of potato-starch, an evanescent pink colour is produced; in case it is present, the colour obtained is dark purple, which in time also disappears.

Among the methods which have been suggested for the detection of such accidental impurities as darnel, ergot, and mildew, are the following :—If pure flour is digested for some time with dilute alcohol, the latter either remains quite clear or it acquires a very light straw-colour ; with flour contaminated with darnel, the alcohol shows a decided greenish tint, and possesses an acrid and disagreeable taste. In case the alcohol used is acidulated with about 5 per cent. of hydrochloric acid, the extract obtained exhibits a purple-red colour with flour containing mildew, and a blood-red colour with flour containing ergot. When flour contaminated with ergot or other moulds, is treated with a dilute solution of aniline violet, the dye is almost wholly absorbed by the damaged granules, which are thus rendered more noticeable in the microscopic examination.

The following test is often used for the detection of alum in flour :—A small quantity of the suspected sample is made into a paste with a little water and mixed with a few drops of an alcoholic tincture of logwood ; a little ammonium carbonate solution is then added. In the presence of alum, a lavender-blue coloured lake is formed, which often becomes more apparent upon allowing the mixture to remain at rest for a few hours. The production of a brown or pink coloration is an indication of the absence of alum. A modification of this test, proposed by Blyth, consists in immersing for several hours in the cold aqueous extract of the flour a strip of gelatine, with which the alum combines ; the gelatine is subsequently submitted to the action of the logwood tincture and ammonium carbonate as above.

For the quantitative estimation of alum in flour, the following processes are usually employed :—A considerable quantity of the sample is incinerated in a platinum dish, the ash is boiled with dilute hydrochloric acid and the solution filtered. The filtrate is next boiled and added to a concentrated solution of pure sodium hydroxide, the mixture being again boiled and afterwards filtered hot. A little sodium diphosphate is now added to the filtrate which is then slightly acidulated with hydrochloric acid, and finally made barely alkaline by addition of ammonium hydroxide. The resulting precipitate, which, in the presence of alum, consists of aluminium phosphate, is brought upon a filter, well washed, and then weighed.

Another method, which is a modification of that of Dupré, is as follows :—The ash obtained by the calcination of the flour (or bread), is fused, together with four times its weight of pure mixed sodium and potassium carbonates, the fused mass treated with hydrochloric acid, the solution evaporated to dryness and the separated silica collected and weighed. A few drops of sodium phosphate solution are added to the filtrate from the silica, then ammonium hydroxide in excess, by which the calcium, magnesium, ferric and aluminium phosphates are precipitated. The two latter are next separated by boiling the liquid with an excess of acetic acid (in which they are insoluble), and brought upon a filter, washed, dried, and weighed. The iron sometimes accompanying the precipitate of aluminium phosphate, can be determined by reduction with zinc and titration with potassium permanganate. If the presence of alum is indicated by the logwood test, and it is quantitatively determined by either of the preceding methods, it has been suggested that an allowance be made for the small proportion of aluminium silicate occasionally found in unadulterated flour or bread, and a deduction from the total alum present of one part of alum for every part of silica obtained is considered proper. The weight of aluminium phosphate found, multiplied by 3·873, or by 3·702, gives respectively the corresponding amounts of potash-alum or ammonia-alum contained in the sample examined.

BREAD.

Bread is usually prepared by mixing flour with water, kneading it into a uniform dough, submitting it to a process of "raising," either by means of a ferment or by the direct incorporation of carbonic acid gas, and finally baking the resulting mass.

Unleavened bread, however, is made by simply kneading flour with water, with the addition of a little salt, and baking.   The oatcake of the Scotch, the passover bread of the Israelites, and the corncakes of the Southern States are the best known varieties of unleavened bread.

The porosity peculiar to raised bread is caused by the generation of a gas, either previous to, or during the process of baking.   In former times (and to some extent at present, notably in Paris), fermented bread was made by the use of *leaven*, which is dough in a state of incipient decomposition ; but in this country, the common agent employed in raising bread is yeast, which consists of minute vegetable cells *(Torula cerevisiæ)* forming either the froth or deposit of fermenting worts.

By the action of these ferments, the gluten of the flour first undergoes a modification and enters into a peculiar combination with the starch-granules, which become more or less ruptured ; the soluble albumen is rendered insoluble, and the starch is transformed, first into sugar, then into carbonic acid and alcohol.   These changes are perfectly analogous to those which occur in the fermentation of the wort in the preparation of fermented liquors.

Other and minor decompositions likewise occur, such as the partial conversion of the starch into dextrine, the sugar into lactic acid, and the alcohol into acetic acid, but the most essential change is the production of alcohol and carbonic acid.   The alcohol formed is mainly volatilised, although an average proportion of $0 \cdot 3$ per cent. of this compound has been found in samples of fresh bread.   The

escape of the carbonic acid is retarded by the gluten, and
to its expansion is due the porous or spongy appearance of
well-made bread.

Of late years, artificial substitutes for the fermentation
process in the production of porous bread have been extensively employed. By the use of these agents, the liberation
of carbonic acid in the dough is accomplished and a slight
gain of weight is effected, as none of the original ingredients
of the flour are lost by fermentation.

"Aërated bread" is made by kneading the flour under
pressure with water highly charged with carbonic acid
gas, which, upon the removal of the pressure, expands, and
gives porosity to the bread. The use of "baking powders"
effects the same result in a more convenient manner, and
is largely practised in families. These compounds generally
consist of sodium bicarbonate (sometimes partially replaced
by the corresponding ammonia salt), and tartaric acid, or
potassium bitartrate, together with rice or other flour. A
more commendable preparation is a mixture of sodium
bicarbonate with potassium or calcium acid phosphates,
the use of which is claimed to restore to the bread the
phosphates lost by the removal of the bran from the flour.
Baking powders are often mixed in the dry state with
flour, and the produce, which is known under the name of
"self-raising flour," only requires to be kneaded with water
and baked to form porous bread. However great the
convenience attending the use of these compounds, they
are often open to the objection that their decomposition
gives rise to the formation of aperient salts, c. g. sodium
tartrate, and that they are very frequently contaminated
with alum.

As a result of the chemical changes which take place in
the fermentation of the flour and the subsequent application of heat, the composition of bread differs materially
from that of the grain from which it is prepared. As
already mentioned, the soluble albuminoids are rendered

insoluble, and the starch is partially transformed into sugar (maltose). The unconverted starch is modified in its physical condition, the ruptured granules being far more readily acted upon by the digestive fluids than before. The proportion of soluble carbohydrates is naturally augmented in bread. The amount of ash is also somewhat increased, chiefly owing to the addition of salt, but it should not exceed a proportion of 2 per cent. The quantity of water in bread varies considerably. Wanklyn fixes 34 per cent. as the standard ; greater proportions have, however, been frequently found. In ten samples of apparently normal bread, examined by E. S. Wood, Analyst to the Massachusetts State Board of Health, the amounts of moisture contained varied from 34 to 44 per cent. The quantity of water decreases very rapidly upon exposure to the air. Thus, Clifford Richardson [*] found that bread which showed 36 per cent. of moisture when freshly baked, contained but 5·86 per cent. after drying for two weeks. Stale bread would seem to contain water in a peculiar molecular condition, and, as is well known, upon heating ("toasting"), it reassumes the porous state.

According to analyses collected by König,[†] the mean composition of bread is as follows :—

	Water.	Nitrogenous substances.	Fat.	Sugar.	Extractive free from Nitrogen.	Cellulose.	Ash.	Dry Substances.	
								N.	Carbo-Hydrates.
	per cent.	per cent.	per cent.	per cent.	per cent.	per cent.	per cent.	per cent.	per cent.
Fine wheat bread ..	31·51	7·06	0·46	4·02	52·56	0·32	1·09	1·75	87·79
Coarse wheat bread ..	40·45	6·15	0·44	2·08	49·04	0·62	1·22	1·65	85·84
Rye bread	42·27	6·11	0·43	2·31	46·94	0·49	1·46	1·69	85·31
Pumpernickel	43·42	7·59	1·51	3·25	41·87	0·94	1·42	2·15	79·74

[*] 'An Investigation of the Composition of American Wheat and Corn.' United States Department of Agriculture, 1883.

[†] 'Die Menschlichen Nahrungs- und Genussmittel,' p. 420. Berlin, 1883.

Clifford Richardson gives the following results of the analysis of ordinary family loaf-bread :—

		Per cent.
Water..	.. ..	37·30
Soluble albuminoids	.. .. ..	1·19
Insoluble "	.. .. ..	6·85
Fat ..	.. ..	0·60
Sugar ..	.. ..	2·16
Dextrine ..	.. ..	2·85
Starch	.. ..	47·03
Fibre ..	.. ..	0·85
Ash ..	.. ..	1·17
		100·00
Nitrogen ..	.. ..	1·29
Total albuminoids	.. ..	8·04

The analysis of bread is conducted essentially in the same manner as that of flour. Under ordinary circumstances, the determinations required are limited to an estimation of the moisture contained in the crumb, the amount of the ash, and special tests for the presence of alum and copper salts. Owing to the broken condition of the starch granules in bread, their identification by the microscope is usually rendered exceedingly difficult. The logwood test for alum in bread is applied by Bell as follows :—About 10 grammes of the crumb are immersed in a little water containing 5 c.c. each of the freshly prepared logwood tincture and solution of ammonium carbonate for about five minutes, after which the liquid is decanted, and the bread dried at a gentle heat. In the presence of alum the bread will acquire the characteristic lavender tint mentioned under Flour. It should be added, that salts of magnesia also produce a lavender lake with alum ; but this fact does not affect the usefulness of the process as a preliminary test to the quantitative determination of the mineral impurities present in the sample under examination. The quantitative examination of alum in bread is made by one of the methods described on p. 93. Bread, free from alum, will sometimes yield 0·013 per cent.

H

of aluminium phosphate, and this amount should therefore be deducted from the weight of the precipitate obtained.

The average of the results obtained by Dr. Edward G. Love, New York State Board of Health, from the examination of the crumb of ten samples of the cheaper varieties of wheaten bread were as follows :—

	Per cent.
Water	42·80
Total ash	1·0066
Silica and sand	0·0056
Aluminium (and ferric) phosphates	0·0053

That the addition of alum to bread is prevalent seems to admit of little doubt. The British Public Analysts, in 1879, tested 1287 samples of bread, of which 95 (or 7·3 per cent.) contained alum. Of 18 samples examined, in 1880, in the city of Washington, 8 were adulterated with the salt. The question of the sanitary effects produced by the use of alumed bread is one which has given rise to very extended discussion. According to some authorities, the conversion of alum into an insoluble salt by the fermentation process, which takes place in bread-making, is regarded as a proof that it remains inert, and is consequently harmless in its effects. Others contend that its action as a preventive of excessive fermentation is at the expense of valuable nutritious constituents of the flour, and that its combination with the phosphates present in the grain results in the formation of an insoluble salt which tends to retard digestion. Experiments have been made by J. West Knights, on the comparative action of artificial gastric juice upon pure and alumed bread, which apparently support this latter view.

Another objection to the use of alum is that it is frequently employed for the purpose of disguising the bad quality of damaged and inferior grades of flour. The presence of copper salts in bread is of rare occurrence. Their detection is accomplished by treating a portion of the crumb with a dilute solution of potassium ferrocyanide acidulated with acetic acid, which, in presence of copper, will impart a reddish-brown colour to the bread. If contained in any appreciable proportion, it can be extracted from the ash obtained by the incineration of the bread, and deposited upon the interior of a weighed platinum capsule by the electrolytic method.

Starch ($C_6H_{10}O_5$).—Starch, which enters so largely into the composition of cereals, is a carbo-hydrate, *i. e.* hydrogen and oxygen are contained in the proportions necessary to form water. In this respect, it is identical with woody fibre, cellulose, and dextrine.

The well-known dark-blue colour produced upon the addition of a solution of iodine to starch-paste forms the usual qualitative test for its presence. This coloration is discharged by alkalies and by a solution of sulphurous acid. The quantitative estimation of starch in mixtures is best effected by heating the dry substance in a closed tube for 24 hours, together with a dilute hot alcoholic solution of potassium hydroxide. The hot liquid is next filtered, the residue washed with alcohol, and the filtrate heated with 2 per cent. solution of hydrochloric acid until it ceases to show the blue coloration when tested with iodine. It is then rendered alkaline, and the proportion of starch originally present, calculated from the amount of sugar formed, as determined by Fehling's solution. Although identical in chemical composition, the various forms of starch met with in the vegetable kingdom vary in size and exhibit characteristic differences in the appearance of the granules. The following are measurements of several varieties of starch granules :—

	Millimetre.		Millimetre.
Wheat ..	·0500	Corn ..	·0300
Rye ..	·0310	Bean ..	·0631
Rice ..	·0220	Potato ..	·1850

The larger granules of potato starch, when suspended

H 2

in water, subside more rapidly than those of wheat starch ; they are also far more readily ruptured.

The identification of the various starches is accomplished by means of the microscope. Starch possesses an orga-nised structure which, fortunately, differs in different plants. Besides varying in size, the granules develope in a different manner and form from centres of growth, and therefore exhibit characteristic conditions and positions. These distinctions, together with their effect upon polarised light, are of great utility in the determination of the source of any particular starch. For this purpose, it is necessary to become familiar with the distinctive microscopical appear-ance of each individual starch. A collection of those most usually met with should be made, and, after careful study, preserved in a dried state for comparative purposes. Polarised light is a very useful adjunct in the examination of starch granules. In the microscopical investigation, a minute portion of the sample is placed upon the glass slide and well moistened with a solution of 1 part glycerine in 2 parts of water ; it is then protected by a thin glass cover, which is put on with gentle pressure. The appearance of various starches, under polarised light, is seen in Plate IX., where the cross lies at the hilum or nucleus of the granule, and the form and relative size is visible in outline. This plate, and Plates VII. and XII. are copied, with permission, from Bulletin No. 11 of the Chemical Division of the U.S. Department of Agriculture. The original negatives (made by Clifford Richardson) were used, but the auto-types are presented in a somewhat modified form.

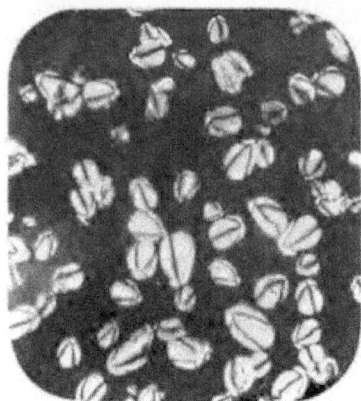

Potato × 145.

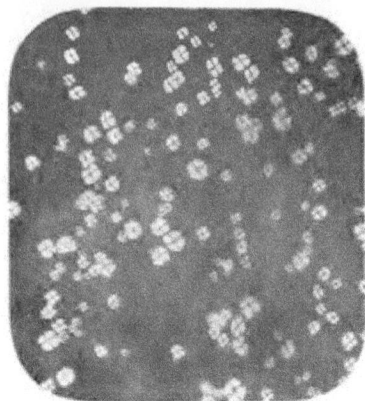

Maize × 145

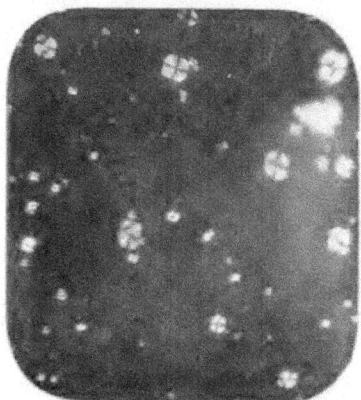

Wheat × 145.

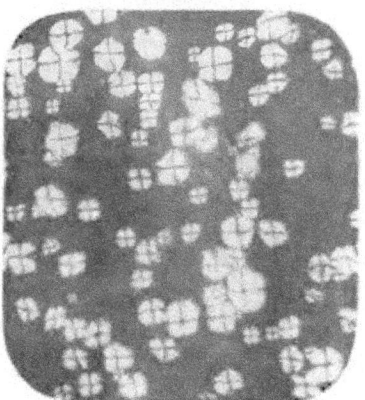

Rice × 450.

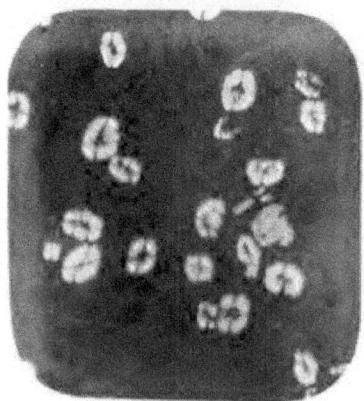

Bean × 145.

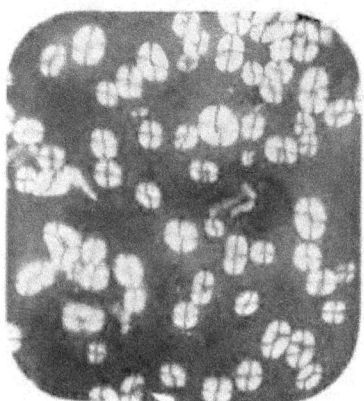

Pea × 145.

BAKERS' CHEMICALS.

THE substances employed for the artificial production of porosity in bread, as already mentioned, are sodium bicarbonate (now termed "saleratus"), potassium bitartrate, tartaric acid, and calcium diphosphate, the various mixtures of these compounds being known as baking powders. Some of the above chemicals are not always used in the pure state, and, in addition to this source of contamination, baking powders are often excessively diluted with flour or starch, and seriously adulterated with alum.

The sodium bicarbonate employed is generally a fairly pure article. Common grades of the salt contain a little sodium chloride, and in some cases as much as 2 per cent. of the corresponding sulphate; it may also prove to be somewhat deficient in the proportion of carbonic acid present. Cream of tartar (potassium bitartrate), is far more liable to adulteration. A certain quantity of calcium tartrate is often found in the commercial article, originating from its method of manufacture, and amounting, on the average, from 6 to 7 per cent. The salt is, moreover, sometimes intentionally mixed with alum, starch, tartaric acid, gypsum, chalk and terra alba.

Occasionally so-called cream of tartar has been found to be wholly composed of starch and calcium diphosphate. In the examination for calcium tartrate and sulphate, a quantitative determination of the total lime and sulphuric acid is made. The quantity of sulphuric acid obtained is calculated to gypsum, any excess of lime left being returned as tartrate. The ash in pure cream of tartar should amount to 36·79 per cent., while that of calcium tartrate is only 21·54 per cent. Naturally, the addition of flour or starch would materially decrease the proportion of ash. The presence of these latter adulterants is recognised by means of the microscope, and by testing the sample with iodine solution. It is generally required that cream of tartar should contain at least 90 per cent. of potassium bitartrate.

Baking powders.—The usual composition of baking powders has already been stated. They all contain sodium bicarbonate, but differ in the acid ingredient present, which may consist of cream of tartar, tartaric acid, calcium diphosphate, or alum. In order to remedy the tendency to deterioration which exists in powders entirely composed of the above salts, it is the practice to add a considerable amount of " filling " (corn-starch, flour, etc.). The quantity of filling employed for this purpose varies from 20 to 60 per cent., but is as a rule, greater than is really necessary. A small proportion of the sodium salt is often replaced by ammonium sesquicarbonate. Alum is a more objectionable constituent of many preparations, and it should be considered an adulteration. The practical value of baking powder is chiefly dependent upon the quantity of carbonic acid it liberates when decomposed, and this is affected by the strength of the acid salt and the amount of " filling " used. The most common varieties of baking powders are :—

(*a*) *Sodium bicarbonate and cream of tartar*, either pure or mixed with starch. In testing this class of powders, it is usual to determine the excessive alkalinity remaining after the decomposition with water, by means of decinormal acid ; this is put down as bicarbonate present in excess. The proportions of sodium bicarbonate and cream of tartar are calculated from the alkaline strength of the ash, minus the excessive alkalinity found.

Impurities originating from the cream of tartar employed are estimated as previously described ; and the amount of starch contained is determined by the usual methods. In some preparations, tartaric acid is substituted for cream of tartar.

The following proportions represent the composition of a baking powder of good quality :—

	Parts.
Cream of tartar	30
Sodium bicarbonate	15
Flour	5

(*b*) *Sodium bicarbonate and calcium diphosphate.*—Calcium sulphate occurs as an impurity in the commercial phosphate and is therefore liable to be met with in phosphate powders. In addition to phosphoric acid, lime, etc., a determination of sulphuric acid and chlorine should be made.

(*c*) *Sodium bicarbonate and alum.*—These constitute the most reprehensible forms of baking powder. The sanitary effects of alum have been referred to under Flour. It may be present either as potash or ammonia alum. The following is a fair example of an alum powder :—

	Per cent.
Alum	26·45
Sodium bicarbonate	24·17
Ammonium sesquicarbonate	2·31
Cream of tartar	None
Starch	47·07

From an exhaustive investigation of baking powders made by Dr. Henry A. Mott, it was found that about 50 per cent. of these preparations were impure, alum being the chief admixture. Of 280 samples of cream of tartar lately examined by various American Health Boards, 100 were adulterated ; of 95 baking powders tested, 16 were adulterated.

SUGAR.

THE sugars of commerce may be conveniently classified
into two varieties. viz., sucrose (cane sugar or saccharose)
and dextrose (grape sugar or glucose). The former, which
is the kind almost exclusively employed for domestic uses,
is chiefly obtained from the sugar cane of the West Indies
and American Southern States (*Saccharum officinarum*),
and, in continental Europe, from the sugar beet (*Beta
vulgaris*). A comparatively small quantity is manufactured
in the United States from the sugar maple (*Acer saccha-
rinum*), and from sorghum (*Sorghum saccharatus*).

Cane Sugar ($C_{12} H_{22} O_{11}$).—Among the more important
chemical properties of cane sugar are the following:—It
dissolves in about one-third its weight of cold water—much
more readily in hot water—and is insoluble in cold absolute
alcohol. From a concentrated aqueous solution it is
deposited in monoclinic prisms, which possess a specific
gravity of 1·580. Cane sugar is characterised by its
property of rotating the plane of a ray of polarised light to
the right ; the rotary power is 66°·6. Upon heating its
solution with dilute mineral acids, it is converted into a
mixture termed "invert sugar," which consists of equal
parts of *dextrose* and *levulose*. The former turns the plane
of polarised light to the right, the latter to the left ; but
owing to the stronger rotation exerted by the levulose, the
combined rotary effect of invert sugar is to the left, *i. e.*,
opposite to that possessed by cane sugar. Invert sugar
exhibits the important property of reducing solutions of
the salts of copper, which is not possessed by pure cane
sugar. Cane sugar melts at 160° ; at a higher temperature

(210°) it is converted into a reddish-brown substance termed *caramel.* When subjected to the action of ferments, cane sugar is first transformed into invert sugar, then into alcohol and carbonic acid, according to the reactions :—

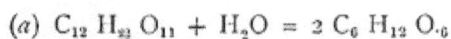

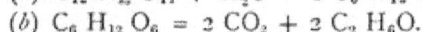

(*a*) $C_{12} H_{22} O_{11} + H_2O = 2 C_6 H_{12} O_6$
(*b*) $C_6 H_{12} O_6 = 2 CO_2 + 2 C_2 H_6O.$

The varieties of cane sugar usually met with in commerce are the following :—

1. Loaf sugar, consisting either of irregular fragments, or (more often) of cut cubes.
2. Granulated sugar.
3. Soft white sugar.
4. Brown sugar, varying in colour from cream-yellow to reddish-brown.

Molasses is a solution of sugar, containing invert sugar, gummy matters, caramel, etc., which forms the mother-liquor remaining after the crystallisation of raw cane sugar; the name "syrup" being commonly applied to the residual liquor obtained in the manufacture of refined sugar.

Dextrose ($C_6 H_{12} O_6$), occurs ready-formed in grape juice, and in many sweet fruits, very frequently associated with levulose; it is also contained in honey, together with a small amount of cane sugar. As already mentioned, it constitutes an ingredient of the product obtained by the action of acids and ferments upon cane sugar. For commercial purposes, glucose is prepared by treating grains rich in starch, with dilute acids. In France and Germany, potatoes are used in its manufacture; in the United States, Indian corn or maize is almost exclusively employed. The processes used consist substantially in first separating the starch from the grain by soaking, grinding, and straining, then boiling it, under pressure, with water containing about 3 per cent. of sulphuric acid, neutralising the remaining acid with chalk, decolorising the solution by means of animal charcoal, and concentrating it in vacuum pans. In the United States thirty-two factories are engaged in the manufacture of glucose, which consume about 40,000 bushels of corn daily, their annual production having an estimated value of 10 millions of dollars. In commerce, the term grape sugar is applied to the solid product, the syrup or liquid form being known as glucose. The chief uses of starch sugar and glucose are in the manufacture of table syrups, and as a substitute for malt in the brewing of beer and ale. Their other most important applications are as a substitute for cane sugar in confectionery, and in the preparation of fruit jellies ; as an adulterant of cane sugar, as an admixture to genuine honey, and as a source for the preparation of vinegar.

Dextrose is soluble in $1\frac{1}{3}$ part of cold water, and is much more soluble in hot water. It has a dextro-rotary power of $56°$. When separated from its aqueous solution, it forms white and opaque granular masses, but from an alcoholic solution, it is obtained in well-defined, microscopic needles, which fuse at $146°$. Two parts of glucose have about the same sweetening effect as one part of cane sugar.* It does not become coloured when mixed with cold concentrated sulphuric acid, which distinguishes it from sucrose ; on the other hand, its solution is coloured dark-brown if boiled with potassium hydroxide, another distinction from cane sugar. Dextrose is capable of directly undergoing vinous fermentation, and, like invert sugar, it possesses the property of reducing alkaline solutions of copper salts, especially upon the application of heat.

* It is of interest in this connection to note the recent discovery of a coal-tar derivative, benzoyle sulphonic imide, $C_6H_4 \underset{SO}{\overset{CO}{<}} > NH$, commercially known as "saccharine." This body possesses about 230 times the sweetening power of cane sugar. It bears, however, no near chemical relation to the sugars, which, for the greater part, constitute hexatomic alcohols. See Amer. Chem. Jour., i. p. 170, and vol. ii. p. 181 ; also, Jour. Soc. Chem. Indus., No. 2, vol. vi. p. 75.

The chief commercial varieties of American glucose are the following :—

1. *Glucose :*

	Per cent. Glucose.
" Crystal H," containing	40
" Crystal B "	45
" Crystal A "	50

2. *Grape Sugar :*

" Brewers' grape	70–75
" A " or " Solid grape "	75–80
" Grained " or " Granulated grape "	80–85

Maltose and *levulose* are isomers of dextrose. The former is prepared by the action of malt or diastase upon starch. It has a dextro-rotary power of 150°, and its property of reducing copper salts is only about 60 per cent. of that of dextrose. It is converted into the latter compound upon boiling with dilute sulphuric acid. Levulose, as previously stated, is formed, together with dextrose, from cane sugar by treatment with dilute acids or with ferments. It turns the plane of a ray of polarised light to the left, its rotary power varying considerably at different temperatures.

Lactose, or milk sugar, has already been referred to under the head of Milk. It is isomeric with cane sugar, possesses a dextro-rotary power (58°·2), and undergoes fermentation when mixed with yeast, and reduces alkaline copper solutions, but in a different degree from glucose.

Many of the substances frequently enumerated as being used to adulterate sugar are at present very seldom employed. The usual list includes " glucose " (often meaning invert sugar), sand, flour, chalk, terra alba, etc. Loaf sugar is almost invariably pure, although its colour is sometimes improved by the addition of small proportions of various blue pigments, such as ultramarine, indigo, and Prussian blue. The presence of ultramarine was detected in about 73 per cent. of the samples of granulated sugar tested in 1881 by the New York State Board of Health. Tin salts * are also occasionally employed in the bleach-

* Of 41 samples of molassan, tested in Massachusetts in 1885, 12 contained tin chloride.

ing of sugar and syrups. Granulated sugar is asserted to be sometimes mixed with grape sugar, and powdered sugar has been found adulterated with flour and terra alba ; but the varieties which are most exposed to admixture are the low grades of yellow and brown sugar, in which, however, several per cent. of invert sugar are normally present. Sand, gravel, and mites form a rather common contamination of raw sugar. From the year 1876 to 1881, 310 samples of commercial sugar were examined by the public health authorities of Canada, of which number 24 were reported as containing glucose, and 11 as of doubtful purity. Of 38 samples of brown sugar recently analysed by Dr. Charles Smart, of the National Board of Health, 9 were adulterated with glucose. From the investigations of A. L. Colby, Analyst to the New York State Board of Health, it was found that of the 116 samples examined, the white sugars were practically pure ; whereas, of 67 samples of brown sugar, 4 contained glucose. Of 16 specimens of brown sugar, tested by a commission appointed by the National Academy of Sciences in 1883, 4 contained about 30 per cent. of this body.* Many varieties of sugar-house syrups, and the various forms of confectionery, are very extensively adulterated with artificial glucose.

The average sugar-house syrup has the following composition :—

	Per cent.
Water	16
Crystallisable sugar	36
Invert sugar	34
Gum, pectose, etc.	10
Ash	4

Dr. W. H. Pitt, in the Second Annual Report of the New

* The average composition of over 100,000 samples of raw cane sugar (mostly Cuban) tested in the United States Laboratory during the past five years, has been as follows :—

	Per cent.
Moisture	3·0
Ash	1·5
Polarisation	96

York State Board of Health, gives the following analysis of grocers' mixed glucose syrup, and of confectioners' glucose :—

American Grape Sugar Co.'s Syrup.

	Per cent.
Ash	0·820
Water	18·857
Dextrine	34·667
Cane syrup	7·805
Glucose	37·851
	100·000

Confectioners' Glucose.

	Per cent.
Ash	0·431
Water	15·762
Dextrine	41·614
Glucose	42·193
	100·000

It is stated that a large proportion of the American maple syrup and maple sugar found on the market, consists of raw sugar, flavoured with the essential oil of hickory-bark, for the manufacture of which letters patent have been granted.

Analysis of Sugar.—The examination of sugar is ordinarily confined to the estimation of the water, ash, and determination of the nature of the organic matters present. The proportion of water contained in a sample is found by drying it for about two hours in an air-bath, at a temperature of 110°. Moist and syrupy sugars, such as muscovadoes, are advantageously mixed with a known weight of ignited sand before drying. The ash is determined either by directly incinerating a few grammes of the sugar in a tared platinum capsule, or by accelerating the process of combustion by first moistening the sample with a little sulphuric acid. In this case the bases will naturally be converted into sulphates, and a deduction of one-tenth is usually made from the results so obtained, in order to reduce it to terms of the corresponding carbonates. The proportion of ash in raw cane sugar varies somewhat, but it should not much exceed 1·5 per cent. Its average composition, as given by Monier, is as follows :—

Calcic carbonate	49·00
Potassium carbonate	16·50
Sodium and potassium sulphates ..	16·00
Sodium chloride	9·00
Alumina and silica	9·50
	100·00

Insoluble mineral adulterants are readily separated by dissolving a rather considerable amount of the sample in water and filtering. In this manner the presence of sand, terra alba, and foreign pigments may be recognised.

The determination of the character of the organic constituents of commercial sugars is effected, either by chemical or by physical tests, and, in some instances, by a combination of these methods. The presence of such adulterants, as flour or starch, is very easily detected upon a microscopic examination of the suspected sample.

If cane sugar, containing grape sugar, is boiled with water, to which about 2 per cent. of potassium hydroxide has been added, the solution acquires a brown colour.

Upon mixing a solution of pure cane sugar with a solution of cupric sulphate, adding an excess of potassium hydroxide, and boiling, only a slight precipitation of red cupric oxide takes place. Under the same conditions, grape sugar at once produces a copious green precipitate, which ultimately changes to red, the supernatant fluid becoming nearly or quite colourless. A very good method for the quantitative estimation of grape sugar when mechanically mixed with cane sugar, is that of P. Casamajor. It is executed by first preparing a saturated solution of grape sugar in methylic alcohol. The sample to be tested is thoroughly dried, and then well agitated with the methylic alcohol solution, in which all cane sugar will dissolve ; any grape sugar present remains behind, and upon allowing the mixture to remain at rest for a short time, forms a deposit which is again treated with the grape sugar solution, and then collected upon a tared filter, washed with absolute methylic alcohol, and weighed.   Glucose and invert sugar are usually quantitatively determined by means of Fehling's solution.

As this preparation is liable to decompose upon keeping, it is advisable to first prepare cupric sulphate solution by dissolving exactly 34,640 grammes of the salt in 500 c.c. of distilled water, and then make up the Rochelle salt solution by dissolving 68 grammes of sodium hydroxide, and 173 grammes of Rochelle salt in 500 c.c. of water, the solutions being kept separate.   When required for use, 5 c.c. each of the copper and Rochelle solutions (corresponding to 10 c.c. of Fehling's solution) are introduced into a narrow beaker, or a porcelain evaporating dish, a little water is added, and the liquid brought to the boiling point. The sugar solution under examination should not contain over 0·5 per cent. of glucose.   It is cautiously added to the hot Fehling's solution from a burette until the fluid loses its blue colour (see p. 37).   The number of c.c. required to completely reduce 10 c.c. of Fehling's solution, represents 0·05 gramme of grape sugar.   The foregoing volumetric method is sometimes applied gravimetrically by adding a slight excess of Fehling's solution to the sugar solution, collecting the precipitated cupric oxide upon a filter and weighing, after oxidation with a few drops of nitric acid ; or, it may be dissolved, and the copper contained deposited by electrolysis, in which case the weight of copper obtained, multiplied by 0·538, gives the equivalent amount of glucose. The proportion of cane sugar in a sample of raw sugar can be determined by first directly estimating the proportion of invert sugar contained by means of Fehling's solution, as just described.   The cane sugar present is then inverted by dissolving one gramme of the sample in about

100 c.c. of water, adding 1 c.c. of strong sulphuric acid, and
heating the solution in the water-bath for 30 minutes, the
water lost by evaporation being from time to time replaced.
The free acid is next neutralised by a little sodium carbonate, its volume made up to 200 c.c., and the invert sugar
now contained estimated by Fehling's solution. The difference in the two determinations represents the glucose
formed by the conversion of the cane sugar; 100 parts of
the glucose so produced is equivalent to 95 parts of cane
sugar.

Commercial cane sugar is, however, generally estimated by
the instrument known as the saccharimeter or polariscope.

In order to convey an intelligent idea of the physical
laws which govern the practical working of the polariscope,
it will first be necessary to refer to the subject of the
polarisation of light. The transformation of ordinary into
polarised light is best effected either by reflection from a
glass plate at an angle of about 56°, or by what is known
as double refraction. The former method can be illustrated
by Fig. 1, Plate X., which represents two tubes, B and C,
arranged so as to allow the one to be turned round within
the other. Two flat plates of glass, A and P, blackened at
the backs, are attached obliquely to the end of each tube at
an angle of about 56°, as represented in the figure. The
tube B, with its attached plate, A, can be turned round in
the tube C without changing the inclination of the plate to
a ray passing along the axis of the tube. If a candle be
now placed at I, the light will be reflected from the plate P
through the tube, and, owing to the particular angle of this
plate, will undergo a certain transformation in its nature,
or, in other words, become "polarised." So long as the
plate A retains the position represented in the figure, the
reflected ray would fall in the same plane as that in which
the polarisation of the ray took place, and an image of the
candle would be seen by an observer stationed at O. But,
suppose the tube B to be turned a quarter round; the

PLATE X.

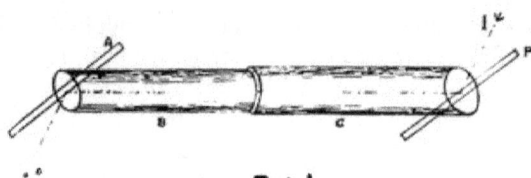

Fig. I.

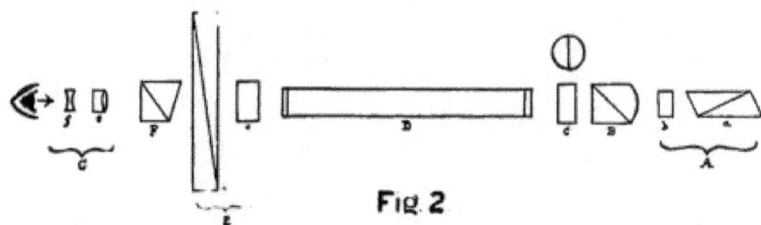

Fig. 2

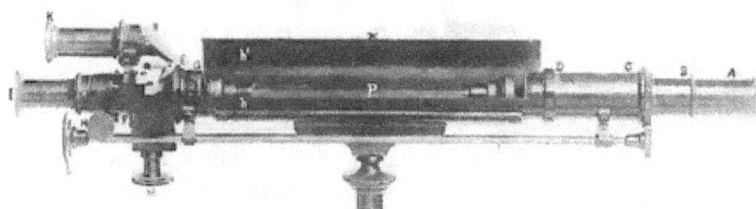

Fig. 3.

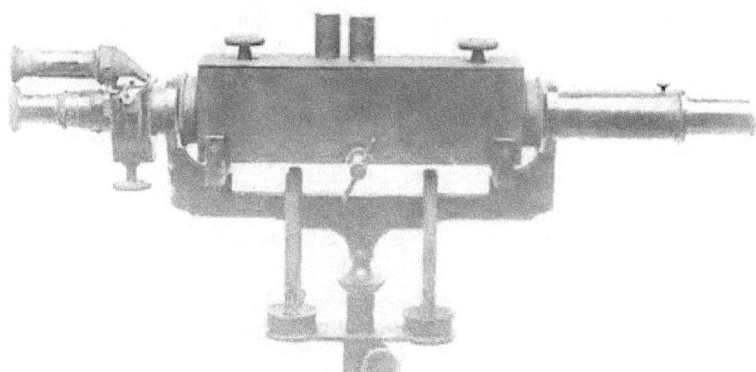

Fig. 4.

Polariscope.

plane of reflection is now at right angles to that of polarisation, and the image will become invisible. When the tube
B is turned half-way round, the candle is seen as brightly
at first ; at the third quadrant it disappears, until, on com-
pleting the revolution of the tube, it again becomes perfectly visible. It is evident that the ray reflected from the
glass plate P has acquired properties different from those
possessed by ordinary light, which would have been reflected by the plate A in whatever direction it might have
been turned.

If a ray of common light be made to pass through certain crystals, such as calc spar, it undergoes double refraction, and the light transmitted becomes polarised. The
arrangement known as Nicol's prism, which consists of
two prisms of calc spar, cut at a certain angle and united
together by means of Canada balsam, is a very convenient
means of obtaining polarised light. If two Nicol's prisms
are placed in a similar position, one behind the other, the
light polarised by the first (or polarising) prism passes
through the second (or analysing) prism unchanged ; but if
the second prism be turned until it crosses the first at a
right angle, perfect darkness ensues. While it would
exceed the limits of this work to enter fully upon the theo-
retical explanations which are commonly advanced concerning the cause and nature of this polarised, or transformed light, it may be well to state here that common
light is assumed to be composed of two systems of beams
which vibrate in planes at right angles to each other,
whereas polarised light is regarded as consisting of beams
vibrating in a single plane only. If, now, we imagine the
second Nicol's prism to be made up of a series of fibres or
lines, running only in one direction, these fibres would act
like a grating and give free passage to a surface like a
knife blade only when this is parallel to the bars, but would
obstruct it if presented transversely. This somewhat crude
illustration will, perhaps, serve to explain why the rays

I

of light which have been polarised by the first Nicol's
prism are allowed to pass through the second prism when
the two are placed in a similar position, and why they are
obstructed when the prisms are crossed at right angles, it
being remembered that in a polarised ray the vibrations of
the beams of light take place in a single plane.

Suppose we place between the two Nicol's prisms, while
they are at right angles, a plate cut in a peculiar manner
from a crystal of quartz, we will discover that rays of light
now pass through the second prism, and that the field of
vision has become illuminated with beautiful colours—red,
yellow, green, blue, etc., according to the thickness of the
quartz plate used. On *turning* the second Nicol's prism
on its axis, these colours will change and pass through the
regular prismatic series, from red to violet, or the contrary,
according to the direction of the rotation produced by the
intervening plate. Quartz, therefore, possesses the remarkable property of rotating the plane of polarisation of the
coloured rays of which light is composed ; and it has been
discovered that some plates of this mineral exert this power
to the right, others to the left ; that is, they possess a right
or left-handed circular polarisation. Numerous other substances, including many organic compounds, possess this
quality of causing a rotation—either to the right or left—
of a plane of polarised light. For example, solutions of
cane sugar and ordinary glucose cause a right-handed rotation, whilst levulose and invert sugar exert a left-handed
rotation. The extent of this power is directly proportional
to the concentration of the solutions used, the length of the
column through which the ray of polarised light passes
being the same. It follows that on passing polarised light
through tubes of the same length which are filled with solutions containing different quantities of impure cane sugar,
an estimation of the amount of pure cane sugar contained
in the tubes can be made by determining the degree of
right-handed rotation produced ; and it is upon this fact

that the application of the polariscope in sugar analysis is based. The optical portions of the most improved form of the polariscope—that known as the Ventzke-Scheibler—are represented by Fig. 2.

The light from a gas burner enters at the extremity of the instrument and first passes through the "regulator A," which consists of the double refracting Nicol's prism *a* and the quartz plate *b*, it being so arranged that it can be turned round its own plane, thus varying the tint of the light used, so as to best neutralise that possessed by the sugar solution to be examined. The incident ray now penetrates the polarising Nicol's prism B, and next meets a double quartz plate C (3·75 millimetres in thickness). This quartz plate, a front view of which is also shown in the figure, is divided in the field of vision, one half consisting of quartz rotating to the right hand, the other half of the variety which rotates to the left hand. It is made of the thickness referred to owing to the fact that it then imparts a very sensitive tint (purple) to polarised light, and one that passes very suddenly into red or blue when the rotation of the ray is changed. Since the plate C is composed of halves which exert opposite rotary powers, these will assume different colours upon altering the rotation of the ray. After leaving the double quartz plate the light, which, owing to its passage through the Nicol's prism B is now polarised, enters the tube D containing the solution of cane sugar under examination ; this causes it to undergo a right-handed rotation. It next meets the "compensator" E, consisting of a quartz plate *c*, which has a right-handed rotary power, and the two quartz prisms *d*, both of which are cut in a wedge shape and exert a left-handed rotation. They are so arranged that one is movable and can be made to slide along the other, which is fixed, thus causing an increase or decrease in their combined thickness and rotary effect. The ray of light then passes through the analysing Nicol's prism F, and is finally examined

by means of the telescope G, with the objective *e* and
ocular *f*. Fig. 3 gives a perspective view of the Ventzke-
Scheibler polariscope. The Nicol's prism and quartz
plate which constitute the "regulator" are situated at A
and B, and can be rotated by means of a pinion connecting
with the button L. The polarising Nicol's prism is placed
at C, and the double quartz plate at D. The receptacle *h*
contains the tube P filled with sugar solution, and is provided with the hinged cover *h'*, which serves to keep out
the external light while an observation is being taken. The
right-handed quartz plate and the wedge-shaped quartz
prisms (corresponding to *c* and *d*, Fig. 2) are situated at G,
and at E and F, and the analysing Nicol's prism is placed
at H. When the wedge-shaped prisms have an equal
thickness coinciding with that of the quartz plate *c* (Fig. 2)
the left-handed rotary power of the former is exactly
neutralised by the right-handed rotary power of the latter,
and the field of vision seen at I is uniform in colour, the
opposing rotary powers of the two halves of the double
quartz plates C (Fig. 2) being also equalised. But if the
tube, filled with a sugar solution, is placed in the instrument, the right-handed rotary power of this substance is
added to that half of the double quartz plate which exerts
the same rotary effect (the other half being diminished in a
like degree), and the two divisions of the plate will now
appear of different colours. In order to restore an equilibrium of colour the movable wedge-shaped quartz plate E
is slid along its fellow F by means of the ratchet M, until
the right-handed rotary power of the sugar solution is
compensated for by the increased thickness of the left-
handed plate, when the sections of the plate C will again
appear uniform in colour. For the purpose of measuring
the extent to which the unfixed plate has been moved, a
small ivory scale is attached to this plate, and passes along
an index scale connected with the fixed plate. The degrees
marked on the scale, which are divided into tenths, are read

by aid of a mirror *s* attached to a magnifying glass K. When the polariscope is in what may be termed a state of equilibrium, *i.e.* before the tube containing the sugar solution has been placed in it, the index of the fixed scale points to the zero of the movable scale.

In the practical use of the Ventzke-Scheibler sacchari-meter the method to be followed is essentially as follows : 26·048 grammes of the sugar to be tested are carefully weighed out and introduced into a flask 100 cubic centi-metres in capacity ; water is added, and the flask shaken until all crystals are dissolved. The solution is next decolorised by means of basic plumbic acetate, its volume made up to 100 cubic centimetres, and a little bone-black having been added if necessary, a glass tube, corresponding to P (Fig. 3) which is exactly 200 millimetres in length, and is provided with suitable caps, is completely filled with the clear filtered liquid. This is then placed in the polari-scope, and protected from external light by closing the cover shown at *k'*. On now observing the field of vision by means of the telescope, it will be seen that the halves into which it is divided exhibit different colours. The screw M is then turned to the right until this is no longer the case, and absolute uniformity of colour is restored to the divisions of the double quartz plate C (Fig. 2). The extent to which the screw has been turned, which corre-sponds to the right-handed rotation caused by the sugar solution, is now ascertained on reading the scale by the aid of the glass K. The instrument under consideration is so constructed that, when solutions and tubes of the concen-tration and length referred to above are used, the reading on the scale gives directly the percentage of pure crystal-lisable cane sugar contained in the sample examined. For instance, if the zero index of the fixed scale points to 96°·5 on the movable scale, after uniformity of colour has been obtained, the sample of sugar taken contains 96·5 per cent. of pure cane sugar. The results given by the polari-

scope possess an accuracy rarely, if ever, attained by any
other apparatus employed in the determination of practical
commercial values.*

The proportion of grape sugar intentionally added to
cane sugar can also be determined by the use of the
polariscope, certain modifications being observed in its
application. As previously stated, cane sugar is converted
into a mixture of dextrose and levulose, termed invert
sugar, by the action of dilute acids. While the rotary
effect of dextrose upon the plane of a ray of polarised light
is constant at temperatures under 100°, that exerted by
levulose varies, it being reduced as the temperature is
increased; hence it follows that at a certain temperature
the diminished levo-rotary power of the levulose will
become neutralised by the dextro-rotary effect of the
dextrose, *i.e.* the invert sugar will be optically inactive.
This temperature has been found to approximate 90°.
Since dextrose is not perceptibly affected by the action of
weak acids, it is evident that by converting cane sugar into
invert sugar and examining the product by the polariscope
at a temperature of about 90°, the presence of any added
dextrose (glucose) will be directly revealed by its dextro-
rotary action. This is accomplished by a method suggested
by Messrs. Chandler and Ricketts,† which consists in sub-
stituting for the ordinary observation tube of the polariscope
a platinum tube, provided with a thermometer, and surrounded by a water-bath, which is heated to the desired
temperature by a gas burner (Plate X. Fig. 4). The sugar
solution to be examined is first treated with a little dilute
sulphuric acid, then neutralised with sodium carbonate,
clarified by means of basic plumbic acetate, filtered, and
the polariscopic reading taken at a temperature of 86° to
90°.

* The foregoing description of the polariscope was embodied in an
article contributed by the author to Van Nostrand's Engineering
Magazine.

† Journ. Amer. Chem. Soc., i. p. 1.

Since the results given by the foregoing method represent pure dextrose, it is necessary to first ascertain the dextro-rotary power of the particular variety of glucose probably employed for the adulteration of the sugar under examination, and then make the requisite correction. This process for the estimation of glucose is especially advantageous, in that the optical effect of the invert sugar normally present in raw cane sugars is rendered inactive.

It is sometimes desirable to determine the relative proportions of the organic constituents which are present in commercial glucose. These usually consist of dextrose, maltose, and dextrine, all of which possess dextro-rotary power, but not in the same degree; that of dextrose being 52, that of maltose 139, and that of dextrine 193. An estimation of the amount of each can be made by first ascertaining the total rotary effect of the sample by means of the polariscope.* This is expressed by the equation

$$P = 52\,d + 139\,m + 193\,d', \qquad (1)$$

in which P is the total rotation observed. Upon now treating the solution of glucose with an excess of an alkaline solution of mercuric cyanide (prepared by dissolving 120 grammes of mercuric cyanide and 25 grammes of potassium hydroxide in 1 litre of water), the dextrose and maltose contained in the sample are decomposed, leaving the dextrine unaffected. A second polariscopic reading is then made, which gives the amount of dextrine present, that is

$$P' = 193\,d', \qquad (2)$$

from which the proportion of dextrine is calculated.

Subtracting the second equation from the first, we have

$$P - P' = 52\,d + 139\,m. \qquad (3)$$

Both dextrose and maltose reduce Fehling's solu-

* Wiley, Chem. News, xlvi. p. 175.

tion, the total reduction (R) being the reducing per cent. of the former (d) added to that of the latter (m). The reducing power of maltose is, however, only 0·62 as compared with dextrine, therefore

$$R = d + 0\cdot62\ m. \qquad (4)$$

Multiplying by 52, we have

$$52\ R = 52\ d + 32\cdot24\ m,$$

and subtract from (3), which gives

$$P - P' - 52\ R = 106\cdot76\ m, \qquad (5)$$

whence

$$m = \frac{P - P' - 52\ R}{106\cdot76}, \qquad (6)$$

$$d = R - 0\cdot62\ m \qquad (7)$$

and

$$d = \frac{P'}{193}.$$

HONEY.

HONEY consists of the saccharine substance collected by the bee (*Apis mellifica*) from the nectaries of flowers, and deposited by them in the cells of the comb. "Virgin honey" is the product of hives that have not previously swarmed, which is allowed to drain from the comb; the inferior varieties being obtained by the application of heat and pressure. As a result of the peculiar conditions of its formation, honey constitutes a rather complex mixture of several bodies; indeed, its exact composition is a matter of some doubt. The chief ingredients are levulose and dextrose, accompanied by a small amount of cane sugar, and inconsiderable proportions of pollen, wax, and mineral matter. According to Dubrunfaut and Soubeiran,* genuine honey contains an excess of levulose mixed with dextrose and some cane sugar. In the course of time the latter is gradually converted into invert sugar, and a crystalline deposit of dextrose forms, the levulose remaining fluid.

The following analyses made by J. C. Brown † and E. Sieben, ‡ show the general composition of pure honey :—

	J. C. Brown.	E. Sieben.
Dextrose	31·77 to 42·02	22·23 to 44·71
Levulose	33·56 „ 40·43	32·15 „ 46·89
Total glucoses	68·40 „ 79·72	67·92 „ 79·57
Sucrose	..	none „ 8·22
Wax, pollen and insol. ..	trace to 2·10	..
Ash	0·07 „ 0·26	..
Water at 100°	15·50 „ 19·80	16·28 to 24·95
Undetermined	4·95 „ 11·00	1·29 „ 8·82

* 'Comptes Rendus,' xxviii. p. 775.   † 'Analyst,' iii. p. 269.
‡ Zeits. Anal. Chem., xxiv. p. 135.

Barth has examined several varieties of genuine honey
with the following results :—

	Per cent.	Per cent.	Per cent.
Water	13·60	15·60	11·06
Dry substance	86·40	84·40	88·94
Ash	0·28	0·24	0·90
Polarisation of 10 per⎱Direct	−4·6°	−5°	+11°
cent. solution (in 200⎰After inver-			
millimetre tube) ⎰ sion	..	−7·5°	+4°
Sugar⎰Original substance	69·60	72·0	60·0
⎱After inversion	69·50	77·0	74·6
Organic matter, not sugar	16·52	7·16	13·44

W. Bishop * obtained the following figures from the
examination of honey of known purity :—

	Hungarian.	Chili.	Italian.	Normandy.
Reducing sugar	67·17	73·05	70·37	79·39
Crystallised sugar	7·58	4·55	5·77	0·
Direct polarisation	−13·70	−14·15	− 8·55	−9·25
Polarisation after inversion	−15·40	−14·85	−12·0	..

The substances said to be employed in the adulteration
of honey are water, starch, cane sugar, and glucose-syrup ;
the last mentioned is undoubtedly most commonly used.
Hager † states that, by treating corn starch with oxalic
acid, a product is obtained which, on standing two or three
weeks, acquires the appearance and taste of genuine honey ;
and samples of commercial honey not unfrequently wholly
consist of this or some other form of artificial glucose.
The season for the collection of honey by bees is a limited
one, and any existing deficiency in their natural source of
supply is sometimes remedied by placing vessels filled
with glucose near the hives. Occasionally the bees are
also supplied with a ready-made comb, consisting, at least
partially, of paraffine. It has been asserted that in some

* Journ. de Pharm. et de Chem., 1884, p. 459.
† Pharm. Centralb. 1885, pp. 303, 327.

instances, this factitious comb is entirely composed of paraffine, but the writer is informed that, if the sophistication is practised to a proportion of over 10 per cent., the bees do not readily deposit the honey in the comb.

Owing to the complex composition of honey and to the rather incomplete character of the analyses of the genuine article at hand, the detection of some of the forms of adulteration resorted to is a matter of considerable difficulty. The presence of starch is best recognised by the microscopic examination of the honey. This will likewise reveal the absence of pollen, which may be regarded as a certain indication of the spurious nature of the sample. There appears to exist a difference of opinion in regard to the presence of cane sugar in genuine honey, but it may safely be accepted that the detection of a considerable proportion of this substance points to its artificial addition. In all cases of suspected adulteration with cane sugar or glucose, the determination of the sugar present by means of the polariscope and by Fehling's method (both before and after inversion) is indispensable. It is commonly stated that unsophisticated honey polarises to the left, and that a sample possessing a dextro-rotary action is necessarily contaminated with glucose or cane sugar; but, while in the great majority of cases this is doubtless the fact, it is equally certain that honey of known purity has been met with which polarised to the right. Upon the inversion of honey containing cane sugar, the dextro-rotation is changed to a levo-rotation.

According to Lenz,* the specific gravity (at $17°$) of a solution of 30 grammes of pure honey in exactly twice the quantity of distilled water is never less than $1·1110$, a lower density indicating adulteration with water. Hehnert† states that the ash of genuine honey is always alkaline, whereas that of artificial glucose is invariably neutral. The proportion of phosphoric acid present in honey varies from

* 'Chemiker Zeitung,' viii., p. 613.　† 'Analyst,' x., p. 217.

0·013 to 0·035 per cent., which is considerably less than the proportion contained in starch sugars. Honey contaminated with starch sugar will generally show about 0·10 per cent. of phosphoric acid, and artificial honey, made from cane sugar, will usually be free from the acid.

The addition of commercial glucose may often be detected by the turbidity produced upon adding ammonium oxalate to a filtered aqueous solution of the sample ; this is due to the presence of calcium sulphate, a common impurity in the commercial varieties of glucose. If the glucose employed for admixture contains much dextrine, as is very often the case, this fact can be utilised in its detection as follows :—2 c.c. of a 25 per cent. solution of the honey are introduced into a narrow glass cylinder, and 0·5 c.c. of absolute alcohol is cautiously added ; with pure honey, the point of contact of the liquids will remain clear or become so upon allowing the mixture to stand at rest, whereas in presence of artificial glucose a milky turbidity will appear between the two strata. Genuine honey may, it is true, contain a small proportion of dextrine and exhibit a slight cloudiness when treated with alcohol, but the difference in the degree of turbidity caused is very considerable, and sufficient to render the test of service.

The test may also be applied by dissolving 20 grammes of the suspected honey in 60 c.c. of distilled water and then adding an excess of alcohol. Under these circumstances pure honey merely becomes milky, while, if commercial glucose is present, a white precipitate of dextrine is formed, which can be collected and weighed. If the sugar in the sample is determined by Fehling's solution, both before and after inversion with a little sulphuric acid, and an estimation of the amount of dextrine present is made by precipitation with alcohol, it often occurs that the quantity of the latter substance is proportional to the difference between the amount of sugar found.

According to the late investigations of Sieben,[*] fairly

* Zeitsch. d. Vereins. f. d. Rübenzucker Ind., p. 837.

satisfactory methods for the detection and determination of glucose syrup in honey are based upon the following facts :—

1st. When genuine honey undergoes fermentation, the substances which remain undecomposed are optically inactive. Glucose, or starch syrup, on the other hand, leaves a considerable amount of dextrine, which is strongly dextrogyrate. The test is made by dissolving 25 grammes of honey in about 160 c.c. of water, and adding 12 grammes of yeast (free from starch). The mixture is allowed to ferment at a moderate temperature for two or three days, after which aluminium hydroxide is added, and the liquid made up to 250 c.c. and then filtered. 200 c.c. of the filtrate are evaporated to a volume of 50 c.c., and a 200 mm. tube is then filled with the concentrated solution and examined by the polariscope.

2nd. The substances remaining unaffected by the fermentation of pure honey are not converted into a reducing sugar by boiling with dilute hydrochloric acid, as is the case with those obtained from starch syrup under the same circumstances. 25 c.c. of the solution employed for the polarisation test, as just described, are diluted with an equal volume of water, 5 c.c. of strong hydrochloric acid added, and the mixture is placed in a flask and heated for an hour over the water-bath. The contents of the flask are neutralised with potassium hydroxide, then diluted to a volume of 100 c.c., and the proportion of reducing sugar estimated in 25 c.c. of the solution. Honey containing different proportions of starch sugar gave the following percentages of reducing sugar :—

Starch-Sugar Present. per cent.	Reducing Sugar Obtained. per cent.
5	1·472
10	3·240
20	6·392
40	8·854

3rd. If the cane sugar originally present in genuine honey has been changed into invert sugar, and the honey

solution is boiled with a slight excess of Fehling's reagent,
no substances capable of yielding sugar when treated with
acids will remain undecomposed.   Starch syrup, when
subjected to this treatment, yields grape sugar in about the
proportion of 40 parts to every 100 parts of the syrup used.
The test is applied as follows :—14 grammes of honey are
dissolved in 450 c.c. of water, and the solution is heated
over the steam-bath with 20 c.c. of semi-normal acid, in
order to invert the cane sugar present.   After heating
for half an hour, the solution is neutralised, and its volume
made up to 500 c.c.   100 c.c. of Fehling's solution are then
titrated with this solution, which may contain about 2 per
cent. of invert sugar (in case the sample examined is pure,
from 23 to 26 c.c. will be required); 100 c.c. of Fehling's
reagent are next boiled with 0·5 c.c. less of the honey solution than was found to be necessary to completely reduce
the copper.   The reduced liquid is then passed through an
asbestos filter, the residue washed with hot water, the filtrate
treated with a slight excess of concentrated hydrochloric
acid, and the solution heated for one hour on the steam-
bath.   Sodium hydroxide is now added, until only a very
little free acid remains unneutralised, and the solution is
made up to 200 c.c.   Upon well shaking the cooled liquid,
a deposit of tartar sometimes separates.   150 c.c. of the
filtered solution are finally boiled with a mixture of 120 c.c.
of Fehling's reagent and 20 c.c. of water, and the proportion
of grape sugar estimated from the amount of metallic copper
obtained. (See p. 111.)   When pure honey is submitted
to the preceding process, the copper found will not exceed
2 milligrammes.   The quantities of copper obtained when
honey adulterated with various proportions of starch sugar
was tested were about as follows :—

Starch Sugar contained. per cent.	Milligrammes of Copper found.	Starch Sugar contained. per cent.	Milligrammes of Copper found.
10	40	50	250
20	90	60	330
30	140	70	410
40	195	80	500

Character of Samples.	Dextrose.	Levulose.	Invert Sugar, by Fehling's Method.	Cane Sugar.	Total Sugar.	Water.	Dry Substance.	Not Sugar.	Polarisation after Fermentation.	Residue of Fermentation when treated with acid gave Grape Sugar:	Milligrammes of Copper found by Method 3.
	per cent.	per cent.	per cent.	per cent.	per cent.	per cent.	per cent.	per cent.	degrees.	per cent.	mgr.
Adulterated with cane sugar : :	..	..	56·39	19·45	76·84	20·85	79·15	2·31	0·0	0·0	0
" " " and water ..	25·63	25·42	51·06	10·62	61·67	36·48	63·52	1·85	0·0	0·0	0
" 15 per cent. glucose syrup	37·20	31·80	69·18	...	69·00	18·54	81·46	12·46	×4·4	4·2	66
" 65 " " "	21·75	19·60	41·30	...	41·35	18·65	81·35	40·00	×25	12·4	366
" 40 " " "	34·61	23·89	58·83	...	58·50	17·81	82·19	23·69	×13	7·6	196
" 40 " " and with cane sugar.	25·47	23·51	49·04	7·06	56·04	19·94	80·06	24·02	×17·4	8·2	192
" 80 per cent. glucose syrup	21·92	12·83	35·00	...	34·75	18·12	81·88	57·13	×34	15·2	492

The tabulation on p. 127 exhibits the results obtained by the application of the foregoing tests to adulterated honey.*

The detection of paraffine in honeycomb is easily accomplished. Genuine bees'-wax fuses at 64°, paraffine usually at a lower temperature. The latter is not affected by treatment with concentrated sulphuric acid, whereas bees'-wax is dissolved by the strong acid, and undergoes carbonisation upon the application of heat. The amount of potassium hydroxide required for the saponification of one gramme of bees'-wax, as applied in Koettstorfer's method for butter analysis (p. 71), widely differs from the quantities consumed by Japanese wax and paraffine. Mr. Edward W. Martin has obtained the following figures :—

	Milligrammes K (O H) required to saponify one gramme.
Bees'-wax	7·0
Japanese wax	212·95
Paraffine	none

18 out of 37 samples of strained and comb honey, examined in 1885 by the Mass. State Board of Health, were adulterated with glucose and ordinary syrup.

---

* 'Jahresberichte,' 1884, p. 1051.

CONFECTIONERY.

PURE white candy should consist entirely of cane sugar with its water of crystallisation, but most of the article commonly met with contains a large proportion of glucose, and in many cases it is wholly composed of this compound (see p. 109). Starch and terra alba (*i. e.* gypsum or kaolin), are the other adulterants sometimes employed to fraudulently increase the bulk and weight of candy.

The substances used for colouring purposes are more liable to be positively deleterious. While such colouring agents as caramel, turmeric, litmus, saffron, beet-juice, indigo, and some of the coal-tar dyes may be considered comparatively harmless, there can be no question in regard to the very objectionable character of certain other pigments which are sometimes employed : these are mainly inorganic, and include plumbic chromate, salts of copper and arsenic, zinc-white, barium sulphate and Prussian blue. Another occasional form of adulteration to which some kinds of confectionery are exposed, is the admixture of artificial flavourings, such as "pear essence" (amylic and ethylic acetates), "banana essence" (a mixture of amylic acetate and ethylic butyrate), and oil of bitter almonds, or its imitation, nitro-benzole. A preparation known as "rock and rye drops," which had acquired a great popularity among school children in several of our large cities, proved upon analysis to consist of a mixture of glucose, flour, and fusel oil.

The examination of candy and other forms of confectionery usually embraces the determinations of glucose, starch, flour, colouring and flavouring agents, terra alba,

K

and mineral admixtures generally. The detection and estimation of glucose has already been described under Sugar.

Starch and flour are readily detected upon treating a minute portion of the suspected candy with a little water and submitting the mixture to a microscopic examination, when, in their presence, the insoluble residue will exhibit the characteristic forms of starch granules. The insoluble portion of the sample may also be tested with a solution of iodine. The proportion of starch can be determined by boiling the matter insoluble in water with dilute sulphuric acid, and estimating the amount of glucose found, by means of Fehling's solution.

Coal-tar and vegetable compounds used for colouring purposes, can often be recognised by means of their behaviour with reducing and oxidising agents, by their solubility in spirits and other menstrua, and by the application of dyeing-tests. Thus vegetable colours may sometimes be identified upon boiling mordanted cotton yarn in a bath prepared from a portion of the sample containing the colouring matter, and slightly acidulated with acetic acid. This process will likewise generally reveal the presence of aniline dyes, unmordanted woollen cloth being substituted for cotton, and a neutral bath being employed. The inorganic pigments used for colouring candy are usually to be sought for in the ash obtained upon incineration.

The presence of copper and lead is detected by the formation of black precipitates upon saturating with sulphuretted hydrogen the solution of the ash in hydrochloric acid; zinc, chromium, etc., are precipitated from the filtered solution upon addition of ammonium hydroxide and ammonium sulphide. It is frequently more convenient to apply special tests for the particular metal thought to be present, either directly to the pigment or to the ash. In this way, arsenic can often be recognised by treating a portion of the colouring matter in a test-tube, when it will sublime and collect upon the cool part of the tube in minute crystals of arsenious acid. Or, an acidulated solution of the detached pigments may be boiled with a piece of polished copper-foil, upon which the arsenic will be deposited as a greyish film : this can be sublimed, and otherwise further examined.

Copper is easily detected and estimated by placing the acid solution of the ash in a tared platinum dish, and reducing the copper by the electrolytic method. Chromium is recognised upon boiling the colouring matter with potassium carbonate solution : in its presence, potassium chromate is formed, which is submitted to the usual distinctive tests for chromium. The colour of Prussian blue is destroyed upon warming it with caustic alkalies : indigo, which remains unaffected by this treatment, forms a blue solution if heated with concentrated sulphuric acid. The presence of terra alba, barium sulphate, etc., is best detected by the examination of the ash. Chalk, or marble-dust, is recognised by its effervescence when treated with an acid, as well as by the presence of a notable proportion of lime in the ash.

Many of the flavouring mixtures added to candy may be separated by treating the sample with chloroform or petroleum naphtha and evaporating the solution to dryness over a water-bath, when their identity is frequently revealed by their odour and other physical properties. Of 198 samples of the cheaper varieties of confectionery examined by Health officials in the United States, 115 were adulterated. Plumbic chromate is a very common addition ; 41 out of 48 samples of yellow- and orange-coloured candy contained this poisonous pigment.

K 2

BEER.

THE name beer is most commonly applied to a fermented infusion of malted barley, flavoured with hops. Its manufacture embraces two distinct operations, _viz._, malting and brewing. Briefly considered, the former process consists in first steeping barley (the seed of _Hordeum distichon_) in water and allowing it to germinate by arranging it in layers or heaps which are subsequently spread out and repeatedly turned over, the germination being thereby retarded ; it is afterwards entirely checked by drying the grain (now known as _malt_) in cylinders or kilns.

The degree of temperature employed in drying and roasting the barley determines the colour and commercial character of the malt, which may be pale, amber, brown or black. In the United States the light-coloured varieties of malt are chiefly made. An important change which takes place during the malting of barley is the conversion of its albuminous constituents into a peculiar ferment, termed _diastase_, which, although its proportion in malt does not exceed 0·003 per cent., exerts a very energetic action in transforming starch, first into dextrine, then into sugar (maltose). The following analyses, by Proust, exhibit the general composition of unmalted and malted barley :—

	Barley.	Malt.
Hordeine	55	12
Starch	32	56
Gluten	3	1
Sugar	5	15
Mucilage	4	15
Resin	1	1
	100	100

The body termed hordeine is generally considered to be an allotropic modification of starch.

In the brewing of beer, the malted grain is crushed by means of iron rollers, and then introduced into the mash-tubs and digested with water at a temperature of about 75°, whereby the conversion of the starch into dextrine and sugar is effected. After standing for a few hours, the clear infusion, or *wort*, is drawn off and boiled with hops (the female flower of *Humulus lupulus*), after which it is rapidly cooled, and then placed in capacious vats where it is mixed with yeast and allowed to undergo the process of fermentation for several days, during which the formation of fresh quantities of yeast and a partial decomposition of the sugar into alcohol and carbonic acid take place. The beer is next separated from the yeast and transferred into clearing-vats, and, later on, into storage casks, where it undergoes a slow after-fermentation, at the completion of which it is ready for consumption. The quality of the water used in the process of mashing and brewing is of great importance, and it is of special moment that it should be free from all organic contaminations. The presence of certain mineral ingredients, notably of calcium sulphate, is believed to exert a beneficial effect on the character of the beer obtained.

In the United States, the best known varieties of malt liquors are ale, porter, and lager beer. The difference between ale and porter is mainly due to the quality of the malt used in their manufacture. Ale is made from pale malt, porter or stout from a mixture of the darker coloured malts, the method of fermentation employed being in both cases that known as the "superficial" (*obergährung*), which takes place at a higher temperature and is of shorter duration than the "sedimentary" (*untergährung*). The latter form of fermentation, which is used in the preparation of Bavarian or lager beer, occurs at a temperature of about 8°, and requires more time for its completion, during which the

beer is, or should be, preserved in cool cellars for several
months before it is fit for use ; hence the common American
name of this kind of beer, from *lager*, a storehouse.   There
are three varieties of Bavarian beer, "lager beer" proper,
or the summer beer, which has been stored for about five
months; "*schenk*," or winter beer, which is fit for use in
several weeks; and "*bock*" beer, which possesses more
strength than the former, and is made in comparatively
small quantities in the spring of the year.   A mild kind of
malt liquor, known as "*weiss*" beer, and prepared by a
quick process of fermentation, is less frequently met with.

   The first brewery in America is said to have been founded
in New York in the year 1644, by Jacobus, who afterwards
became the first burgomaster of the city, then New
Amsterdam.   Subsequently, William Penn established a
brewery in Bucks Co., Pa., and a century later, General
Putnam engaged in the manufacture of beer in the State of
Connecticut.   The brewing of lager beer in the United
States began to assume prominence about thirty-five years
ago.   It is estimated that, at the present time, over 2000
breweries are devoted to the preparation of this form of
malt liquor, with an invested capital of at least 60 millions
of dollars, the annual production exceeding 15 millions of
barrels.*   The industry is chiefly carried on in New
York, Brooklyn, Philadelphia, Milwaukee, St. Louis, and
Cincinnati.

   The composition of beer naturally varies according to
the kind of grain from which it is made and the process of
fermentation employed.   The chief ingredients are alcohol,
carbonic acid, sugar (maltose), dextrine, the oil and bitter
principle of hops (lupuline), albuminoids, lactic, acetic,
succinic and propionic acids, inorganic salts, and traces of
glycerine.   The term "extract" is applied to the non-

   * The total production of all kinds of malt liquors in the United
States was, for the fiscal year 1886, 20 millions of barrels ; it is assumed
that at least three-quarters of this amount consisted of lager beer.

Variety.	Specific Gravity.	Carbonic Acid. per cent.	Alcohol (by weight). per cent.	Extract. per cent.	Albuminoids. per cent.	Sugar. per cent.	Dextrine. per cent.	Acid. per cent.	Ash. per cent.	Phosphoric Acid. per cent.
Porter	1·0207	0·16	5·4	6·0	0·83	..	7·72	0·24	0·40	..
Scotch ale	..	0·15	8·5	10·9	0·77	0·34	2·50	0·19	..	..
Burton ale	1·0106	..	5·9	14·5	0·57	..	3·64	0·32	..	..
Munich (Salvator)	1·0129	0·18	4·6	9·4	0·67	..	..	..	..	0·024
„ (Bock)	1·0118	0·17	4·2	9·2	..	0·80	..	0·14	0·22	..
„ (Schenk)	..	..	3·8	5·8	..	..	6·17	..	..	..
„ (Lager)	1·0110	0·15	5·1	5·0	0·83	0·35	..	0·20	0·21	..
Berlin	..	..	3·1	5·8	..	..	..	..	0·21	..
„ (Tivoli)	..	..	4·35	5·14	..	..	..	0·23	0·19	..
Erlanger	..	..	4·56	4·81	..	0·40	1·44	..	0·48	..
Thüringer (common)	..	..	2·00	..	..	0·31	7·71	0·16	..	..
Culmbacher	1·0228	..	4·00	7·38	0·53	1·52	..	0·19	..	..
American lager, average 19 samples	1·0162	..	2·78	6·05	..	..	..	..	0·305	0·105
American ale	1·0150	..	4·69	6·50	0·74	4·96	..	..	0·353	0·080
American lager, maximum 474 samples	1·0370	..	8·99	9·54	..	..	..	..	0·46	0·166
minimum	0·999	..	0·68	1·28	..	..	..	..	0·10	0·028
According to König maximum	1·034	0·500	7·3	11·24	1·98	2·45	7·85	0·40	0·48	0·09
minimum	1·0100	0·100	1·00	2·60	0·02	0·10	1·46	0·08	0·14	0·02

volatile constituents, which include the sugar, dextrine, albuminoids, ash, etc. The foregoing table, collated from the analyses of various chemists, gives the general composition of some of the best known brands of malt liquor, as well as the minimum and maximum proportions that have been found.

The composition of beer ash is evidently affected by the character of the water used in the brewing process. Blyth gives the following as the average composition of the ash of English beers:—

	Per cent.
Potash	37·22
Soda	8·04
Lime	1·93
Magnesia	5·51
Ferric oxide	traces
Sulphuric acid	1·44
Phosphoric acid	32·09
Chlorine	2·91
Silica	10·82

The following results were obtained by the writer from the analysis of the ash of American lager beer of fair quality :—

	Per cent.
Silica	9·97
Alumina and ferric oxide	0·46
Lime	3·55
Magnesia	7·27
Soda	13·81
Potassa	19·59
Sulphuric acid	3·25
Chlorine	4·40
Phosphoric acid	37·70
	10·000
Percentage of ash	0·274

Strictly speaking, normal beer consists solely of the product of malt and hops, and the presence of any ingredients other than these should be regarded as an adulteration. It is maintained by brewers, and with justice, that the term "malt" is not necessarily restricted to barley, but includes other varieties of malted grain, such as wheat, corn, and rice. The old English law, while permitting the addition of wholesome bitters, prohibits the use of various other substances, but in the United States, no legal definition of pure beer has, as yet, been formulated, and the necessity for such a measure is being experienced.* The past literature of beer adulteration makes mention of very numerous substances which, in former times, have been resorted to as admixtures. Among these the following are the most prominent :—

1st. *Artificial bitters.*—Picric acid, picrotoxine, aloes, gentian, quassia, and wormwood. Several years ago the author had occasion to examine two samples, imported under the name of "hop substitutes," both of which proved to consist of *salicine*, the bitter principle of the willow. The fruit of the hop tree (*Ptelea trifoliata*), has also been employed as an artificial bitter for beer.

2nd. *Flavourings.* — For flavouring purposes, cayenne pepper, "grains of paradise," cloves, orris root, coriander seeds, the oils of anise, nutmegs, and carraway, are stated to have been used.

3rd. *Malt substitutes.*—These mainly consist of corn, rice, and glucose.

A substitute for malt, of rather recent origin, and commercially known as "cerealine," is prepared by subjecting hulled and coarsely ground Indian corn to the action of steam, the product being subsequently pulverised by means of hot rollers. It is said to have the following average composition :—

Water..	9·98
Insoluble starch	61·43
Soluble starch, dextrine, and maltose ..	17·79
Albuminoids	9·07
Oil	1·22
Cellulose	0·23
Mineral matter..	0·28

* In Bavaria the use of all malt and hop substitutes is legally prohibited.

In addition to the foregoing, several chemical compounds, such as ammonium carbonate, tartaric acid, alkaline phosphates, boric and salicylic acids and glycerine are,
or at least have been, employed as accessories in the
manufacture of beer. From the investigations of the New
York State Board of Health, it appears that the present
adulteration of American beer—more especially of "lager
beer"—is limited, so far as the brewer is concerned, to the
use of various substitutes for malt, the addition of salt, and
of sodium bicarbonate.

The proportion of diastase obtained by the germination
of barley, or other cereals, is largely in excess of the
amount required to convert into sugar the starch actually
present in the grain treated ; hence the brewer can add
other forms of amylaceous substances, such as corn or rice,
to malted barley with decided economy, and the majority
of New York brewers employ such substitutes, usually in
a proportion of 25 per cent. The brewer may likewise
advantageously add glucose syrup to the malt infusion,
since, by its use, he arrives at the same end, *i. e.* instead of
obtaining all of his sugar as the result of the malting process,
he directly provides himself with the same body, at least
so far as it possesses value to him as a source of alcohol.
The question of the sanitary effects of the use of artificial
glucose as an adulterant of sugar and syrups, and as a
substitute for malted grain in the manufacture of beer, has
given rise to extensive controversy. In this regard, one
fact seems to have been demonstrated. Glucose, as it is
now to be found on the market, is free from any appreciable
amount of deleterious contamination. The discovery of
its artificial production has given birth to a very important
branch of industry, and, according to all available reports,
the commercial product at present met with is for many
purposes an economical and harmless substitute for cane
sugar, the chief objection to its application as such being
the fact that it possesses considerably less sweetening power.

The United States National Academy of Sciences, after having carefully investigated the sanitary aspects of the glucose question, arrived at the following conclusion: [*] "That, though having at best only about two-thirds the sweetening power of cane sugar, yet starch sugar is in no way inferior to the cane sugar in healthfulness, there being no evidence before the committee that maize-starch sugar, either in its normal condition or fermented, has any deleterious effect upon the system, even when taken in large quantities." In regard to the use of glucose as a substitute for malt in beer-making, it is asserted by some authorities that dietetic advantages to be derived from pure malt will be to some extent wanting in the extractive matters of beer manufactured partially from the artificial product. A distinction between glucose and maltose, to the advantage of the latter, is also made. The brewer, on the other hand, claims that sugar is sugar, whether obtained from the malting of grain or from the conversion of starch by the aid of acids. Regarding these bodies merely as sources of alcohol, attempts to differentiate between them are of little service. The superiority claimed for barley malt over its substitutes would rather appear to be due to its greater richness in certain soluble constituents, more especially those containing nitrogen and phosphoric acid.[†] A proposed law to prohibit the use of all malt substitutes has recently been rejected by the German Reichstag. In the English Beer Adulteration Act (1886), however, it is directed that, in

---

[*] 'Report of the National Academy of Sciences,' 1883, p. 88.

[†] Hanemann has made the following determinations of fermented worts prepared from pure malt and from malts containing 40 per cent. of each substitute :—

	Pure Malt.	Maize Malt.	Rice Malt.	Starch Malt.
Alcohol	2·71	2·76	2·90	3·19
Extract	6·59	6·48	6·25	5·91
Proteids	0·43	0·39	0·33	0·28

case beer (ale or porter) made from other substances than hops and barley-malt is offered for sale, the fact shall be mentioned on a prominent placard, stating the nature of the foreign ingredients.

The addition of sodium bicarbonate is resorted to in order to increase the effervescing power of the beverage, and, possibly in some instances, to neutralise the acids formed by the souring of new and hastily prepared beer.* One of the chief objections to which certain inferior varieties of American lager beer are open is that they are not allowed to "age" properly. The apparent gain to the brewer of such beer consists in an economy of time and ice ; he is also enabled to turn over his invested capital sooner than the more scrupulous manufacturer, who is thus placed in a disadvantageous position so far as trade competition is concerned. It is stated that some of the beer made in the neighbourhood of New York is sent out for consumption two weeks after its brewing.† Beer of this character would be apt to contain abnormally large proportions of dextrine, dextrose, etc., as well as be contaminated with unchanged yeast and other products of imperfect fermentation. It is said to be the practice to submit it to a process of clarification by means of isinglass and cream of tartar, and then impart additional life to the product by adding sodium bicarbonate, which is used in the form of cartridges or pills, and in a proportion of two ounces of the salt to the keg of beer.‡ Such a beverage obviously

---

* The writer is assured by a prominent New York brewer, that the addition of sodium bicarbonate is resorted to, not so much as a remedy for poor beer, as for the purpose of satisfying the vitiated taste of the public, who demand a lively and sparkling beverage. The proportion employed is claimed not to exceed one ounce to the keg of beer.

† 'Annual Report Brooklyn Board of Health,' 1885, p. 89.—The accuracy of this statement is denied by the brewers. A blending of new and old beer is, however, occasionally practised with, it is said, no deleterious effects.

‡ Ibid.

possesses very little claim to the name "lager" beer. It is, perhaps, to this reprehensible practice that many of the deleterious effects on the digestive organs which sometimes follow the consumption of considerable quantities of *poor grades* of lager beer are to be ascribed ; and it is often asserted to be the fact that beer drinkers who have daily drunk from 20 to 25 glasses of German beer with apparent impunity, experience disagreeable results from the habitual consumption of much smaller quantities of some varieties of American lager.

It should be remarked, in this connection, that the brewer is by no means responsible for all of the sophistications to which beer is exposed, as after it leaves his hands it may be watered by the retailer as well as allowed to deteriorate in quality by careless methods of preservation. From all procurable information, it would appear that the only questionable features of beer brewing, as now generally carried on in the United States, are the following :—

1st. The use of corn and other meals, and of artificial glucose as substitutes for malted barley.

2nd. The use of sodium bicarbonate, to impart additional life to the beer, and the occasional use of common salt.

Concerning the alleged employment of artificial bitters in beer it should be stated, that a few years since, when a very marked increase occurred in the price of hops, other bitter preparations were advertised and offered for sale in the market ; unfortunately, but little authentic data can be secured in regard to the extent of their use. At present, this form of adulteration has apparently been discontinued. It is worthy of notice, that the addition of hops to beer was originally considered a falsification, and was prohibited in England by legal enactments. In regard to the manufacture and sale of partially fermented beer, the question of the prevalence of this practice must be regarded as undetermined. No objection exists to the proper use of isinglass or other forms of gelatine for the clarification of beer.

Of 476 samples of beer tested by Dr. F. E. Engelhardt, of the New York State Board of Health, about one-quarter gave evidence of the use of malt substitutes in their manufacture, but no sample was conclusively shown to be adulterated with bitters other than hops.

The examination of beer properly includes an inspection of its physical characteristics, such as taste, colour, and transparency, the determination of the specific gravity, quantitative estimations of the proportions of alcohol, carbonic acid, extractive matter, sugar, organic acids, ash and phosphoric acid, and qualitative tests for the detection of the presence of artificial substitutes for malt and hops.

When of good quality, beer exhibits a bright and transparent colour, a faint but not disagreeable aroma, and a clean and slightly bitter taste. It should be free from any signs of viscosity, the appearance of which is usually an indication of the presence of unchanged yeast.

The specific gravity of beer is determined by first removing the excess of carbonic acid by repeatedly agitating the sample in a capacious glass flask, or by pouring it from one beaker into another several times, and then filling a specific gravity bottle with the liquid and allowing it to stand at rest until all air or gas bubbles have escaped ; the weight of the bottle and its contents is now taken at 15°. In order to determine the proportion of alcohol present, 100 c.c of the beer are introduced in a suitable flask which is connected with a Liebig's condenser and subjected to distillation until about one-half of the quantity taken has passed over. The distillate is then made up to its original volume by the addition of water, and its density ascertained by means of the specific gravity bottle, from which the percentage of alcohol present (by weight and by volume) is readily obtained upon referring to the alcoholometric table on p. 144. The frothing of beer and the volatilisation of the free acids present are best obviated by the addition of a little tannic acid and baryta-water to the sample before the distillation. An indirect method for the determination of alcohol in beer is also frequently employed. It is accomplished by first ascertaining the density of the liquor, next removing the alcohol present by evaporation over the water-bath, subsequently adding sufficient water to restore the original volume and again taking the specific gravity of the product. The density of spirit of equal strength to the beer taken ($\times$) is obtained by the formula, $\dfrac{D}{D'} = \times$, in which D is the original gravity of the sample, and D' the gravity of the de-alcoholised liquor when made up to its first volume. The following table (see p. 144) from 'Watts' Dictionary of Chemistry' gives the percentages of alcohol by volume and weight, corresponding to different densities at 15°.

The amount of carbonic acid is conveniently found by introducing 100 c.c. of the *well-cooled* beer into a rather large flask, provided with a delivery-tube which connects, first with a wash-bottle containing concentrated sulphuric acid, next with a U-tube, filled with fused calcium chloride. The latter is connected with a Liebig's bulb containing a solution of potassium hydroxide, then with a U-tube containing solid potassium hydroxide, both of which have previously been tared. The flask is heated over a water-bath until the evolution of carbonic acid ceases, after which, the gas remaining in the apparatus is caused to traverse the potash bulb by drawing air through it. This is done by means of a tube attached to the flask and reaching below the surface of the beer. At its other extremity, it is drawn out to a fine point and connected with a small potash bulb (for the retention of atmospheric carbonic acid), by aid of a rubber tube, which permits of breaking the glass point before drawing air through the apparatus. The amount of carbonic acid present in the sample is ascertained by the increase of weight found in the larger potash bulb and U-tube.

ALCOHOLOMETRIC TABLE FOR BEER, ETC.

Volume per cent.	Weight per cent.	Specific Gravity.	Volume per cent.	Weight per cent.	Specific Gravity.
1·0	0·80	0·99850	4·5	3·60	0·99350
1·1	0.88	0·99835	4·6	3·68	0·99336
1·2	0·96	0·99820	4·7	3·76	0·99322
1·3	1·04	0·99805	4·8	3·84	0·99308
1·4	1·12	0·99790	4·9	3·92	0·99294
1·5	1·20	0·99775	5·0	4·00	0·99280
1·6	1·28	0·99760	5·1	4·08	0·99267
1·7	1·36	0·99745	5·2	4·16	0·99254
1·8	1·44	0·99730	5·3	4·24	0·99241
1·9	1·52	0·99715	5·4	4·32	0·99228
2·0	1·60	0·99700	5·5	4·40	0·99215
2·1	1·68	0·99686	5·6	4·48	0·99202
2·2	1·76	0·99672	5·7	4·56	0·99189
2·3	1·84	0·99658	5·8	4·64	0·99176
2·4	1·92	0·99644	5·9	4·72	0·99163
2·5	2·00	0·99630	6·0	4·81	0·99150
2·6	2·08	0·99616	6·1	4·89	0·99137
2·7	2·16	0·99602	6·2	4·97	0·99124
2·8	2·24	0·99588	6·3	5·05	0·99111
2·9	2·32	0·99574	6·4	5·13	0·99098
3·0	2·40	0·99560	6·5	5·21	0·99085
3·1	2·48	0·99546	6·6	5·30	0·99072
3·2	2·56	0·99532	6·7	5·38	0·99059
3·3	2·64	0·99518	6·8	5·46	0·99046
3·4	2·72	0·99504	6·9	5·54	0·99033
3·5	2·80	0·99490	7·0	5·62	0·99020
3·6	2·88	0·99476	7·1	5·70	0·99008
3·7	2·96	0·99462	7·2	5·78	0·98996
3·8	3·04	0·99448	7·3	5·86	0·98984
3·9	3·12	0·99434	7·4	5·94	0·98972
4·0	3·20	0·99420	7·5	6·02	0·98960
4·1	3·28	0·99406	7·6	6·11	0·98949
4·2	3·36	0·99392	7·7	6·19	0·98936
4·3	3·44	0·99378	7·8	6·27	0·98924
4·4	3·52	0·99364	7·9	6·35	0·98912
			8·0	6·43	0·98900

The proportion of malt extract in beer can be directly determined by the evaporation of 5 or 10 c.c. of the sample in a capacious platinum dish over the water-bath and drying the residue until constant weight is obtained.* It should be allowed to cool under a bell-jar over calcium chloride, before weighing. Usually the estimation is made by an indirect process, which consists in removing the alcohol by evaporation, bringing the liquid up to its original volume by the addition of water, and then taking its specific gravity and determining the percentage of malt extract by means of the following table :—

SPECIFIC GRAVITY AND STRENGTH OF MALT EXTRACT.

Specific Gravity.	Per Cent. Malt Extract.	Specific Gravity.	Per Cent. Malt Extract.	Specific Gravity.	Per Cent. Malt Extract.
1·000	0·000	1·024	6·000	1·048	11·809
1·001	0·250	1·025	6·244	1·049	12·047
1·002	0·500	1·026	6·488	1·050	12·285
1·003	0·750	1·027	6·731	1·051	12·523
1·004	1·000	1·028	6·975	1·052	12·761
1·005	1·250	1·029	7·219	1·053	13·000
1·006	1·500	1·030	7·463	1·054	13·238
1·007	1·750	1·031	7·706	1·055	13·476
1·008	2·000	1·032	7·950	1·056	13·714
1·009	2·250	1·033	8·195	1·057	13·952
1·010	2·500	1·034	8·438	1.058	14·190
1·011	2·750	1·035	8·681	1·059	14·428
1·012	3·000	1·036	8·925	1·060	14·666
1·013	3·250	1·037	9·170	1·061	14·904
1·014	3·500	1·038	9·413	1·062	15·139
1·015	3·750	1·039	9·657	1·063	15·371
1·016	4·000	1·040	9·901	1·064	15·604
1·017	4·250	1·041	10·142	1·065	15·837
1·018	4·500	1·042	10·381	1·066	16·070
1·019	4·750	1·043	10·619	1·067	16·302
1·020	5·000	1·044	10·857	1·068	16·534
1·021	5·250	1·045	11·095	1·069	16·767
1·022	5·500	1·046	11·333	1·070	17·000
1·023	5·750	1·047	11·595		

The sugar contained in beer is best determined by taking 50 c.c. of the sample, adding 10 c.c. of plumbic basic acetate solution, and making the volume of the mixture

* The albuminoids in beer may be estimated by diluting 1 c.c. of the sample with water and then submitting it to Wanklyn's process for water analysis (see p. 211). The albuminoid ammonia thus obtained, multiplied by 5·2, gives the proteids in the beer taken.

L

up to 300 c.c. with distilled water. After standing for
some time the solution is passed through a dry filter. It
is then examined by cautiously adding it from a burette to
10 c.c. of Fehling's solution (diluted with 40 c.c. of distilled
water and brought to the boiling-point), until the blue
colour of the latter disappears (see p. 111). It should be
borne in mind that, while 10 c.c. of Fehling's solution
are reduced by 0·05 gramme of glucose, it requires
0·075 gramme of maltose to effect the same reduction.

In order to estimate the dextrine, 10 c.c. of the beer are
reduced by evaporation to about 4 c.c., and heated with
1 c.c. of dilute sulphuric acid to 110° by means of an oil-
bath in a strong hermetically closed glass tube for five
hours. At the completion of this operation the solution is
neutralised with sodium hydroxide, diluted, and the total
glucose determined by Fehling's reagent, as just described.
The glucose due to the conversion of the dextrine is found
by deducting the amount of maltose (expressed in terms
of glucose) previously obtained from the total glucose ;
10 parts of glucose represent 9 parts of dextrine.

The organic acids (acetic and lactic) are estimated as
follows :—(a) *Acetic acid*, by distilling 100 c.c. of the sample
almost to dryness, and titrating the distillate with decinormal soda solution ; (b) *Lactic acid*, by dissolving the
residue remaining after the distillation in water, and either
determining its acidity by decinormal soda, or by treating
the residue with water and a little sulphuric acid, adding
barium carbonate to the mixture, heating in the water-bath
and filtering, the precipitate being thoroughly washed with
hot water. The filtrate is then concentrated to a syrup by
evaporation, and agitated in a test-tube with a mixture of
1 part each of sulphuric acid, alcohol, and water, and
10 parts of ether. After standing at rest for some time,
the ethereal solution is separated by means of a pipette and
evaporated to dryness in a tared capsule. The residue
(impure lactic acid) can be weighed, or it is dissolved in

water, the solution treated with zinc carbonate, and the lactic acid determined as zinc lactate, which contains 54·5 per cent. of the anhydrous acid.

Phosphoric acid may be estimated in the beer directly by first expelling the carbonic acid, then adding a small quantity of potassium acetate, heating, and titrating with a standard solution of uranium acetate, using potassium ferrocyanide as the indicator. It can also be determined gravimetrically in the ash.

The estimation of the ash is made by evaporating 100 c.c. of the sample in a weighed platinum dish to dryness, and incinerating the residue at a rather moderate heat, so as to avoid volatilisation of the chlorides. The amount of ash in normal beer should never exceed 0·5 per cent., the usual proportion being about 0·3 per cent.; this would naturally be increased by the addition of sodium bicarbonate or sodium chloride to the beer. The complete analysis of the ash is seldom necessary, but it is often of importance to estimate the amount of sodium chloride contained. This is effected by dissolving the ash-residue in distilled water and precipitating the chlorine from an aliquot portion of the solution by silver nitrate; one part of the precipitate obtained represents 0·409 part of common salt. The proportion of sodium chloride in pure beer is very inconsiderable, but it may be added to the beverage either to improve the flavour or to create thirst. For the determination of phosphoric acid, a weighed portion of the ash is dissolved in nitric acid, the solution evaporated to dryness, and the residue boiled with water containing a little nitric acid. It is then filtered, concentrated by evaporation, an excess of ammonium molybdate solution added, and the mixture set aside for about ten hours, after which the precipitate formed is separated by filtration and dissolved in ammonium hydroxide. A solution of magnesium sulphate (mixed with a considerable quantity of ammonium chloride) is now added, and the precipitated ammonio-magnesium phosphate collected, washed, ignited, and weighed. 100 parts of this precipitate contain 64 parts of phosphoric anhydride (P_2O_5).

The positive detection of the presence of artificial substitutes for malt in beer is a matter of considerable difficulty. According to Haarstick, a large proportion of commercial glucose contains a substance termed *amylin*, which exerts a strong dextro-rotary effect upon polarised light, but is not destroyed by fermentation, and upon these facts is based a process for the identification of starch-sugar in beer. It is executed by evaporating 1 litre of the sample to the consistency of a syrup and separating the dextrine present by the gradual addition of 95 per cent. alcohol.* After standing at rest for several hours the liquid is filtered, the greater portion of the alcohol removed from the filtrate by distillation, and the residual fluid evaporated to dryness over the water-bath. The solid residue is then diluted to about a litre, yeast added, and the sugar present decomposed by allowing fermentation to take place for three or four days, at a temperature of 20°. It was found that, under these conditions, pure beer afforded a solution which was optically inactive when examined by the polariscope, while beer prepared from artificial glucose gave a solution possessing decided dextro-rotary power. The use of rice and glucose in the manufacture of beer is also indicated when there is a deficiency in the proportion of phosphoric acid in the ash, and of the extract, which applies, although to a somewhat less extent, if wheat or corn meal has been substituted for barley malt.

The following conclusions were reached by a commission of chemists appointed in Germany to determine standards for beer :—A fixed relation between the quantity of alcohol and extract in beer does not invariably exist. As a rule in Bavarian and lager beer, for 1 part by weight of alcohol

* The dextrine can also be removed by subjecting the beer to dialysis (see p. 183).

a maximum of 2 parts and a minimum of 1·5 parts of extract should be present. In case malt has been replaced by glucose, or other non-nitrogenous substances, the percentage of nitrogen in the extract will fall below 0·65. The acidity should not exceed 3 c.c. of normal alkali solution for 100 c.c. of beer. The ash should not exceed 0·3 per cent. The maximum proportion of glycerine should not exceed 0·25 per cent. For clarification, the following means are permissible: Filtration, the use of shavings, etc., and of isinglass or other forms of gelatine ; for preservation, carbonic acid gas, and salicylic acid may be employed— the latter, however, only in beer which is intended for exportation to countries where its use is not prohibited.

Several samples of so-called "beer preservatives" examined by the author, consisted of a solution of sodium salicylate and borax, dissolved in glycerine. Salicylic acid is employed in order to prevent fermentation in beer, which is exposed to great variations in temperature. Its presence is detected by the following process, suggested by Röse,* which is equally applicable to wine :—The beer (or wine) is acidulated with sulphuric acid, and well shaken with its own volume of a mixture of equal parts of ether and petroleum naphtha. After standing at rest, the ethereal layer is removed by a pipette, and evaporated or distilled until reduced to a few c.c. A little water and a few drops of a dilute ferric chloride solution are then added, and the liquid filtered : in presence of salicylic acid, the filtrate will exhibit a violet colour. In the case of wines, where the presence of tannic acid might interfere with the salicylic acid reaction, the filtrate is re-acidulated, then diluted, and the treatment with the ether mixture and iron chloride repeated. The second residue will now show the violet coloration, even in wines rich in tannin, and containing but 0·2 milligramme of salicylic acid per litre. The tannin can also be removed by precipitation with

* Chem. Centralb., 1886, p. 412.

gelatine, and the colour test for salicylic acid subsequently applied. Glycerine is likewise sometimes used as
a preservative of beer, and is also added to render the
liquor richer in appearance, by communicating a viscosity
to the froth which causes it to adhere longer to the sides of
the glass. It can be quantitatively estimated by evaporating 100 c.c. of the sample in a capsule at a temperature
of 75°, until the carbonic acid has been expelled, then adding
about 5 grammes of magnesium hydroxide, and thoroughly
stirring the mixture until it forms a homogeneous, semifluid
mass. The contents of the dish are allowed to cool, and
are then well digested with 50 c.c. of absolute alcohol, and
the fluid portion afterwards separated by decantation, the
residual mass being again treated with 20 c.c. of absolute
alcohol, and the alcoholic solution thus obtained added to
the first. The malose, parapeptone, etc., present in the
solution are now precipitated by adding (with constant
stirring) 300 c.c. of anhydrous ether, after which the liquid
is filtered, and the filtrate concentrated, at first by spontaneous evaporation, subsequently by heating over the
water-bath, until it assumes the consistency of a syrup,
when it is placed in an exsiccator which connects with an
air-pump, where it is allowed to remain for twenty-four
hours. The syrupy residue is then digested with 20 c.c.
of absolute alcohol and filtered, the filtrate being collected
in a tared capsule, which is again exposed to the heat of
the water-bath, and allowed to remain in the exsiccator for
twelve hours, after which it is weighed. The increase in
weight gives approximately the amount of glycerine contained in the beer examined.*

It is certain that many of the poisonous substances
which in former times have been detected in beer, such as
strychnine, hyoscyamine, picric acid, and picrotoxine, are
not used at present. It is much more probable that such
bitters as gentian and quassia may be met with, especially

* Griessmayer ; Corresp. Blatt. d. Ver. Anal. Chem. No. 4, Feb. 1880.

at times when hops are dear. These latter far exceed hops in bitterness, and do not exert deleterious effects upon health. Willow bark, or its active principle, salicine, has also been employed. The detection of some of the most apocryphal substitutes for hops is effected, according to Wiltstein,* by the following method : One litre of the beer is concentrated over the water-bath to a syrupy liquor, which is introduced into a rather capacious tared cylinder and weighed. The gum, dextrine, and mineral salts are first separated by adding to the syrup five times its weight of 95 per cent. alcohol, with which it is thoroughly mixed, and allowed to digest for twenty-four hours. The clear, supernatant solution is now drawn off, and the residue treated with a fresh quantity of alcohol, which is afterwards united with the solution first obtained, the whole being then evaporated until the alcohol is expelled. A small portion of the residue is dissolved in a little water, and tested for picric acid, as described later on. The remainder is repeatedly shaken with about six times its weight of pure benzol, which is subsequently removed by decantation, the operation being then repeated with fresh benzol, the two solutions added and evaporated to dryness at a very moderate temperature. The residue thus obtained is divided into three portions, which are placed in small porcelain dishes and tested as follows :—

To one portion a little nitric acid (sp. gr. 1·330) is added; if a red coloration ensues, *brucine* is present ; if a violet colour, *colchicine.* A second portion is treated with concentrated sulphuric acid ; the production of a red colour indicates the presence of *colocynthine.* To a third portion, a few fragments of potassium dichromate and a little sulphuric acid are added ; if a purple-violet coloration takes place, *strychnine* is present.

The portion of the syrup which has remained undissolved by benzol is first dried over the water-bath, and

* Archiv. der Pharm., Jan. 1876.

then agitated with pure amylic alcohol, by which treatment
picrotoxine and aloes, if present, will go in solution, and
impart a bitter taste to the liquid.

The solution can be examined as subsequently directed
for picrotoxine ; the presence of aloes is best recognised by
the characteristic saffron-like odour possessed by this body.
The syrup which remains after the successive treatments
with benzol and amylic alcohol is next freed from any
remaining traces of the latter compound by means of blot-
ting-paper, and then thoroughly agitated with anhydrous
ether, which is afterwards removed and allowed to spontaneously evaporate. If the residue now obtained exhibits
a wormwood-like aroma, and gives a reddish yellow solution, which rapidly changes to a deep blue when treated
with concentrated sulphuric acid, *absinthine* is present. The
syrup insoluble in ether may still contain quassine, gentipicrine, and menyanthine, and the presence of any of these
bodies is indicated if it possesses a bitter taste, since the
bitter principle of hops would have been removed by the
foregoing treatment with solvents. The syrup is dissolved
in a little warm water, the solution filtered and divided
into two portions. To one a concentrated ammoniacal
solution of silver nitrate is added, and the mixture heated :
if it remains clear, quassine is probably present ; the forma-.
tion of a metallic mirror points to the presence of either
gentipicrine or menyanthine. A second portion of the
aqueous solution is cautiously evaporated in a small
porcelain capsule, and a few drops of strong sulphuric acid
are added to the residue : if no change takes place in
the cold, but upon applying heat a carmine-red coloration
appears, *gentipicrine* is present ; if a yellowish brown colour,
which afterwards changes to a violet, is produced, the
presence of *menyanthine* is probable.*

* A comprehensive scheme for the detection of foreign bitters in
beer, suggested by Dragendorff, will be found in the Archiv. der
Pharm. [3] iii. 295 ; iv. 389.

Picric acid can be detected by means of the following tests :—

1. Upon shaking pure beer with animal charcoal, it becomes decolorised, whereas beer containing picric acid retains a lemon-yellow colour after this treatment.

2. The bitter taste of normal beer is removed by treatment with a little plumbic diacetate and filtering, which is not the case with the flavour imparted by the use of picric acid.

3. Unbleached wool or pure flannel will acquire a decided yellow colour if boiled for a short time in beer adulterated with picric acid, and afterwards washed.

4. Upon agitating 20 c.c. of the suspected beer in a test-tube with 10 c.c. of amylic alcohol, allowing the mixture to remain at rest, and then removing the amylic alcohol, a solution is obtained which contains any picric acid present in the sample treated. It is evaporated to dryness, the residue dissolved in a little warm distilled water, and the aqueous solution submitted to the following tests :—

(*a*) To one portion a concentrated solution of potassium cyanide is added; in presence of picric acid, a blood-red colour is produced, due to the formation of iso-purpuric acid.

(*b*) A second portion is treated with a solution of cupric-ammonium sulphate ; if picric acid be present, minute greenish crystals of cupric-ammonium picrate will be formed.

(*c*) To a third portion, a little ammonium sulphide, containing free ammonium hydroxide, is added ; in presence of picric acid, picramic acid is produced, the formation of which is accelerated by the application of heat, and is made evident by the appearance of an intensely red colour.

The detection of *cocculus indicus*, or its poisonous alkaloid, *picrotoxine*, may be effected by first agitating the beer with plumbic acetate, filtering, removing the lead from the filtrate by means of sulphuretted hydrogen, and again filtering. The filtrate is first boiled, then carefully evaporated until it possesses a thickish consistency, when it is shaken up with animal charcoal, which is afterwards brought upon a filter, washed with a very little cold water, and dried at 100°. The picrotoxine possibly present is then extracted from the animal charcoal by boiling it with strong alcohol, from which the alkaloid separates on evaporating the solution, either in quadrilateral prisms or in feathery tufts.

Again reverting to beer adulteration, Prof. H. B. Cornwall has lately made an interesting report in this regard.* Several years ago, in reply to a circular issued by the "Business Men's Moderation Society of New York City," the "Association of United Lager Beer Brewers" asserted that the only substitutes for barley malt employed were corn starch, corn meal, rice, glucose, and grape sugar, no artificial bitters being used. The addition of glucose and grape sugar, the association stated, was not necessarily on account of economy, but had for its object an increase in the strength of the wort, without resorting to concentration and the production of beer of desirable flavour and colour. Rüdlinger † denies that beer is subjected to injurious adulteration in Germany. He states substantially as follows : "Cases of sickness, frequently claimed to be caused by the beer, are due either to excess or to the consumption of the new and incompletely fermented beverage. It has been affirmed that brewers often economise in hops by the use of other and deleterious bitters, and that picric acid and strychnine have been employed for this purpose. Nonsense, once written, is frequently copied by hundreds, and in this way circulates among the masses. The maximum amount of hops used in beer is really inconsiderable, and there exists no necessity for resorting to foreign substitutes, even in seasons when the price of hops is abnormally high, since the proportion of this ingredient could

* Reports of Am. Health Assoc., vol. x.
† 'Bierbrauerei,' 1876.

be slightly decreased without incurring the danger of detection which would follow the use of artificial bitters." On the other hand, it is certain that, *in past years*, such injurious additions as cocculus indicus, picric acid, aloes, etc., have actually been discovered by chemists of high standing in bitter ale and other forms of beer. A. Schmidt,* asserts that glycerine, alum, and sodium bicarbonate are added to beer, and states that beer, poor in extractive and alcoholic constituents, is liable to become sour, a defect which is remedied by the use of alkalies and chalk, the resulting disagreeable taste being disguised by means of glycerine. The same authority deprecates the use of glucose on account of the absence of nutritious albuminoids and phosphates in this substance. It would certainly appear obvious that the direct addition of starch-sugar to the wort, which results in augmenting the alcoholic strength of beer without correspondingly increasing the proportion of valuable extractive matter, is of doubtful propriety. Grains are less open to this objection. Of these, maize is generally regarded as the best substitute for barley malt, both on account of its similarity in composition and its cheapness. The International Congress of Medical Sciences, held at Brussels in 1875, adopted the following resolutions :—

1. Genuine beer should be made from grain and hops.

2. No other substances should replace these, either wholly or partially.

3. All substitutes should be considered as adulterations, and should come under the penalty of the law, even if not deleterious to health.

The German Brewers' Association, at its Frankfort meeting, defined wholesome beer as the produce of malt, hops, yeast, and water with a partial substitution of the malt by starch meal, rice, maize, and glucose, and regarded the use of some malt substitutes as permissible on scientific and hygienic grounds. It recommended, however, that,

* Archiv. der Pharm., xii. 392.

in case such substitutes are employed, the beer so prepared should be designated by a distinctive name, such as "rice beer," "sugar beer," etc.

The darker varieties of beer are sometimes artificially coloured by the addition of caramel, and, although the result reached is virtually the same as that caused by the over-roasting of malt, the practice is prohibited in Germany unless the product is designated as "coloured beer." * According to Guyot, some of the Bavarian beer sold in Paris is coloured with methyl orange.† Licorice is employed in beer brewing in Germany, both on account of its sweetening power and for clarifying purposes.

In regard to the use of artificial preservatives, such as salicylic acid and sodium bisulphite, it is very probable that articles of food which have been treated with these preparations are not readily digested. Their use, moreover, should be unnecessary, if due care has been exercised in the manufacture of the beer. This is especially applicable to beer intended for home consumption.

* Deutsch. Reichsanzeiger, July 31, 1885.
† Répert. de Pharm., xii. p. 513.

WINE.

WINE is the fermented juice of the grape of *Vitis vinifera*. In its preparation, the fully matured grapes are usually (but not always) first separated from the stalks, and then crushed, the *marc* so obtained being afterwards placed in butts provided with perforated sides, through which the expressed juice or *must* percolates. It is next introduced into vats, and allowed to undergo a process of fermentation, which is very analogous to that of beer wort. The addition of yeast is, however, in this case unnecessary, as the fermentation of grape-juice is spontaneous, it being due to the generation of the fungus *Penicillium glaucum*, which is the product of the action of atmospheric germs upon the albuminoid matters contained in the must. The most important constituents of grape-juice are glucose (10 to 30 per cent.), organic acids (0·3 to 1·5 per cent.), and albuminous substances. During the fermentation the glucose is converted into alcohol and carbonic acid, the latter being evolved in bubbles; a deposit of potassium bitartrate and yeast-cells, forming the *lees*, likewise occurring. This first fermentation ceases after the lapse of several days, the period being indicated by the cessation of escaping gas. In order to prevent the oxidation of the alcohol to acetic acid, the liquid is removed from the lees and transferred into casks, in which a slow after-fermentation and a further separation of potassium bitartrate take place. The wine is subsequently stored for a considerable time in fresh

casks, during which it "ages," and acquires its characteristic flavour.

The more common varieties of wine are classified according to the country of their production—into French
(claret, burgundy, champagne, etc.), German (Rhine),
Spanish (sherry and port), and Italian.

The production of American wine has experienced a
noteworthy increase during the past twenty-five years.
While, in 1860, less than two millions of gallons of native
wine were consumed in the United States, in the year
1884 the quantity used exceeded seventeen millions of
gallons.* Aside from the general distinction of red and
white, wines are classified by their characteristic properties,
as dry, sweet, and cordial. In dry wines, such as those of
the Gironde and Rhenish districts, considerable free acid,
and but little or no sugar are contained, whereas in sweet
wines (Madeira, port, etc.) a certain proportion of the
sugar remains undecomposed. Cordial wines are distinguished by their sweetness and comparatively heavy body.
The nature of wines is materially affected by the proportion
of glucose and acids contained in the original must, as
well as by the environments of their manufacture, such
as climate and temperature. From a chemical point of
view, the most important constituents of wine are the
primary products of fermentation—alcohol, succinic acid,
and glycerine, but its market value is far more dependent
upon the flavour and bouquet, which are chiefly due to the
formation of secondary products, usually included under
the name "oenanthic ether," and consisting of the ethers
of caproic, caprylic, and other organic acids.

The following table exhibits the constituents of some
of the best known varieties of wine, according to results
obtained by different authorities :—

* During the year 1886 the total production of Californian wine
approximated 19½ million gallons, of which 3½ million gallons were
consumed in the manufacture of brandy, and 5 million gallons
exported.

Kind of Wine.	Specific Gravity.	Alcohol, by Weight.	Fixed Acids (as Tartaric).	Volatile Acids (as Acetic).	Total Acids.	Real Tartaric Acid.	Total Residue.	Sugar.	Ash.	Potass (KOH).	Potassium Carbonate.	Sulphates and Chlorides.	Phosphoric Acid.
		per cent.	per cent.	per cent.	per cent.	per cent.	per cent.	per cent.	per cent.	per cent.	per cent.	per cent.	per cent.
French (red) *	0·9950	12·00	0·430	0·170	0·590	0·180	2·43	0·200	0·220		0·060	0·10	0·03
French (white)	0·9922	10·84	0·435	0·169	0·604	0·102	1·257	0·880	0·197				0·031
Vin Ordinaire		6·99	0·610	0·110	0·720		5·04	0·110	0·450	0·13			
St. Julien (1858)		9·84	0·510	0·140	0·650		2·67	0·250	0·400				
Frousac		10·74	0·450	0·270	0·720		2·36	0·370	0·270				
Champagne	0·9934	7·95					12·41	10·63	0·25		0·07		0·080
Rhenish*		9·26	0·420	0·110	0·530	0·250	1·850	0·012	0·170		0·07	0·07	0·040
Rüdesheimer		13·32		0·6100	0·630		1·840	0·017	0·170				0·050
Alsatian *		10·38							0·178				0·03
Würtemberg		7·09	0·87						0·230	0·09			0·0253
Sherry *	0·9940	17·20	0·270	0·150	0·420	0·018	2·22	2·56	0·450		0·001	0·36	0·02
Port *	1·0040	18·56	0·310	0·080	0·390	0·022	4·20	4·33	0·280		0·05	0·130	0·03
Madeira *	0·9940	17·75	0·330	0·160	0·490	0·03	7·55	2·08	0·39		0·03	0·25	0·04
Marsala *	0·9960	16·71	0·190	0·110	0·300		4·35	3·24	0·22		0·02	0·15	0·02
Red Vœslauer		10·25	0·480	0·060	0·540		4·98	0·29	0·32				
Lachryma Christi		9·70	0·460	0·110	0·560		23·63	18·91	0·48				
White Capri		10·40	0·480	0·190	0·650		1·96	0·48	0·29	0·14			
Cyprus		10·09		0·120	0·600		23·81	23·12	0·53	0·10			
Greek *	0·9931	13·89	0·233	0·177	0·710	0·03	2·55	0·36	0·37	0·11	0·02	0·24	0·04
Hungarian*	0·9921	8·54	0·530	0·150	0·700	0·067	1·82	0·06	0·17	0·11	0·01	0·08	0·02

* These figures denote the weight in grammes of the ingredients contained in 100 c.c. of the wine ; otherwise, percentages are expressed.

Two varieties of Californian wine, examined by J. L. de Fremery,* had the following composition :—

Grammes in 100 c.c.	Gutedel (White).	Zinfandel (Red).
Alcohol	10·45	9·80
Extract	2·0908	2·1270
Mineral matter..	0·1978	0·2218
Volatile acids (as acetic)	0·0804	0·0972
Fixed acids (as tartaric)..	0·4845	0·4110
Potassium bitartrate	0·1579	0·1428
Free tartaric acid	0·0060	..
Other free acids (as tartaric)	0·5850	0·5325
Sulphuric acid	0·0384	0·0168
Phosphoric acid	0·0220	0·0193
Chlorine	0·0036	0·0054
Lime	0·0056	0·0084
Magnesia	0·0170	0·0160
Glycerine	0·6133	0·5647
Sugar	0·0165	0·0276
Polarisation	+0·2	..
Succinic acid	0·0068	0·0097
Malic acid	0·0324	0·0922

According to analyses made by R. Fresenius and R. Borgmann,† natural wine has the following *average* composition :—

Grammes in 100 c.c.

Alcohol	7·71
Extract	2·75
Free acids	0·73
Mineral matter..	0·23
Glycerine	0·79
Sulphuric acid	0·038
Phosphoric acid	0·040
Lime	0·018
Magnesia	0·018
Potassa	0·092
Chlorine	0·004
Potassium bitartrate	0·200

Natural wines are frequently subjected to various processes of treatment, designed to remedy certain defects

---

* Berichte der Deutsch. Chem. Gesell., 1885, p. 426.

† Zeit. f. Anal. Chem., 1885, p. 44.

existing in the original must. While these do not, perhaps, all properly come under the head of adulteration, it is certain that many of the practices resorted to affect the dietetic quality of the wine in a deleterious manner. The most common modes of treatment, generally considered harmless, are the following :—

Pasteuring, which consists essentially in heating the wine to 60°, with a limited supply of air, and effects the artificial ageing and better conservation of the product. Wines which exhibit ropiness and other diseases are restored by destroying the fungi present. This is accomplished by subjecting the well-filled and corked bottles to a temperature of from 45° to 100° for several hours.

A process of freezing is likewise employed for the improvement of wine. It results in the removal of much of the cream of tartar, colouring matter, and nitrogenous substances contained, and also causes an increase in the alcoholic strength of the wine, thereby considerably decreasing its tendency to undergo an after-fermentation.

The proportions of sugar and acid best adapted to the production of wine of good quality are at least 20 per cent. of the former to not more than 0·5 per cent. of the latter. As these conditions do not always obtain in grape-juice, artificial methods are employed to supply the necessary constituents. Of these, the most rational consists in diluting the must until the amount of acid is reduced to 0·5 per cent., and increasing the sugar to a proportion of 20 per cent. by the addition of glucose. In a somewhat similar process, due to Petiot, the marc is repeatedly mixed with water containing 20 per cent. of sugar, and then subjected to fermentation. In other methods, the removal of the excess of free acid is effected by neutralisation with pulverised marble or neutral potassium tartrate. The use of these agents results in the formation and subsequent separation of insoluble salts—in the latter case, of

M

potassium bitartrate.   Another process for the improvement
and preservation of natural wine, proposed by Scheele,
consists in the addition of glycerine, in a maximum pro-
protion of 3 per cent., after the first fermentation has taken
place.

R. Kayser [*] has made a very exhaustive investigation
of wine-must of different sources, and of the wine prepared
therefrom, both in its natural state and after having been
subjected to various "processes of improvement." The
following table shows the results obtained from the analysis
of Franken must and wine (both natural and "improved"),
made from Riessling grapes in 1880 :—

	Must.	Natural Wine.	Gall's Process (Cane Sugar added).	Gall's Process (Grape Sugar used).	Chaptal's Process (Calcium Carbonate added).	Plastered.	Petiot's Process (Cane Sugar added to grape husks).
	per cent.	per cent.	per cent.	per cent.	per cent.	per cent.	per cent.
Alcohol	..	6·60	12·20	9·10	6·60	6·70	10·40
Extract	17·87	2·53	2·11	5·91	2·19	2·80	1·98
Ash	0·33	0·26	0·10	0·17	0·28	0·29	0·16
Sulphuric acid ..	0·010	0·006	0·002	0·010	0·006	0·077	0·002
Phosphoric acid.	0·031	0·024	0·020	0·021	0·023	0·025	0·017
Lime	0·012	0·009	0·007	0·018	0·027	0·039	0·006
Magnesia	0·012	0·011	0·012	0·009	0·012	0·012	0·008
Free acid (as tar-taric)	1·365	1·275	0·765	0·802	0·660	1·297	0·488
Total tartaric acid	0·501	0·342	0·120	0·140	0·014	0·260	0·150
Free tartaric acid	0·188	0·012	..	..	..	0·160	..
Malic acid	0·720	0·715	0·400	0·388	0·710	0·716	0·165
Succinic acid ..	..	0·110	0·140	0·114	0·112	0·101	0·127
Glycerine	..	0·650	1·150	0·800	0·600	0·700	0·900
Sugar	13·90	0·210	0·180	0·340	0·200	0·180	0·300
Potassa	0·156	0·117	0·051	0·081	0·134	0·127	0·093

Magnier de la Source [†] has recently made some investigations concerning the difference in chemical composition

* Repert. Anal. Chem., 1882, ii., p. 1.
† 'Comptes Rendus,' xcviii. p. 110.

of natural and plastered wine ; he gives the following constituents of 1 litre of wine :—

	Natural.	Plastered.
	gr.	gr.
Tartar	1·94	0
Sulphuric acid	2·58	3·10
Potassium	1·12	2·46
Calcium (in soluble portion of ash)	0	0·037
Calcium (in insoluble portion of ash)	0·179	0·151

Adulteration of Wine.—Although there may be some question in regard to the moral status of the foregoing methods of improvement of natural wine, numerous other practices are resorted to concerning which no doubt can exist. The more common forms of wine adulteration include plastering, sulphuring, fortification, blending, flavouring, colouring, and the manufacture of fictitious imitations.

The "plastering" of wines consists in the addition of plaster of Paris (often mixed with lime), either to the unpressed grapes or to the must. The process, which is rather hypothetically claimed to aid in the preservation of the wine and correct any excessive acidity, is very objectionable, in that it determines the formation of free sulphuric acid and acid sulphates, as well as of calcium tartrate and potassium sulphate. The lime salt, being insoluble, is deposited with the lees ; the potassium sulphate, however, remains in solution, and as it exerts a decided purgative effect, its presence in wine cannot fail to be detrimental. In France, the sale of wine containing over 0·2 per cent. of potassium sulphate is prohibited. The plastering of wine is chiefly carried on in Spain, Portugal, and southern France. The ash of pure wine does not exceed 0·3 per cent., but in the samples of sherry usually met with it reaches a proportion of 0·5 per cent., and is almost entirely composed of sulphates. The "sulphur-

ing " of wines is also extensively practised. It is effected
either by burning sulphur in the casks or by conducting
sulphurous acid through the wine itself, the object sought
being to preserve the product and impart to it the ripe-
ness naturally acquired by age. Sulphured wines, while
not necessarily showing an increase in the amount of
ash, can often be recognised by the abnormally large
proportion of sulphates present.

The strength and preservative qualities of wine are
frequently augmented by the addition to it of inferior
sorts of brandy. Port wine usually receives an addition
of about 30 per cent., and sherry is invariably fortified, if
not to so great an extent. By the Customs regulations
in England, 10 per cent. of brandy is allowed to be
added to wines in bond, while, in France, the sophistication is equally permitted in wines intended for export,
provided the total amount of alcohol in the fortified
article does not exceed 21 per cent.

Doubtless the mixing or blending of wines constitutes
the most frequent form of their sophistication. Natural
wines of the same manufacture vary to some extent from
year to year in colour, flavour, and other characteristic
properties, and mixing is resorted to in order to supply
the trade with a product always possessing nearly identical qualities. In many cases, the flavour of wines is
improved by blending, and their intoxicating effects are
also increased, both results being due to the formation of
compound ethers. Common instances of wine mixing are
the addition of Hermitage and Rousillon wines to clarets ;
of Malaga and Teneriffe to port ; of *solaras* (a mixture
of Amontillado and Manzanilla) to sherry ; and of a liqueur
composed of sugar, some kind of full, rich wine, and
brandy, to champagne. The flavour and bouquet of expensive wines are frequently imparted to inferior grades
by the addition of various substances, among which are
elderflowers, orris root, cherry water, essential oil of al-

monds, sweet briar, and numerous perfumes, such as orange-
flower water, neroli, *essence de petit grain*, violet petals, etc.
The tincture of raisin seeds is said to communicate a
genuine port flavour to poor wines, and a grain of amber-
gris, triturated with a little sugar, is stated to impart a
much esteemed bouquet to a hogshead of claret. Numerous tinctures, as those of strawberry root, raspberries, and
walnuts, are likewise used. Sweet and liqueur wines are
extensively imitated at Cette and Montpelier. The following recipes* will serve to illustrate the general character
of the mixtures employed :—

For *Lachryma Christi* :—

Bagnols (dry)	85 litres.
Gum kino	50 grammes.
Infusion of walnuts	1 litre.
Syrup of raisins	6 litres.
Alcohol (85°)	8 „

For *Madeira* :—

Picardan (dry)	60 litres.
Tavel (old and strong)	25 „
Infusion of walnuts	2 „
Infusion of bitter almonds	2 „
Rock candy	1½ kilos.
Brandy (58°)	10 litres.

For *Malaga* :—

Bagnols (old)	80 litres.
Syrup of raisins	10 „
Infusion of walnuts	2 „
Alcohol (85°)	8 „

For *Tokay* :—

Bagnols	80 litres.
Syrup of raisins	10 „
Dried elder flowers	300 grammes.
Infusion of white raspberries	2 kilos.
„ „ walnuts	1 kilo.
Alcohol	6 litres.

Port is frequently flavoured with a mixture of elderberry
juice, grape juice, brown sugar, and crude brandy known
as "*Jerupiga.*" Sherry often consists of Cape wine mixed

* *Vide* 'Spon's Encyclopædia.'

with honey, bitter almonds, and brandy. Astringency is
conveyed to wines, deficient in this quality, by means of
tannin ; and the property of forming a crust on the interior of the bottle is produced, especially in port, by the
admixture of cream of tartar and gum. "Dryness" is
also obtained by artificial methods. A preparation met
with in the trade, and used for this purpose, has the following composition : *—

						Per cent.
Glucose	..	..	..	..	..	28·72
Glycerine	..	..	..	..	..	38·40
Tannin	..	..	··	..	..	4·10
Dextrine	..	..	..	..	..	3·14
Boracic acid	..	..	..	..	..	4·27
Cream of tartar	..	..	..	..	..	trace
Moisture and ash	..	..	..	..	..	21·37
						100·00

The colour of white wines is caused by the oxidation of
the tannin present, but it is sometimes increased by the
addition of the concentrated juice of highly - coloured
grapes, or by means of a small proportion of caramel. The
colour of natural red wine is due to the presence of *oeno-
cyanin*, a bluish-black compound, chiefly contained in the
grape skins, which is insoluble in water, but dissolves in
acidulated alcohol. In Spain and southern France, a wine
prepared from a vine known as the *Teinturier*, and possessing an intense bluish-red colour, is extensively employed
for colouring of wines. There appears to be no doubt but
that elderberries, black cherries, mulberries, and hollyhock
are also frequently used as colouring agents. Souberian †
mentions a mixture, termed *liqueur de fismes*, composed
of elderberries, but also containing about 5 per cent. of
alum, which is occasionally employed. The general use
of several deleterious dyes, such as logwood, cochineal,
and the aniline colours, is far more problematical. In re-

* Jay, Bullet. de la Soc. Chim., xlii. p. 217.
† Dict. des Falsifications.

gard to the last-mentioned agents, it has, however, been asserted,* that in a commune near Beziers, of 1800 inhabitants, magenta, to the value of 30,000 francs, is annually consumed in the adulteration of wine.

It is also worthy of remark that an aniline preparation used in Spain for the artificial colouring of wine has recently been found to contain 1·62 per cent. of arsenic acid.†

Owing to the ravages of the phylloxera, a very considerable decrease in the source of natural wines has taken place during the past few years. Between 1883 and 1884 no less than 22 thousand acres of vineyards were entirely destroyed in the Gironde district alone, and it is stated, upon good authority, that the total production of wines in France in 1884 was 220 millions of gallons less than the average of the previous ten years.‡ There is no doubt but that this decrease has greatly stimulated the manufacture of imitation wines. These occasionally contain a certain proportion of genuine wine as the basis, but more frequently they consist entirely of factitious constituents. The following recipe furnishes a fair example of those of the first class :—

Rousillon wine	50 litres.
Water	85 „
Common brandy	20 „
Vinegar	1 „
Tartaric acid	300 grammes.
Powdered orris	20 „
Wood charcoal	500 „

Agitate thoroughly, add the white of two eggs, with constant stirring ; allow to settle, and draw off.

* 'Les Mondes, Revue Hebd. des Sciences,' No. 4, 1876.
† Bullet. de la Soc. de Chim., xlii. pp. 167 and 207.
‡ Recent reports of the vintage in France for the year 1886, indicate that, while a decided improvement has been experienced in the Champagne, Burgundy, Hérault, and Rousillon districts, this has failed to be the case in Charentes and Gironde, where the phylloxera has again seriously injured the crops.

Of late years, the production of wine from dried fruit has assumed very extensive proportions in France. The product, which is generally known as "*vin de raisins secs*," is claimed by its manufacturers to be wholesome.* A wine said to possess the qualities of a fair claret, is made by submitting to fermentation the following mixture :—

White sugar	5 kilos.
Raisins	5 ,,
Sodium chloride	125 grammes.
Tartaric acid	200 ,,
Brandy	12 litres.
Water	95 ,,
Gall nuts	20 grammes.
Brewer's yeast	200 ,,

Another recipe for Bordeaux wine is :—

Orris root	1 lb.
Water	5 galls.
Raspberry juice	1 ,,
Pure spirit	10 ,,
Essence of claret	½ lb.
Sugar syrup	1 gall.
Colour with cochineal.	

It is authentically stated that in the year 1881, 52 millions of gallons of factitious claret wine were made in France, and the industry has certainly not diminished in extent since this date. It is a significant fact that the importation of Spanish raisins into France has undergone a

---

* F. Schaffer (Zeits. Anal. Chem., xxiv. p. 559) has made the following analyses of artificial wine (grammes in 100 c.c.) :—

Alcohol (by volume) ..	8·05	9·55	7·02
Extract .. .. ,, ..	2·395	1·962	1·797
Sugar	0·330	0·409	0·321
Ash	0·209	0·135	0·160
Acidity (as tartaric) ..	0·743	0·501	0·772
Free tartaric acid	—	traces	traces
Cream of tartar	0·264	0·227	0·471
Sulphuric anhydride ..	0·0374	—	—
Phosphoric anhydride ..	0·0196	0·0135	0·0172

remarkable increase during the past few years. Nor is this species of sophistication confined to foreign wines. Establishments are in active operation in New York City and elsewhere in this country, where imitations of Californian hock and claret are made from fermented infusions of dried fruit (often charged with salicylic acid), and offered for sale at less than thirty cents per gallon, with more than the usual trade discount.* According to a reliable estimation, less than one-tenth of the wine sold as champagne is actually the product of that district, the remainder being fabricated from other wines or from cider.

Analysis of Wine.—The analysis of wine comprises the following estimations :—Specific gravity, alcohol, extract, sugar, polarisation, glycerine, total free acids, volatile acids, free tartaric acid, potassium bitartrate, malic acid, succinic acid, tannin, ethers, ash, chlorine, sulphuric and phosphoric acids, and colouring matters.

Specific gravity.—The density is determined by means of the gravity bottle, at a temperature of $15°$.

Alcohol.—The proportion of alcohol is ascertained by the distillation of 50 or 100 c.c. of the wine in a suitable flask, which is connected with a Liebig's condenser, until about half of the liquid has passed over. The distillate is made up to the original volume with water, and its specific gravity taken, from which the amount of alcohol (by weight) present is calulated by aid of the usual alcoholmetric tables (see p. 196). The result (as well as the proportions of the other constituents) is preferably stated in grammes per 100 c.c. of wine. The determination may also be made by first removing the alcohol by evaporation, adding distilled water to restore the original volume, and then estimating the density of the liquid (see under Beer, p. 142). In unfortified wines the alcoholic strength ranges

---

* It is asserted by a prominent wine merchant in New York that the monthly production of two manufacturers of artificial wine in this city exceeds 30,000 gallons.

from 6 to 12 per cent., and in wines which have received an addition of spirit, it may vary from 12 to 22 per cent.

Extract.—The extract is conveniently determined by evaporating 50 c.c. (measured at 15°), in a platinum dish over the water-bath, the residue being dried for 2½ hours in the steam-oven. In case a wine rich in sugar (containing, say, over 0·5 grammes per 100 c.c.) is under examination, 20 c.c. will suffice for the determination. The indirect method used in the estimation of the malt extract in beer may also be employed. According to Girardin and Pressier, it is possible to detect the watering of certain wines, the average composition of which is known, by means of the proportions of extract and alcohol present. For example, in genuine Bordeaux wines the proportion of extract ranges from 20 to 20·8 grammes per 1000 c.c., and the amount of alcohol is also very constant, it being a mean of 100 grammes per 1000 c.c. Should a sample of Bordeaux wine show an extract of 14·5 grammes per litre, the proportion of genuine wine present would be 72·5 per cent., for $\dfrac{1000 \times 14\cdot5}{20} = 725\cdot00$, the remainder being water and alcohol. In order to estimate the amount of spirits artificially added, the alcohol contained in 72·5 parts of the wine is determined. If, for instance, it is found to be 11 parts, then, (11 − 7·25 =) 3·75 parts of alcohol have been added.* The quantity of extract in pure natural wine varies from 1·5 to 3 per cent., but in sweet and fortified wines, it may reach 10 per cent. or more.

Sugar.—The sugar in wine consists of a mixture of fruit and grape sugar, usually in the proportion of 3 parts of the former to 1 part of the latter. The amount of sugar is best estimated by Fehling's solution (see p. 111). In the case of white wines, it is advisable to employ 100 c.c. for the determination ; with sweet rich wines 25 c.c. are sufficient. The alcohol is first removed by evaporation over the water-

* Blyth, op. cit., p. 445.

bath, and the diluted liquid is next decolorised by means of bone-black or plumbic acetate, filtered, and made alkaline by addition of sodium carbonate. It is then made up to a volume of 200 c.c. and gradually added to 10 c.c. of Fehling's solution. It is always well to test the wine by the polariscope, and, whenever the presence of cane sugar is indicated, to invert 100 c.c. of the sample by heating with a few drops of hydrochloric acid, and again make a sugar determination with Fehling's reagent after neutralisation with sodium carbonate.

Polarisation.—The optical examination of wine is conducted by adding 20 c.c. of plumbic acetate solution to 100 c.c. of the sample, shaking the mixture, allowing it to stand for a short time, and passing it through a filter. If necessary the filtrate is further decolorised with animal charcoal and again filtered. The polariscope tube is then filled with the clear solution and the reading made. The majority of wines exhibit a left-handed polarisation, which is due to the fact that, as a rule, the proportion of fruit sugar present predominates over that of grape sugar; moreover, ½ part of fruit sugar will neutralise the dextro-rotary action of 1 part of grape sugar. In case the presence of an excess of grape sugar is indicated by the polariscopic examination, it is often assumed that this body has been directly added to the wine. It sometimes occurs, however, that, in the fermentation process, more grape sugar remains undecomposed than fruit sugar, under which circumstances the preponderance of the former body in the resulting wine would not prove sophistication; but, under ordinary conditions, the presence of an excessive proportion of grape sugar may safely be regarded as strongly pointing to the artificial addition of must syrup.

Glycerine.—100 c.c. of the wine are reduced by evaporation on the water-bath to 10 c.c., some pure sand added, and then milk of lime to decided alkaline reaction, after which the mixture is evaporated nearly to dryness. When

cold, the residue is thoroughly agitated with 50 c.c. of
96 per cent. alcohol, next heated to boiling on the water-
bath, and then passed through a filter. The insoluble
residue is repeatedly washed with more hot alcohol, the
washings being added to the first filtrate. The solution is
now evaporated until it assumes a viscous consistency.
The residue is taken up with 10 c.c. of absolute alcohol, and
15 c.c. of ether are added, the mixture being shaken and
allowed to stand at rest in a well-stoppered flask until it
becomes clear. The solution is subsequently filtered into
a tared glass capsule, then carefully evaporated to a syrupy
condition over the water-bath, and the residue dried in the
steam-oven for one hour, and finally weighed. According
to Pasteur, 112·8 parts of grape sugar yield 3·6 parts of
glycerine; in natural wine, therefore, the glycerine should
amount to about $\frac{1}{14}$th part of the alcohol present.

Acids.—The acids in wine consist of acetic, tartaric,
malic, tannic, succinic, racemic, formic, and propionic.

Total free Acids.—These are determined by titrating 10 c.c.
of the sample with $\frac{1}{10}$th normal soda solution, litmus paper
or tincture of logwood being employed as the indicator.
Wines containing free carbonic acid should be repeatedly
well-shaken before making the estimation. The free acids
are expressed in terms of tartaric acid $(C_4H_6O_6)$. If
sulphuric acid or potassium bisulphate is present, a piece
of filter paper will be rendered brittle when immersed
in the wine for some time, and afterwards cautiously
dried.

Volatile Acids.—The volatile acids are estimated by
slowly evaporating 10 c.c. of the wine to the consistency of
a syrup, and repeating the titration with $\frac{1}{10}$th normal alkali
solution. The difference in acidity represents the proportion of volatile acids present, which is stated in terms of
acetic acid $(C_2H_4O_2)$. It is evident that the non-volatile
acids can be calculated' by deducting from the total
amount of free acids, the tartaric acid corresponding to

the acetic acid found. The proportion of volatile acid in genuine wine varies from 0·3 to 0·6 per cent. According to Dupré, in white wine, one-fourth of the total acidity should be due to volatile acids, and in fortified and red wine, they should not exceed a proportion of one-third.

Free Tartaric Acid and Potassium Bitartrate.—In the presence of a small amount of free acids, the detection of a considerable proportion of free tartaric acid may fairly be considered as strong evidence that the wine is artificial. Nessler recommends the following qualitative test:—20 c.c. of the sample are repeatedly shaken with a little freshly prepared and finely ground cream of tartar. After standing one hour, the solution is filtered, 3 or 4 drops of a 20 per cent. solution of potassium acetate are added, and the mixture is allowed to remain at rest for twelve hours, when, in presence of free tartaric acid, a precipitation will take place. The quantitative estimation of free tartaric acid and potassium bitartrate is made by Berthelot's method, as follows :—Separate portions of the wine (20 c.c. each) are introduced into two flasks, a few drops of 20 per cent. solution of potassium acetate being added to the second flask. 200 c.c. of a mixture of equal parts of alcohol and ether are then added to both flasks, their contents repeatedly shaken and finally set aside for eighteen hours at a temperature between 0° and 10°. The separated precipitates are now removed by filtration, washed with the ether-alcohol mixture, and then titrated with $\frac{1}{10}$th normal alkali solution. That formed in the first flask corresponds to the potassium bitartrate originally contained in the wine; the second represents the total tartaric acid present. The addition of a small quantity of clean sand will assist in the separation of the precipitates.

Malic Acid.—A slight excess of lime-water is added to 100 c.c. of the wine, and, after standing for some time the

solution is filtered, concentrated by evaporation to one-half
its original volume, and treated with an excess of absolute
alcohol. The resulting precipitate (consisting of calcium
malate and sulphate) is collected upon a filter, dried and
then incinerated. The proportion of malic acid contained
is now estimated by volumetrically determining the amount
of calcium carbonate present by means of a normal acid
solution : 1 part of calcium carbonate represents 1·34 parts
of malic acid ($C_4H_6O_5$).

Tannic Acid.—10 c.c. of the sample are taken, the free
acids present neutralised with normal alkali solution, and
a few drops of concentrated sodium acetate solution (40 per
cent.) added. A solution of ferric chloride (10 per cent.)
is then added, drop by drop, carefully avoiding an excess.
A single drop of the iron solution represents 0·05 per
cent. of tannic acid. The method of tannin determination
described under Tea (see p. 22) can also be applied.

Succinic Acid.—500 c.c. of the wine are decolorised with
bone-black, filtered, the filtrate evaporated over the water-
bath nearly to dryness, and the residue repeatedly treated
with alcohol-ether. The solution thus obtained is concentrated, carefully neutralised with lime-water, evaporated to
dryness, and the glycerine present removed by washing
with the alcohol-ether mixture. The remaining residue is
now treated with 80 per cent. alcohol, in order to dissolve
the calcium succinate contained, every 100 parts of which
represent 75·64 parts of succinic acid ($H_6C_4O_4$). Thudichum and Dupré state that one litre of pure wine contains
from 1 to 1·5 grammes of succinic acid.

Ethers.—The compound ethers in wine are volatile
and fixed, and exist in but minute proportions. Of the
former class, ethylic acetate $C_2H_3(C_2H_5)O_2$ is the most
important. As already mentioned, the aroma of wine is
largely influenced by the presence of the ethers of the fatty
acids, butyric, caprylic, etc. Dupré determines the proportion of both kinds of ethers indirectly as follows :—250 c.c. of

the wine are distilled until 200 c.c. have passed over. Water
is then added to the distillate to a volume of 250 c.c. 100 c.c.
are first titrated with $\frac{1}{10}$th normal soda solution. Another
100 c.c. of the distillate are next heated with a known
quantity of alkali (by which the ethers are decomposed into
their corresponding acids and alcohol), and the titration
is repeated. The amount of *volatile* ethers is then calculated
from the increased acidity shown by the second titration.
In order to determine the proportion of *fixed* ethers, 500 c.c.
of the sample are evaporated over the water-bath to a
small volume which is made alkaline, and then subjected to
distillation. The distillate is acidulated with sulphuric acid
and again distilled. The alcohol present in the second distillate is now oxidised to acetic acid by means of potassium
dichromate, and the amount of this acid found estimated
by titration. According to Berthelot, the proportion of ethers
in genuine wine bears a fixed relation to the amounts of
alcohol and acids present: he suggests the following formula
for calculating the amount of alcohol contained in the
compound ether of one litre of wine, when etherification is
complete :—

$$y = 1 \cdot 17\,A + 2 \cdot 8$$

$$x = \frac{y \times a}{100},$$

where A is the percentage, by weight, of alcohol; a the
amount of alcohol equivalent to the total free acid in one
litre of wine (assuming this to be acetic acid); y, the proportion per cent. of a present as compound ether in one
litre of wine, when the alcoholic strength of the wine is A ;
and x, the amount of alcohol present in the compound ether
of one litre of wine.

The Ash.—100 c.c. of the wine are evaporated to dryness
in a platinum dish, over the water-bath, and the residue is
incinerated at a rather low temperature and weighed. By
this process, the tartrates and malates contained in the wine

are converted with carbonates. The ash of normal wine consists of potassium sulphate, carbonate, phosphate and chloride, sodium chloride, calcium carbonate, etc., but, in many samples, it will be found to be largely if not entirely composed of sulphates, which is due to the practice of sulphuring and plastering.* Generally speaking, the proportion of ash in genuine wine ranges from 0·15 to 0·30 per cent.

Chlorine.—100 c.c. of the sample are neutralised with sodium carbonate, evaporated to dryness, and the residue gently ignited. It is then extracted with boiling water, filtered, and the chlorine determined by means of silver nitrate, either volumetrically or gravimetrically.

Sulphuric Acid.—100 c.c. are acidulated with hydrochloric acid, the liquid heated to boiling, and the sulphuric acid precipitated by barium chloride. The precipitate is well washed, dried, and weighed. 100 parts represent 42·49 parts H_2SO_4. Pure wine contains from 0·109 to 0·328 gramme of monohydrated sulphuric acid per litre (corresponding to 0·194 to 0·583 gramme potassium sulphate). The presence of an excess of this maximum amount indicates that the wine has been plastered.

Phosphoric Acid.—100 c.c. of the wine are evaporated, the residue ignited, dissolved in a little water, acidulated with nitric acid, and then added to an excess of solution of ammonium molybdate. After standing over night the separated precipitate is dissolved in ammonia and the phosphoric acid determined by means of an ammoniacal solution of magnesium sulphate. 100 parts of the precipitate thus obtained correspond to 63·96 parts of phosphoric acid. The former belief that the best qualities of

* According to J .Carter Bell ('Analyst,' vi. pp. 197, 221), the average composition of the ash of pure grape-juice is as follows :—

K_2O	Na_2O	CaO	MgO	Fe_2O_3 & Al_2O_3	SiO_2	P_2O_5	SO_3	Cl
42·14	3·37	11·48	9·67	0·75	0·29	9·60	9·14	1·09

wine contain the largest proportion of phosphoric acid does not appear to be invariably correct.

Salicylic Acid.*—The determination of this acid is accomplished as follows :—100 c.c. of the sample are repeatedly agitated with chloroform, which is subsequently separated and evaporated to dryness. The residue is re-crystallised from chloroform and weighed ; its identity can be established by dissolving it in water and adding solution of ferric chloride (see p. 149).

Sulphurous Acid.—For the detection and estimation of sulphurous acid, the following methods have been recommended :—500 c.c. of the wine are placed in a flask, the exit-tube of which dips into a test-tube which is suitably cooled, and subjected to distillation. When about 2 c.c. have distilled, a few drops of a *neutral* solution of silver nitrate are added to the distillate : in presence of sulphurous acid, a white curdy precipitate will be formed, which differs from silver chloride in being soluble in nitric acid. According to Haas,† this test is not invariably decisive, as pure wine may cause the precipitation under certain conditions ; moreover, acetic acid is said to render silver nitrate turbid in strong alcoholic solutions. Sulphurous acid can be quantitatively determined by adding phosphoric acid to 100 c.c. of the wine, and distilling it in an atmosphere of carbonic acid gas. The distillate is received in 5 c.c. of normal iodine solution. When one-third of the sample has passed over, the distillate (which should still contain an excess of free iodine), is acidulated with hydrochloric acid, and the sulphuric acid formed precipitated with barium chloride.

---

* Curtman (Jour. Pharm., xiv. p. 523) states that salicylic acid can be detected by adding to 4 c.c. of the wine (or beer) 2 c.c. of methylic alcohol and 2 c.c. of sulphuric acid. Shake the mixture, heat gently for two minutes, then allow to cool. Next heat to boiling, when, in presence of the acid, the odour of oil of wintergreen will be perceptible.

† Zeit. f. Anal. Chem., xxi. p. 3, 1882.

Colouring matters.—Very numerous processes have been published for the detection of foreign and artificial colouring matters in wine. Among those suggested are the following :—

1. A few drops of the sample are placed in succession on the smooth surface of a piece of white calcined lime, and notice taken of the tint produced. The following colours are stated to occur with pure and artificially coloured wine :—

Natural red wine		.. ..		yellowish brown.
Wine coloured with fuchsine		..	..	rose colour.
,,	,,	,,	Brazil wood	..	,, ,,
,,	,,	,,	logwood	.. ..	reddish violet.
,,	,,	,,	black hollyhock		yellowish brown.
,,	,,	,,	poke-berries	..	yellowish red.

2. If ammonium hydroxide be added to the suspected sample to distinct alkaline reaction, then a little ammonium sulphide and the liquid filtered, the filtrate from genuine wine will possess a green tint, whereas that obtained from artificially coloured wine will exhibit other colours, such as red, blue, violet, or brown.

3. 100 c.c. of the wine are evaporated to about one-half of the original volume, ammonium hydroxide added to alkaline reaction, and the liquid thoroughly shaken. Ether is then added, and the mixture again well shaken. It is next introduced into a separator, and allowed to stand at rest until the ether has risen to the surface, when the lower stratum is drawn off, and the residual ether washed by agitation with water, which is subsequently removed. The ethereal solution is now transferred to a flask connected with a Liebig's condenser, a piece of white woollen yarn introduced into the liquid, and the contents of the flask distilled at a gentle heat : in presence of the smallest amount of fuchsine, the wool will acquire a very perceptible reddish hue.

4 A slight excess of ammonium hydroxide is added to

50 c.c. of the wine, a piece of white woollen fabric introduced, and the liquid boiled until the alcohol and ammonia are expelled. By this treatment it will be found
that most aniline colouring matters, if present, become
attached to the wool. Their presence can be corroborated
by removing the fabric, washing and pressing it, and then
dissolving it, with constant stirring, in a hot solution of
potassium hydroxide. When solution has taken place,
the liquid is allowed to cool, and one-half its volume of
alcohol is added, then an equal volume of ether. The
mixture is vigorously shaken, and, after remaining at
rest for some time, the supernatant ethereal solution is
removed, introduced into a test-tube, and a drop or
two of acetic acid added. In presence of fuchsine, its
characteristic colour will now become apparent. Methyl
violet and aniline blue are separated by an analogous
process.

5. Logwood and cochineal may be detected by agitating
100 c.c. of the suspected wine with manganic peroxide,
and filtering. The filtrate afforded by pure wine will be
colourless.

6. In Dupré's process,* cubes of jelly are first prepared
by dissolving 1 part of gelatine in 20 parts of hot water,
and pouring the solution into moulds to set. These are
immersed in the wine under examination for 24 hours, then
removed, slightly washed, and the depth to which the
colouring matter has permeated is observed : pure wine
will colour the gelatine very superficially; the majority
of other colouring principles (e.g. fuchsine, cochineal, logwood, Brazil wood, litmus, beetroot, and indigo) penetrate
the jelly more readily and to a far greater degree. Dilute
ammonium hydroxide dissolves from the stained cake the
colouring matter of logwood and cochineal, but not that
derived from fuchsine or beetroot.

7. The colouring principle of genuine wine when sub-

* Journ. Chem. Soc., xxxvii. p. 572.

N 2

jected to dialysis, does not pass through the animal membrane to any decided extent, while that of logwood, cochineal, and Brazil wood easily dialyses.

8. Many of the foreign dyes added to wine are precipitated by a solution of basic plumbic acetate. The precipitate obtained upon treating 10 c.c. of the sample with 3 c.c. of this reagent is collected on a filter and washed with a 2 per cent. solution of potassium carbonate, which dissolves cochineal, sulphindigotic acid and aniline red. The latter is separated upon neutralising the solution with acetic acid, and shaking with amylic alcohol, which, in its presence, will acquire a rose colour. The liquid is next acidulated with sulphuric acid, and again agitated with amylic alcohol, by which the carminamic acid, originating from cochineal, is isolated. Any remaining indigo (as well as the carminamic acid) is to be subsequently identified by means of its spectroscopic reactions. Upon treating the portion of the plumbic acetate precipitate which remains undissolved by potassium carbonate with a dilute solution of ammonium sulphide, the colouring matter of pure wine and of logwood is dissolved. If, in presence of logwood, the original sample is shaken with calcium carbonate mixed with a little calcium hydroxide solution and filtered, the filtrate will exhibit a decided red tint, but, if the wine treated be pure, little or no coloration will be produced.

9. An artificial colouring for wine, known as *rouge végétale*, is not uncommonly employed. According to Amthor,* its presence can be recognised as follows :— 100 c.c. of the wine are distilled until all alcohol is removed. The residual liquid is strongly acidulated with sulphuric acid, and agitated with ether. Some woollen yarn is next introduced into the ethereal solution, which is then evaporated over the water-bath. In presence of *rouge végétale*,

* Schweizer Wochenschrift, xxii. p. 143.

the wool will acquire a brick-red colour, which turns violet upon treatment with ammonium hydroxide.

10. Cauzeneuve and Lepine * state that acid aniline red, "naphthol-yellow S," and roccelline red are harmless, whereas safranine and ordinary Martius' yellow are decidedly poisonous.

The presence of "Bordeaux red"† is recognised by first adding sodium sulphate to the suspected wine, then a solution of barium chloride : the artificial dye is carried down with the precipitated barium sulphate, from which it can be extracted by means of sodium carbonate solution. The brownish-red liquid thus obtained acquires a deep red colour if acidulated with acetic acid, which it readily communicates to silk upon boiling. Natural red wine fails to produce a coloration under the same circumstances.

For the detection of the presence of artificial colouring matter the following process is used in the Municipal Laboratory in Paris :—Preliminary tests are made—

1st. By soaking pieces of chalk in an aqueous solution of egg-albumen ; these are dried and applied for use by dropping a little of the wine upon them, and noting the coloration produced. Natural coloured wine usually causes a greyish stain, which, in highly coloured varieties, may verge to blue.

2nd. Baryta water is added to the wine under examination until the mixture acquires a greenish hue, after which it is shaken with acetic ether or amylic alcohol. If the wine be pure, the upper layer remains colourless, even after acidulation with acetic acid ; whereas, in presence of *basic* coal-tar dyes, such as fuchsine, amidobenzole, safranine, chrysoidine, chrysaniline, etc., characteristic colorations will be obtained.

3rd. A few c.c. of the sample are made alkaline by the

* 'Comptes Rendus,' 101, pp. 823, 1011, 1167.
† Répert de Pharm. xii. p. 504.

addition of dilute potassium hydroxide, some mercuric acetate added, and the mixture agitated and filtered. With pure wines, the filtrate is colourless; in the presence of *acid* coal-tar derivatives, it is red or yellow.

The general character of the artificial dye contained in the wine having been ascertained by the foregoing tests its more precise nature is determined as follows :—

In case the foreign colouring is *basic*, the supernatant layer obtained in the second test is separated, and divided into two portions ; one portion being evaporated with pure woollen yarn, the other with filaments of silk. The dyed threads are then subjected to the following tests :—

(*a*) *Rose-aniline or safranine* affords a red coloration ; safranine usually attaches itself only on silk.

(*b*) *Soluble aniline violet* produces coloured threads which become green upon treatment with hydrochloric acid, the primitive colour reappearing upon dilution with water.

(*c*) *Mauve-aniline* gives a colour which turns blue upon addition of the acid.

(*d*) *Chysotoluidine* causes a coloration which is only slightly affected by the acid, but which is discharged upon boiling with zinc powder ; upon protracted exposure to the air the colour reappears.

(*e*) *Chrysoidine* and *Amidonitrobenzole* produce yellow colours, the former turning poppy-red if treated with sulphuric acid, the latter, scarlet. A general characteristic of dyes, similar to rose-aniline, is that they are decolorised by treatment with sodium bisulphite.

If the presence of an *acid* coal-tar dye is indicated by the third preliminary test, the following special methods of procedure are employed :—

Two portions of the wine are saturated respectively with hydrochloric acid and with ammonium hydroxide water, and each portion is strongly agitated with acetic ether. The ethereal layers are removed by means of a pipette, then mixed together, evaporated to dryness, the residue obtained treated with a drop of concentrated sulphuric acid, and observations made of the colour obtained :—

(a) Roccelline	affords a	violet colour.
(b) Bordeaux, R. and B.	„	blue „
(c) Panceau R., R.R., R.R.R.	„	scarlet „
(d) Panceau, B.	„	red „
(e) Biebrich red	„	green to violet colour.
(f) Tropeoline, O.O.O.	„	red colour.
(g) Tropeoline, O., and Chrysoidine	„	orange-yellow colour.
(h) Tropeoline, O.O.	„	violet-red „
(i) Eosine	„	yellow „

The method employed in the Paris Municipal Laboratory for the detection of dried fruit wine, or of added commercial glucose, is substantially the following :—A little beer-yeast is added to 300 c.c. of the suspected wine, and the mixture is allowed to undergo fermentation at a temperature of about 30°. When the fermentation is completed, the filtered liquid is introduced into a dialyser, the outer water of which is automatically renewed. The process of dialysis is continued until the outer water ceases to show a rotary effect when examined by the polariscope, after which it is neutralised with calcium carbonate and evaporated to dryness over the water-bath, with constant stirring. The residue obtained is treated with 50 c.c. of absolute alcohol and filtered, the insoluble matters being twice washed with 25 c.c. of alcohol. The alcoholic filtrates are next decolorised by means of animal charcoal, and evaporated to dryness, and the solid residue is dissolved in 30 c.c. of water and polarised. Genuine claret, when tested in this manner, fails to exhibit a rotary power, or is but slightly dextrogyrate, whereas fruit wines, and those containing artificial starch sugar, strongly rotate respectively to the left or to the right.

The following are some of the conclusions arrived at by a commission, appointed by the German Government, to inquire into uniform methods for wine analysis, and establish standards of purity for genuine wine.*

(*a*) After deducting the non-volatile acids, the extract in natural wine should amount to at least 1·1 gramme per 100 c.c. ; after deducting the free acids, to at least 1 gramme per 100 c.c.

(*b*) Most natural wines contain one part of ash to every 10 parts of extract.

(*c*) The free tartaric acid should not exceed ⅙th of the total non-volatile acids.

(*d*) The relation between the alcohol and glycerine varies in natural wines between 100 parts alcohol to 7 parts glycerine, and 100 parts alcohol to 14 parts glycerine. These proportions do not apply, however, to sweet wines.

(*e*) Genuine wines seldom contain less than 0·14 gramme of ash, nor more than 0·05 gramme of sodium chloride per 100 c.c.

According to the analyses of Moritz, the maximum and minimum relative proportions of the constituents of natural wine are as follows :—The extract (after deducting the free acids) ranges from 1·10 to 1·78 per cent. ; the proportion of ash to extract varies from 1 : 19·2 to 1 : 6·4; that of phosphoric acid to ash ranges from 1 : 12·3 to 1 : 10·49 ; that of alcohol to glycerine, from 100 : 12·3 to 100 : 7·7.† From the investigations of Dr. Dupré, it would appear that in genuine unfortified wines, the amount of alcohol present varies from 6 to 12 per cent. by weight. A wine containing less than 6 per cent. would be unpalatable, and more than 13 per cent. cannot well be present, since natural grape-

---

* Reichsanzeiger, 1884, No. 154.

† R. Borgman (loc. cit.) gives the follow average relations of ingredients in pure wine :—

Alcohol : glycerine	= 100 : 10·5
Extract : acidity	= 1000 : 16·6
Acidity : ash	= 10 : 3·4
Ash : extractives	= 1 : 11·2
Phosphoric acid : ash	= 1 : 6·8

juice does not contain the quantity of sugar requisite for the production of a greater amount of alcohol ; moreover, an excess of this proportion would retard, if not entirely stop, the process of fermentation. Pure wines contain a greater proportion of volatile than fixed ethers, but in fortified wines the reverse is frequently the case. In natural wines, which are not over a few years old, the sugar present rarely amounts to 1 per cent., generally it is much less. Fortified wines, in which fermentation has been checked by the addition of alcohol, often contain 5 per cent. of sugar ; champagnes usually show from 4 to 10 per cent., and, in some liqueur wines, a maximum of 25 per cent. has been found. In natural wines, the total dry residue generally ranges from 1·5 to 3 per cent., while in fortified wines the addition of sugar and other substances may increase its proportion to 10 per cent., or even more. At the Paris Municipal Laboratory the following standards are adopted : The amount of added water in all wines, not sold as of a special or abnormal character, is calculated on a basis of 12 per cent. of alcohol (by volume) and 24 grammes of dry extract per litre. The proportion of potassium sulphate in unplastered wines must not exceed 0·583 gramme per litre. The use of salicylic acid is prohibited.

LIQUORS.

THE ordinary forms of liquors (namely, whisky, rum, and gin), are prepared by the distillation of alcoholic infusions. The process of distillation is preceded either by the conversion of the amylaceous constituents of grain, first into sugar, then into alcohol, or by the fermentation of saccharine bodies into alcohol, or, as in the case of brandy, it may be directly applied to a solution containing alcohol.

Brandy.—When genuine, brandy is the product of the distillation of various sorts of rich, light-coloured wines. The most esteemed quality is prepared in the neighbourhood of Cognac, in the Deux Charentes district, and in Armagnac ; but numerous inferior grades are manufactured in Rochelle and Bordeaux and in other parts of Southern France, as well as in Spain and Portugal. In the United States, a considerable quantity is produced by the distillation of California and Ohio wine. The fermented marc and lees of grapes are also extensively utilised in the manufacture of brandy. Most of the liquor known in commerce under this name, however, is made from the spirit obtained by the distillation of potatoes, corn, and other grains, which is subsequently rectified, deodorised, and then suitably flavoured. In France, the different grades of brandy are known as *eau-de-vie supérieure* (the best quality of Cognac); *eau-de-vie ordinaire* (common, sp. gr. 0·9476); *eau-de-vie de marc* (chiefly used for mixing purposes) ; *eau-de-vie seconde* (weak and inferior) ; *eau-de-vie à preuve de Hollande* (sp. gr. 0·941) ; *eau-de-vie à preuve d'huile* (sp. gr. 0·9185) ; *eau-de-vie forte* (sp. gr. 0·8390) ; and *esprit-de-vin* (sp. gr. 0·8610).

The characteristic taste and bouquet of the original wine are to a considerable extent communicated to the resulting brandy, and upon these qualities its value is greatly dependent. Many of the remarks made in regard to the ageing, flavouring and blending of wines equally apply to brandy, and need not be repeated in this place. When freshly distilled, it is colourless, its amber tint being either due to the casks in which it has been stored, or to added caramel. The normal constituents of genuine brandy are water, alcohol (including small amounts of butylic, propylic and amylic), various ethers (acetic, oenanthic, butyric, and valerianic), aldehyde, acetic and tannic acids, and traces of sugar and the oil of wine. The specific gravity usually approximates $0 \cdot 9300$ (equivalent to 52 per cent. of alcohol by volume), it may, however, range from $0 \cdot 9134$ to $0 \cdot 9381$ (from 60 to 48 per cent. of alcohol). Owing to the presence of acetic acid, genuine brandy usually shows a slightly acid reaction. According to Blyth, the constituents vary as follows:—total solids, from 1 to $1 \cdot 5$ per cent.; ash, from $\cdot 04$ to $\cdot 2$ per cent.; acids (estimated as tartaric), from $\cdot 01$ to $\cdot 05$ per cent.; sugar from 0 to $\cdot 4$ per cent. A partial examination of brandy, by König,[*] furnished the following percentages:—specific gravity, $0 \cdot 8987$; alcohol (by weight), $61 \cdot 70$; extract, $0 \cdot 645$; ash, $0 \cdot 009$. The ingredients found in twenty-five samples of brandy tested for the New York State Board of Health varied as follows:— specific gravity, $0 \cdot 9297$ to $0 \cdot 9615$; alcohol (by weight) from $25 \cdot 39$ to $42 \cdot 96$; extract, from $0 \cdot 025$ to $1 \cdot 795$; ash, from $0 \cdot 002$ to $0 \cdot 014$.

The majority of these samples were certainly abnormal in composition. Ordonneau[†] has quite recently determined by careful fractional distillation the proportions of the more important constituents of cognac brandy twenty-five years old, with the following results, the quantities being stated in

[*] 'Nahrungs u. Genussmittel,' 1st part, p. 187.
[†] 'Comptes Rendus,' 102, p. 217-219.

grammes per hectolitre :—aldehyde, 3 ; ethylic acetate, 35 ; acetal, traces ; normal propylic alcohol, 40 ; normal butylic alcohol, 218·6; amylic alcohol, 83·8 ; hexylic alcohol, 0·6; heptylic alcohol, 1·5 ; propionic, butyric and caproic ethers, 3 ; oenanthic ether, 4 ; amines, traces. The large proportions of normal butylic and amylic alcohols obtained are very significant. It was found that commercial alcohol, prepared from corn, potatoes and beetroot, while containing isobutylic alcohol, was entirely free from normal butylic alcohol, and the difference in flavour between genuine brandy and brandy distilled from grains would appear to be mainly due to this fact. Normal butylic alcohol is obtained when fermentation takes place under the influence of elliptical or wine yeast, whereas the iso-alcohol is the product of fermentation induced by means of beer yeast ; and it was shown that, by fermenting molasses, etc., with the aid of wine yeast, a spirit was obtained which much resembled brandy in colour and flavour.

Whisky.—Whisky is the spirituous liquor prepared by distilling fermented infusions of barley, wheat, corn, and other grains. Spirits that contain over 60 per cent. of alcohol are known as "high wines," or common spirits ; those containing 90 per cent. of alcohol are often termed " cologne spirits," the name whisky being usually given to the product of a former distillation, containing about 50 per cent. by weight of alcohol. In Great Britain, the largest amount of whisky is made in Scotland and Ireland ; in the United States, the principal supply comes from the States of Illinois, Ohio, Indiana, Kentucky (Bourbon Co.), and Pennsylvania (Monongahela Co.). The grains taken differ greatly in composition. In Scotland and Ireland, malted barley (pure, or mixed with other grain) is extensively employed ; in the preparation of Bourbon, partially malted corn and rye are taken, while, for Monongahela whisky, only rye (with 10 per cent. of malt) is used. The essential features of whisky-making are, first, the conversion of the starch of the grain into dextrine and glucose, which takes place in the process of *mashing*, the change being due to the action of the nitrogenous principle, *diastase* (formed during the germination of the gain) ; then, the transformation of the sugar into alcohol and carbonic acid by fermentation, which is induced by the addition of yeast ; and, finally, the concentration of the alcohol by distillation. The quality of whisky is much affected by the nature of the grain from which it is prepared, and by the care exercised in its manufacture, more particularly in the process of distillation. The most injurious ingredient in distilled spirits is commonly known as " fusel oil," which term comprises several products of alcoholic fermentation, possessing a higher boiling point than ethylic alcohol, and consisting chiefly of amylic alcohol, accompanied by small proportions of butylic and propylic alcohols. Several varieties of fusel oil exhibiting distinctive properties are met with, but that obtained from potato-spirit is the most common. As a rule, the spirits prepared from malted grain contain the smallest proportion. In the manufacture of whisky, a danger of promoting the formation of fusel oil is incurred by carrying on the distillation to the furthest point, in order to obtain the greatest possible quantity of alcohol. In Great Britain, the fermented mash is removed from the remaining grain before its introduction into the still ; but in this country the entire mash is occasionally taken, by which means a larger yield of alcohol is supposed to be effected. This practice is evidently open to the objection that the solid matters of the wort are liable to suffer destructive distillation, and engenders the formation of fusel oil. Another result, sometimes experienced, is the imparting of a smoky flavour to the product, which was originally intentionally communicated to the famous "poteen" whisky of Ireland, by using malt dried by means of burning turf. This quality is said to be still artificially obtained by the use of creosote. Genuine whisky, when recently made, is nearly colourless; but, if preserved in casks, it gradually acquires a brownish colour. It contains minute quantities of tannic acid, and ethylic and amylic acetates and valerianates. The specific gravity generally ranges between 0·9220 and 0·9040, corresponding to 48 and 56 per cent. of alcohol. The solid extract in whisky is usually below 1 per cent., and the total volatile acids under 0·1 per cent. In regard to the average composition of whisky, chemical literature furnishes but very meagre data. The examination of a large number of samples of ordinary American whisky in 1881, for the New York State Board of Health, gave the following results:—Specific gravity ranged from 0·9018 to 0·9645; alcohol (by weight) from 23·75 to 52·58; solid residue, from 0·100 to 0·752; ash, from 0·0020 to 0·0280. Several samples of rye whisky, examined by Mr. Green,[*] showed alcohol (by weight) from 32·50 to 51·20; tannic acid, 0·0003; acetic acid, ·0012 to 0·002; sugar, 0·002 to 0·005; solid residue, 0·160 to 0·734.

Rum.—Rum is obtained by the distillation of the fermented juice of sugar-cane or of molasses; a very considerable proportion of the article bearing this name is, however, made from grain spirit. In France and Germany the mother-liquor remaining after the extraction of beet-sugar, is utilised in the manufacture of a spirituous liquor greatly resembling rum in properties. The characteristic odour and taste of the liquor are mainly due to the presence of ethylic butyrate, and are frequently factitiously communicated to its imitations by the direct addition of this ether or of butyric acid. Grain spirit is also sometimes treated with pineapples, which likewise impart the distinctive flavour. Rum is chiefly produced in the West Indies, and in North America. The specific gravity ranges from 0·874 to 0·926; alcohol, from 50 to 70 per cent.; solid residue, from 0·7 to 1·50 per cent.; ash, under 0·10 per cent.[†]

[*] Am. Chem. 1876, p. 46.   [†] Blyth, op. cit.

The following are the results obtained by Berkhurts, from the analysis of various samples of genuine and artificial Jamaica rum :*—

Source.	Specific Gravity.	Alcohol by Weight.	Total Solids.	Ash.
London	0·885	61·38	0·668	0·023
Glasgow	0·875	61·38	4·800	0·089
Bremen	0·875	74·07	0·568	0·031
Directly imported	0·910	51·33	2·047	0·098
Artificial	..	38·94	0·469	0·033
Artificial	..	58·86	0·926	0·021

The variations in the composition of commercial rum would seem to be so great that little information of value concerning its authenticity is to be derived from analyses of a general character.

Gin.—Genuine Holland gin is a spirit prepared by the distillation of fermented grain infusions (rye and malted barley), flavoured with juniper berries, or oil of turpentine. Formerly the flavouring was directly introduced into the still together with the mash, but the more recent practice is to add salt, water, and juniper berries to the distilled grain spirit, and then re-distil the mixture. Numerous other aromatic substances are likewise employed in the manufacture of gin, among which are coriander, cardamom, and caraway seeds, orris, angelica, and calamus roots, cassia, bitter-almonds, sweet fennel, etc. Cayenne pepper, sugar, and acetic acid, are said to be also frequently added to gin. Gin doubtless possesses more of an artificial character than any other spirit. It is safe to assert that the great bulk of the drink sold under the name is simply grain-spirits flavoured with some of the preceding aromatics. On the other hand, the flavouring agents employed are not, as a rule, harmful in their effects, so that the quality of the liquor is mainly dependent upon the extent to which the

* 'Wieder die Nahrungsfälscher,' 1881, p. 105.

spirits used have been rectified.   It is difficult to define
"pure gin," since, owing to its compound character, it
varies in composition according to the method of manufacture followed by each individual distiller.   The variations found from the examination of twenty-five samples of
the commercial article, tested by the New York State Board
of Health, were as follows : *—Specific gravity, from 0·9302
to 0·9694; alcohol (by weight), from 18·64 to 44·33;
solid residue, from 0·018 to 0·772 ; ash, from 0·001 to
0·019.

Adulteration of liquors.—Although it is notorious that
the more common varieties of spirituous liquors are
sophisticated, the practices resorted to are unfortunately
usually of a character that does not permit of positive
detection, and, unless an actual adulteration, such as the
addition of some substance foreign to the genuine liquor,
has been made, a chemical examination alone is frequently
inadequate to distinguish between the true and the factitious article.   In fact, the ordinary physical qualities, such as
odour and taste, are often of greater service in determining
the genuineness of distilled spirits than more scientific tests.
The most prevalent form of sophistication with brandy,
rum, and gin, is their artificial imitations ; the direct addition of substances deleterious to health being of comparatively unfrequent occurrence.   It is usual to employ a
certain proportion of the genuine liquor in the fabrication
of its imitation.   An apparent objection to this species of
adulteration is that grain spirits are liable to be used as the
basis of the fictitious product, which is therefore apt to be
contaminated with fusel oil, a compound producing toxic
effects in a proportion fifteen times greater than ordinary
ethylic alcohol.

In the United States, whisky is probably less subjected to
serious sophistication than other spirituous drinks.   While

* See Report by Dr. F. E. Engelhardt, New York State Board of
Health, 1882.

the blending of this liquor (i. e. the mixing of new and old grades) is almost universally practised by the refiner, and while the retail dealer often reduces its alcoholic strength by the addition of water, there is very little ground for the belief that, in this country, whisky is subjected to noxious admixture to any great extent.

A very large number of recipes have been published for the manufacture of spurious liquors ; the following are characteristic, and will indicate their general nature :—

For Brandy :—

Cologne spirits (reduced to proof) ..	40 galls.
Oil of cognac	$\frac{1}{6}$ oz.
Burnt sugar colouring	$1\frac{1}{2}$ pint.
Tannin	$\frac{1}{4}$ oz.
Brandy essence..	1 part.
Alcohol	1000 parts.
Water	600 ,,

The compound known as " Brandy essence " consists of oil of grapes, 5 parts ; acetic ether, 4 parts ; tincture of allspice, 1 part ; tincture of galls, 3 parts ; and alcohol, 100 parts. " Oil of cognac " is a mixture of amylic alcohol and oenanthic ether.

According to M. Duplais, the best imitation of Cognac is the following :—

Alcohol (85 per cent.)	54 litres.
Rum (good quality)	2 ,,
Syrup of raisins	3 ,,
Infusion of green walnut hulls	2 ,,
Infusion of the shells of bitter almonds ..	2 ,,
Catechu, in powder	15 grammes.
Balsam of tolu	6 ,,
Pure water	37 litres.

Mix and colour with caramel.

New Cognac, Montpellier, Saintonge, and other brandies are aged and improved by adding to every 100 litres : old

O

rum, 2 litres ; old kirsch, 1¾ litres ; infusion of green walnut
hulls, ¾ litre ; syrup of raisins, 2 litres.

A compound sold as " London Brandy Improver " consists of sugar syrup, acetic ether and essence of cayenne,
coloured with caramel.

Whisky :—

(Rye) Proof spirit	50 galls.
Pelargonic ether	2 oz.
Pear oil	1 ,,
Oil of wintergreen (dissolved in alcohol)	10 drops.
Acetic ether	4 oz.
Oil of cloves (dissolved in acetic ether)	4 drops.
(Scotch) Alcohol (95 per cent.)	46 galls.
Scotch whisky	8 ,,
Water	18 ,,
Honey (3 lbs. in 1½ gall. water)	
Creosote	5 drops.
Acetic acid	2 oz.
Pelargonic ether	1 ,,
Ale	1 gall.
(Irish) Spirits	30 galls.
Irish whisky	5 ,,
Old ale	½ ,,
Creosote (dissolved in acetic acid) ..	4 drops.
Pelargonic ether	1 oz.

The preparation met with in commerce under the name
of "pelargonic ether" appears to be identical with oenanthic
ether.

Rum :—

Rectified spirits	6 quarts.
Jamaica rum	22 ,,
Rum essence	1½ oz.
Vanilla essence	1/10 ,,
Water	2 quarts.
St. John's bread	1½ oz.
Raisins	1½ ,,
Proof spirits	40 galls.
Rum essence	½ pint.
Sugar colouring	¼ ,,
Sugar syrup	1 quart.

"Rum essence" is composed of butyric ether, 15 parts; acetic ether, 2 parts; vanilla tincture, 2 parts; essence of violets, 2 parts; and alcohol, 90 parts.

Gin :—

Corn spirits	80 galls.
Oil of turpentine	1 pint.
Oil of juniper	8 oz.
Salt	21 lbs.
Water..	35 galls.
Oil of caraway	½ oz.
Oil of sweet fennel	¼ „
Cardamoms	8 „

Distil over, 100 galls.

The chemical examination of distilled spirits is ordinarily limited to a determination of the alcohol, solid residue, ash, and volatile acids, coupled with special qualitative and quantitative tests for any particular adulterants, the presence of which may be suspected.

(*a*) *Alcohol.*—In properly distilled liquors, a fairly approximate estimation of their alcoholic strength is effected by the specific gravity determination, which is best made by means of the special gravity bottle. In the case of spirituous liquors which contain extractive matters, it is necessary to first separate the alcohol present by the process of distillation, and then determine the density of the distillate when made up to the volume originally taken. The following table gives the percentages of alcohol by weight and by volume, and of water by volume, for specific gravities at 15°. *

The percentages of alcohol in the table are calculated for the temperature of 15°. The necessary correction for differences of temperature at which the determination is made is obtained by multiplying the number of degrees above or below 15° by 0·4, and adding the product to the percentage shown by the table, when the temperature is lower than 15°, and deducting it when it is above.

* Hager's 'Untersuchungen.'

Percentage of alcohol, by weight and by volume, and of water by volume, for specific gravity at 15°; water at same temperature being the unit :—

Specific Gravity.	Percentage By Weight. Alc.	By Volume. Alc.	By Volume. Water.	Specific Gravity.	Percentage By Weight. Alc.	By Volume. Alc.	By Volume. Water.	Specific Gravity.	Percentage By Weight. Alc.	By Volume. Alc.	By Volume. Water.
1·0000	0·	0	100·	0·9607	28·14	34	69·04	0·8954	60·38	68	35·47
0·9985	0·80	1	99·05	0·9595	29·01	35	68·12	0·8930	61·43	69	34·44
0·9970	1·60	2	98·11	0·9582	29·88	36	67·20	0·8905	62·50	70	33·39
0·9956	2·40	3	97·17	0·9568	30·75	37	66·26	0·8880	63·58	71	32·35
0·9942	3·20	4	96·24	0·9553	31·63	38	65·32	0·8855	64·64	72	31·30
0·9928	4·00	5	95·30	9·9538	32·52	39	64·37	0·8830	65·72	73	30·26
0·9915	4·81	6	94·38	0·9522	33·40	40	63·42	0·8804	66·82	74	29·20
0·9902	5·61	7	93·45	0·9506	34·30	41	62·46	0·8778	67·93	75	28·15
0·9890	6·43	8	92·54	0·9490	35·18	42	61·50	0·8752	69·04	76	27·09
0·9878	7·24	9	91·62	0·9473	36·09	43	60·58	0·8725	70·16	77	26·03
0·9867	8·06	10	90·72	0·9456	37·00	44	59·54	0·8698	71·30	78	24·96
0·9855	8·87	11	89·80	0·9439	37·90	45	58·61	0·8671	72·43	79	23·90
0·9844	9·69	12	88·90	0·9421	38·82	46	57·64	0·8644	73·59	80	22·83
0·9833	10·51	13	88·00	0·9403	39·74	47	56·66	0·8616	74·75	81	21·76
0·9822	11·33	14	87·09	0·9385	40·66	48	55·68	0·8588	75·91	82	20·68
0·9812	12·15	15	86·19	0·9366	41·59	49	54·70	0·8559	77·09	83	19·61
0·9801	12·98	16	85·29	0·9348	42·53	50	53·72	0·8530	78·29	84	18·52
0·9791	13·80	17	84·39	0·9328	43·47	51	52·73	0·8500	79·51	85	17·42
0·9781	14·63	18	83·50	0·9308	44·41	52	51·74	0·8470	80·72	86	16·32
0·9771	15·46	19	82·60	0·9288	45·37	53	50·74	0·8440	81·96	87	15·23
0·9761	16·29	20	81·71	0·9267	46·33	54	49·74	0·8409	83·22	88	14·12
0·9751	17·12	21	80·81	0·9247	47·29	55	48·74	0·8377	84·47	89	13·01
0·9741	17·96	22	79·92	0·9226	48·26	56	47·73	0·8344	85·74	90	11·88
0·9731	18·79	23	79·09	0·9205	49·24	57	46·73	0·8311	87·04	91	10·76
0·9721	19·63	24	78·13	0·9183	50·21	58	45·72	0·8277	88·37	92	9·62
0·9711	20·47	25	77·23	0·9161	51·20	59	44·70	0·8242	89·72	93	8·48
0·9700	21·31	26	76·33	0·9139	52·20	60	43·68	0·8206	91·08	94	7·32
0·9690	22·16	27	75·43	0·9117	53·19	61	42·67	0·8169	92·45	95	6·16
0·9679	23·00	28	74·53	0·9095	54·20	62	41·65	0·8130	93·89	96	4·97
0·9668	23·85	29	73·62	0·9072	55·21	63	40·63	0·8089	95·35	97	3·77
0·9657	24·70	30	72·72	0·9049	56·23	64	39·60	0·8046	96·83	98	2·54
0·9645	25·56	31	71·80	0·9026	57·25	65	38·58	0·8000	98·38	99	1·28
0·9633	26·41	32	70·89	0·9002	58·29	66	37·54	0·7951	100·00	100	0·00
0·9620	27·27	33	69·96	0·8978	59·33	67	36·51				

(b) *Solid residue.*—This is determined by evaporating

100 c.c. of the liquor in a tared platinum dish, until constant weight is obtained.

(c) *Ash.*—The proportion of ash is found by the incineration of the solid residue. If the presence of poisonous metallic adulterants (such as copper or lead) is suspected, a further examination of the ash is necessary.

(d) *Acids.*—The acidity of distilled liquors is generally due to minute quantities of acetic acid, and can be estimated by means of $\frac{1}{10}$th normal soda solution.

Any mineral acid (*e.g.*, sulphuric acid) supposed to be present is to be sought for in the residue remaining, after the distillation process employed in the determination of alcohol.

The presence of fusel oil in liquors is sometimes quite readily detected, by first removing the ethylic alcohol by gentle evaporation, and then inspecting the odour and taste of the still warm residue. The suspected liquor may also be agitated with an equal volume of ether, water added, and the ethereal stratum removed by means of a pipette, and concentrated by evaporation ; the residue is to be examined for amylic alcohol. When distilled with a mixture of sulphuric and acetic acids, amylic alcohol is converted into amylic acetate, which may be recognised by its characteristic pear-like odour ; or, the amylic alcohol can be transformed into valerianic acid (which also possesses a distinctive odour) by oxidation with sulphuric acid and potassium dichromate. Another simple qualitative test for fusel oil consists in first decolorising a small quantity of the liquor under examination with animal charcoal, adding a few drops of hydrochloric acid, and then a little freshly distilled and colourless aniline oil, when, in presence of fusel oil, it will be observed that the aniline compound acquires a perceptible rose tint as it falls to the bottom of the liquid. The quantitative determination of fusel oil presents some difficulties. A very ingenious method has been suggested by Marquardt.* It consists

* 'Berichte,' 1882, pp. 1370, 1661.

essentially in first agitating the sample with chloroform, draining off the solution obtained, washing it by repeated shaking with water, and then treating it at 85° with a mixture of 5 parts potassium dichromate, 2 parts sulphuric acid, and 30 parts of water. The valerianic acid thus formed is now separated by distilling the mixture of water and chloroform. The distillate is digested with barium carbonate, next concentrated by evaporation, and then filtered, and divided into two equal portions. One portion is evaporated to dryness, the residue taken up with water containing a little nitric acid, and the amount of barium present determined by precipitation with sulphuric acid. In the other portion, the chlorine originating from a partial oxidation of the chloroform, is to be estimated. The amount of barium combined with the chlorine, is deducted from the total quantity obtained; the remainder represents the proportion in combination with the fatty acids formed by oxidation. Of these, valerianic acid largely predominates; and the amount of barium valerianate $[Ba_2(C_2H_3O_2)]$ found is calculated to its equivalent in amylic alcohol. Capsicum, creosote, etc., are isolated by treating the sample with ether or benzole, and testing the odour and taste of the evaporated solutions so prepared.

Creosote gives a blue colour with ferric chloride solution; and the exceedingly pungent vapours evolved upon heating a residue containing capsicum are equally characteristic. The presence of tannin in distilled spirits, which is mostly derived from their preservation in casks, is recognised by the formation of a bluish-black colour upon the addition of ferric solutions. The identification of the various ethylic and amylic ethers used in the preparation of factitious liquors is a matter of some difficulty. Their presence is most readily detected by means of their characteristic odour, which is developed upon adding a little sodium hydroxide to the sample, evaporating the mixture over the water-bath almost to dryness, and then adding a small quantity of sulphuric acid. Another means of ascertaining the nature of the organic ethers present in spirits is to first remove the ethylic alcohol contained by a partial distillation with an alkaline solution, and then acidulate the remaining liquid with sulphuric acid, and repeat the distillation, when the volatile fatty acids originally contained in the ethers will be found in the distillate ; their identity is to be established by means of their characteristic properties. Nitrous ether (which compound is not contained in genuine liquors) may be detected by partially distilling the sample and adding a mixture of potassium iodide, starch paste, and acetic acid to the first portion of the distillate, the production of a blue colour indicating its presence. As previously remarked, the exercise of the ordinary senses is frequently of greater value in judging the quality of liquors than the results of chemical tests. Many of the organic ethers employed in the manufacture of artificial liquors are identical with those contained in the genuine article, and it is obvious that, in such instances, no distinction can be made between them.

WATER.

THE subject of the purity of potable waters possesses the highest degree of importance in its sanitary relations, and particular attention has been bestowed upon methods of analysis that would serve to indicate the character and significance of existing impurities. The earlier processes of examination, which chiefly consisted in the determination of the mineral constituents of water, while of use in furnishing an idea of the general nature of the water regarded as an inorganic solution, almost totally failed to reveal the presence of the more subtle and important organic contaminations which are now known to exert an active influence in the propagation of zymotic diseases. During the past few years, decided progress has been attained in the analytical methods employed. Little is known of the exact nature of the organic constituents present in water that has received sewage contamination. They may be either of vegetable or animal origin, and it appears to be very probable that they constitute organised germs. But, although we are still unable to determine the constitution of these deleterious ingredients, it is at present possible to approximately ascertain the hygienic character of drinking water, and to distinguish, with a fair degeee of accuracy, between a good and a bad sample. In arriving at a conclusion regarding the sanitary quality of water, it is, however, also needful to take into consideration the origin and surrounding conditions which affect the chances of contamination. Most of the more recent methods of water analysis are based upon the fact, that the putrefactive decomposition of harmful organic matter is attended by the genesis of certain compounds (such as ammonia, nitrites, and nitrates), of which quantitative estimations can be made. For the purpose of ascertaining the character of a potable water, the following determinations are usually necessary :—

1. Colour, odour, and taste.
2. Total solid matter and loss on ignition.
3. Organic matter in solution.
4. Chlorine.
5. Ammonia, free and albuminoid.
6. Nitrogen, as nitrites and nitrates.

Certain precautions should be observed in the collection of samples of water intended for examination. It is indispensable for this purpose to employ scrupulously clean glass stoppered bottles, which are washed out several times with the water previous to being filled. If a well or stream is to be sampled, the bottle should be entirely immersed in the water some distance from the sides of the stream, and, if taken from a pump or pipe, the latter should be cleansed by first running a considerable quantity of the water before charging the bottle.

1. *Colour, odour, and taste.*—The colour is best determined by filling a glass cylinder, about 2 feet in height, with the sample, placing it upon a white surface and observing the tint produced ; or, by the use of a coloured glass tube of the same length, which is provided with glass plates attached at each end, and is filled with the sample and viewed when held towards a sheet of white paper.

As a rule, pure water exhibits a light-bluish tint, a yellowish hue being generally considered a suspicious indication ; but it frequently occurs that a perfectly colourless water is bad, and one possessing a decided colour may prove to be at least, fair in quality. The odour of the sample is ascertained by placing a corked bottle, one-half filled with the water, in a warm place (at about 38°) for some time, and then shaking the bottle, withdrawing the stopper and immediately testing the odour. Pure water should be free

from much perceptible odour of any kind, and more especially from one of a disagreeable nature. The same
remark applies to the taste. Water should be practically
tasteless, even when warmed. It frequently happens, however, that a water may be highly contaminated with deleterious organic impurities, and still remain devoid of any
marked unpleasant taste. There are few simple tests of
any value which will reveal at once the sanitary quality of
drinking water. One, sometimes employed, is to fill a
clean quart bottle about three-fourths full with the suspected sample, and dissolve in it a teaspoonful of fine
granulated white sugar. The bottle is then corked and
allowed to remain in a warm place for two days, when,
in the presence of sewage contamination, it will become
cloudy or milky.* According to Wanklyn and Chapman,† if a brownish colour or precipitate is produced
upon the addition of 1·5 c.c. of Nessler's reagent (see p. 208)
to 100 c.c. of the water, it should be considered unfit for
domestic use.

2. *Total solid residue and loss on ignition.*—500 c.c. of the
water under examination are introduced, in small portions
at a time, into a tared platinum dish, and evaporated to
dryness over the water-bath, the residue being subsequently
dried for three or four hours in an air-bath at 100°. The
solid residue obtained, multiplied by 200, represents parts
in 100,000 : or, by 140, grains per imperial gallon. It is
usually considered that, unless the proportion of total solids
exceeds 40 grains per Imperial gallon (32 grains per U.S.
gallon, or about 56·5 parts per 100,000), the water need
not be objected to for drinking purposes on this ground
alone. The volatile and organic matters are determined by
igniting the solid residue, which is afterwards allowed to
cool. It is then moistened with a little carbonic acid water

* This test presupposes the existence in the water of the substances
necessary for the support of vegetable growth.

† 'Water Analysis.'

or solution of ammonium carbonate, dried to constancy at
130°, and the organic matter estimated by the decrease in
weight. Formerly, this process was chiefly depended upon
for determining the proportion of organic substances contained in water. It is open to numerous serious objections,
among which are, that it may afford a result either below
or above that correctly representing the quantity of organic
ingredients present in the sample. The first case takes
place when a portion of the organic matter is decomposed
during the process of evaporation, and is quite liable to
occur ; the second case takes place when the water contains
nitrates, which would be decomposed upon ignition. The
method, however, possesses some value, and is still often
resorted to as affording a general idea of the proportion of
organic contamination present, the degree of blackening of
the solid residue during the process of ignition being, at
least, a useful qualitative indication.

3. *Organic matter in solution.*—A method frequently employed for this determination is based upon the supposition
that the amount of potassium permanganate required to
oxidise the organic constituents contained in water would
serve as a criterion of its sanitary value. It is generally
known as the "Forchammer" or "oxygen" process, and,
although of undoubted service in comparing the quality of
samples of very impure water, it is defective in the following important respects : Different organic substances are
not affected to an equal extent by potassium permanganate ; albumen, for instance, being far less easily oxidised
than other compounds, and the value of the results afforded
is vitiated by the presence of certain inorganic bodies,
such as nitrites, sulphuretted hydrogen, ferrous salts, etc.
It has been stated, that the more deleterious and putrescent
organic ingredients of water are those most readily affected
by the permanganate solution. As modified and improved
by Miller * and by Tidy,† the process consists substantially

* Jour. Lond. Chem. Soc., xviii. p. 117.　　† Ibid., xxxv. p. 67.

in adding an excess of a standard solution of potassium permanganate to a measured quantity of the water under examination (acidulated with sulphuric acid), and then determining the excess of permanganate used by means of sodium hyposulphite and potassium iodide. The following solutions are required :—

Potassium Permanganate.—0·395 gramme of the salt is dissolved in 1 litre of distilled water ; 10 c.c. of this solution represent 0·001 gramme of available oxygen.

Sodium Hyposulphite.—One gramme of the salt is dissolved in a litre of water.

Starch solution.—One gramme of starch is triturated with about 20 c.c. of boiling water, and the mixture allowed to stand at rest over night, after which the clear supernatant solution is drawn off.

Pure distilled Water.—This is prepared by digesting 10 litres of distilled water with 10 grammes of potassium hydroxide and 2 grammes of potassium permanganate in a still provided with an inverted condenser at 100° for twenty-four hours, after which the water is distilled, separate portions being frequently tested with Nessler's solution ; the distillate is not reserved for use until this reagent ceases to produce a brownish coloration.

The determination proper is executed as follows :—Two flasks are first thoroughly cleansed by washing with concentrated sulphuric acid, and subsequently with water ; 250 c.c. of the water to be examined are introduced into one, and the same volume of the pure distilled water, prepared as above, is placed in the other. 10 c.c. of dilute sulphuric acid (1 part pure acid and 8 parts distilled water) and 10 c.c. of the potassium permanganate solution are now added to each flask, both then being put aside for three hours. Two drops of a 10 per cent. solution of potassium iodide are next added to the flasks, and the amount of iodine liberated (which is equivalent to the quantity of permanganate unacted upon by the water) is determined by titration with the sodium hyposulphite solution. The precise end of the reaction is ascertained by means of a few drops of the starch paste, the hyposulphite being added to each flask until the blue colour produced by the starch disappears. The quantities of solution used in each titration are then read off.

The amount of permanganate consumed is equal to $A - B$, where A represents the hyposulphite used with the distilled water, and B, that used with the sample under examination, and the proportion of oxygen which is consumed by the water tested, can be calculated by the formula :—

$$\frac{(A - B)\,a}{A}$$

in which a is the available oxygen in the added permanganate. For example, if 10 c.c. of permanganate ($= 0.001$ gramme available oxygen) are added to the 250 c.c. ($= \frac{1}{4}$ litre) contained in each flask, and the distilled water required 35 c.c., the sample 15 c.c., of the hyposulphite solution, the proportion of oxygen consumed by the $\frac{1}{4}$ litre of water, would be

$$\frac{(35 - 15) \times .001}{35}$$

$= .000571$, which represents .228 parts of oxygen in 100,000 parts of water.

In applying the preceding test, it is requisite that the flasks should be kept at a particular temperature, such as 27°. The presence of putrescent and readily oxidised organic matter or nitrites, which indicates dangerous contamination, is recognised by the absorption of any considerable proportion of oxygen in the space of two minutes. According to Dr. Tidy, 100,000 parts of water of various degrees of purity, absorb the following amount of oxygen in three hours :—

		Part Oxygen.
1. Great organic purity	.. .. ..	0 to 0.05
2. Medium purity	.. ..	0.05 „ 0.15
3. Doubtful ..	.. ..	0.15 „ 0.21
4. Impure	.. ..	over 0.21

4. *Chlorine.*—The importance attached to the estimation
of chlorine in potable waters is derived from the fact that this
element enters largely into the food of men and animals,
and is thrown off in their excreta. This, naturally, contri-
butes to the sewage contamination to which water is often
exposed. Water, however, may take up a certain proportion of chlorides from the geological strata through which
it passes, and it is of importance to bear this fact in mind
in forming a conclusion as to the significance of the results
afforded by this determination. It is, likewise, to be
remembered that vegetable organic pollution would escape
detection were the quantity of chlorine contained alone
taken into consideration. The determination is conveniently
made as follows :—50 c.c. of the water are introduced into a
beaker, a drop or two of a concentrated and neutral solution of potassium chromate added, and then a standard
solution of silver nitrate very cautiously added from a
burette, drop by drop, until a faint but permanent red tint
is produced. If the silver solution is prepared by dissolving 2·394 grammes of the nitrate in 1 litre of distilled
water, the number of c.c. required to cause the reddish
coloration directly indicates the parts of chlorine present
in 100,000 parts of the water examined. According to
Frankland, 100,000 parts of water from various sources
contain the following proportions of chlorine :—

Rain water	0·22
Upland surface water	1·13
Springs	2·49
Deep wells	5·11

Watts' ' Dictionary of Chemistry ' quotes the proportions
below :—

Thames, at Kew	1·21
Thames, at London Bridge	6·36
Loch Katrine	0·56
Rhine, at Basle	0·15
Rhine, at Bonn	1·45

Lake of Geneva	..	..	..	..	..	..	..	0·67
Elbe, near Hamburg		..	..	..	..	..	..	3·94
Loire, at Orleans		..	..	..	..	..	..	0·29

The amount of chlorine contained in sewage is stated to range from 6·5 to 21·5 parts, the average being 11·54 parts.* It is generally considered that a proportion in excess of 5 parts in 100,000 parts of a drinking water, which is not liable to be affected by mineral admixture, is to be ascribed to organic contamination.

5. *Ammonia, free and albuminoid.*—It has already been mentioned that the decomposition of the nitrogenous organic impurities present in polluted water results in the production, first, of ammonia, then of nitrites and nitrates, and, as it is commonly asserted that the deleterious character of water is mainly due to the putrefactive processes taking place, which are probably directly proportionate to the quantity of ammonia produced, it is evident that the determination of this compound is of considerable importance. The proportion of albuminous and allied constituents in a sample can, moreover, be measured by the quantity of ammonia produced when the water is boiled with an alkaline solution of potassium permanganate. Upon the foregoing facts, Messrs. Wanklyn, Chapman, and Smith † have based a method for the determination of the sanitary quality of potable waters, which is in very general use. It involves, first, an estimation of the ammonia generated upon distilling the water with sodium carbonate ("free" ammonia); second, the quantity given off by boiling with alkaline potassium permanganate ("albuminoid" ammonia). In case the water tested is contaminated with urea, which is not improbable, this compound will be decomposed into ammonia by the treatment with sodium

* Sixth Annual Report, Rivers Pollution Commission, "Blue Book."

† Jour. Lond. Chem. Soc. 1867, xx. p. 445.

carbonate. The following solutions are employed in the execution of the test :—

Ammonium Chloride.—Dissolve 1·5735 grammes of the dry and pure salt in 1 litre of distilled water. When required for use, dilute 100 c.c. of the solution to 1 litre ; 1 c.c. of this diluted solution contains ·00005 gramme of N H$_3$.

Pure Sodium Carbonate.—The ordinary pure reagent is freed from any ammonia possibly contained by heating it in a platinum capsule.

Pure distilled Water.—This is obtained as directed on p. 204.

Nessler's Reagent.—This is a strong alkaline solution of mercury biniodide. It may be prepared by first dissolving 62·5 grammes of potassium iodide in 250 c.c. of hot distilled water (reserving 10 c.c. of the solution), and adding a concentrated solution of mercury bichloride, with constant shaking, to the remainder, until a permanent precipitate remains undissolved ; this is then brought in solution by means of the 10 c.c. of iodide solution, set aside, and the addition of mercury bichloride is carefully continued until a slight precipitate reappears. A concentrated solution of potassium hydroxide (200 grammes dissolved in water) is now added, and the volume of the whole made up with distilled water to 1 litre. The solution is then allowed to subside, after which it is decanted and preserved in a well-stoppered bottle.

Permanganate solution.—Dissolve 8 grammes of potassium permanganate and 200 grammes of potassium hydroxide in 1 litre of water, and boil to expel any ammonia present.

The estimation of free and albuminoid ammonia is made as follows :—100 c.c. of the water to be examined are introduced into a glass retort, which connects with a Liebig's condenser, and has previously been thoroughly cleansed by boiling with distilled water ; one gramme of pure

sodium carbonate is added, and the water distilled until
40 c.c. have passed over, the distillate being separately
collected in four 10 c.c. cylinders or tubes. About 10 c.c.
of the alkaline solution of potassium permanganate is then
added to the remaining contents of the retort, and the
distillation continued almost to dryness. The second
distillate is likewise collected in fractions of 10 c.c. each.
It is advisable to so regulate the process of distillation,
that only about 10 c.c. pass over in the space of eight
minutes. The two sets of distillates are then separately
tested by adding 0·5 c.c. of the Nessler solution to each
cylinder, well stirring the mixture, and setting it aside for
at least five minutes. A series of comparison tubes
(10 c.c. in capacity) are prepared by adding ·001, ·003,
·005 up to ·01 gramme of ammonium chloride, and filling
to the 10 c.c. mark with pure distilled water; 0·5 c.c. of
the Nessler reagent being added to each. The degree of
coloration exhibited in the cylinders containing the two
sets of distillates is then matched by the comparison
cylinders.

It is evident, that from the data thus obtained, the
amount of ammonia obtained by the first distillation with
sodium carbonate (free ammonia), and by the second distillation with alkaline potassium permanganate (albuminoid ammonia), can be determined. It has been previously mentioned that urea evolves ammonia when boiled
with sodium carbonate; the amount of ammonia obtained
by the first process of distillation will therefore include
that actually contained as such in the water, and that
generated by the decomposition of any urea possibly
present. As the presence of this body is incompatible
with a good drinking water, this fact is of little real importance. In case, however, it be desired to make an
estimation of the free ammonia really present, 500 c.c.
of the water to be tested are treated with 1 or 2 c.c. of
calcium chloride solution, then with a slight excess of

P

potassium hydroxide, and the liquid filtered. It is next distilled as directed above, and the remaining contents of the retort made up to 500 c.c. 200 c.c. of the original sample are then subjected to the same treatment with calcium chloride and potassium hydroxide, and filtered. The second solution, which contains all the ammonia originally present in the water, is now tested with Nessler's reagent, the solution first obtained by diluting the contents of the retort being employed, instead of pure distilled water, for comparison.

The proportions of free and albuminoid ammonia found in the preceding operations are usually expressed in parts per 100,000 of the water. Wanklyn gives the following amounts of free and albuminoid ammonia contained in 100,000 parts of several kinds of water :—

```
Deep spring water  ..    ..    ..    ..    not over 0·001
    ,,      ,,     ,,    mixed with surface water  0·005
Filtered water ..    ..    ..    ..    ..    0·005 to 0·010
Imperfectly filtered water    ..    ..    0·01  ,,  0·02
Sewage    ..    ..    ..    ..    ..    ..    ..    ..    0·30
```

The same authority makes the following classification of potable water, reference being made to parts of albuminoid ammonia present in 100,000 parts :—

```
Extraordinary purity            ..        0 to 0·005
Satisfactory purity ..          ..    0·005 ,, 0·010
Dirty ..    ..    ..    ..       ..        over 0·010
```

The presence of any considerable proportion of free ammonia is usually indicative of recent sewage contamination. In the absence of free ammonia, a water need not be rejected unless the albuminoid ammonia exceeds 0·010 part, but a water containing over 0·015 part of albuminoid ammonia should be condemned under all circumstances.

6. *Nitrogen as nitrites and nitrates.*—It is quite generally accepted that the presence in water of the oxidation

products of nitrogen, is to be ascribed to the oxidation of nitrogenous organic matter, unless they are the result of percolation through soil containing nitrates, and, for this reason, considerable importance attaches to the quantitative estimation of the nitrogen present in the state of nitrates, and, in some cases, nitrites. One of the most reliable methods for this determination is the eudiometric process of Frankland, which is based upon that of Crum,[*] and consists in agitating the concentrated water with mercury and strong sulphuric acid, and measuring the volume of nitric oxide formed by the reduction of nitrates and nitrites. Owing, however, to the necessity of employing gas apparatus, this method is not in very general use. Wanklyn's process is the following:—100 c.c. of the sample are made alkaline with pure sodium hydroxide, evaporated to about one-fourth of its original volume, next made up to 100 c.c. by adding pure distilled water, and introduced into a flask which connects with a U-tube filled with powdered glass moistened with hydrochloric acid. A piece of aluminium foil is then added to the contents of the flask, and the mixture is allowed to stand at rest for six or seven hours. The contents of the U-tube are now transferred to the flask, the latter is connected with a Liebig's condenser and the liquid distilled. The proportion of ammonia contained in the distillate is determined by Nessler's reagent as previously described, from which the amount of nitrogen present as nitrates and nitrites is calculated.

Griess[†] has suggested a very useful process for the determination of nitrous acid and nitrites in potable waters. It is executed by placing 100 c.c. of the filtered water in a glass cylinder, and adding a few drops of dilute hydrochloric acid, and 1 c.c. of a solution of sulphanilic acid and naphthylamine hydrochloride. In the presence of nitrites, a beautiful rose-red colour (due to the formation of azobenzol-

[*] Phil. Mag., xxx. p. 426.
[†] Ber. der Deutsch. Chem. Gesell. xii. p. 427.

naphthylamine sulphonic acid), will be produced. The
proportion of nitrites contained in the water, is ascertained
by simultaneously subjecting a solution of potassium nitrite,
of known strength, to the same treatment, and matching
the degree of colour obtained, as in the Nessler process.
This solution can be prepared by dissolving 0·406 gramme
of dry silver nitrite in hot water, and adding a slight
excess of potassium chloride.   After cooling, the solution is
made up to one litre, the silver chloride allowed to settle,
and the clear liquid filtered.   If 100 c.c. of the filtrate are
further diluted to one litre, each c.c. will contain 0·00001
gramme of nitrous acid.

In Ditmar's method, the residue obtained by the
evaporation of the water, is first mixed with pure sodium
hydroxide, and placed in a small silver boat.   It is next
introduced into a combustion tube and burned in a current
of hydrogen, the evolved gases being received in an
absorption apparatus filled with very dilute hydrochloric
acid.   In this method the amount of ammonia formed, is
likewise estimated by means of Nessler's solution.   The
proportion of *organic nitrogen* is found by deducting the
free ammonia present in the water and multiplying the
remainder by $\frac{14}{17}$.

Messrs. Dupré and Hake * determine the *organic carbon*
in water essentially as follows :—The residue of the evaporation of the water is obtained in a very thin silver dish,
which can be rolled up and introduced into a combustion
tube filled three-fourths of its length with cupric oxide.
The residue is then burned in a stream of oxygen.   The
evolved carbonic acid is absorbed in a solution of barium
hydroxide, the precipitate formed being collected upon a
filter, washed, dried, and weighed ; its weight, divided by
19·4, gives the amount of organic carbon present in the
sample.   The carbonates and nitrates originally contained
in the water can be removed by boiling with a saturated

* Chem. Soc. Journ., March, 1879.

solution of sulphurous acid before the preliminary evaporation.

Frankland gives the following average proportions of nitrogen, as nitrates, occurring in 100,000 parts of various kinds of water :—

Rain water	0·007
Upland surface water	0·009
Deep wells and springs	0·400
Surface water (cultivated districts)	0·250
Shallow wells (no average), 2 to 5 parts common.	

Other authorities regard the presence of more than 0·6 part of nitrogen as nitrates per 100,000 parts of water as indicating dangerous pollution.

At the International Pharmaceutical Congress held in Brussels,* the following standards of purity for potable water were recommended :—

1st. A water should be limpid, transparent, colourless, without smell, and free of matter in suspension.

2nd. It should be fresh, with a pleasant taste, and its temperature should not vary much, and certainly not be higher than 15°.

3rd. It should not contain noxious animal or vegetable matter, and especially none of these substances in a state of decomposition.

4th. It should not contain more than 6 to 10 mgrms. of organic matter per litre, expressed in terms of oxalic acid. It should not contain nitrogenous matter.

5th. The nitrogenous organic matter, oxidised with an alkaline solution of potassium permanganate, should not yield more than 0·01 part of albuminoid ammonia per 100,000.

6th. It should not assume a disagreeable smell after having been kept in an open or closed vessel.

7th. It should not contain white algæ, nor numerous infusoria, bacteria, etc.

* Pharm. Zeit., 1885, No. 76.

8th. It must hold air in solution, which should contain a larger proportion of oxygen than ordinary air.

9th. It should not contain, per litre, more than :—

0·5 gramme	.. .. ..	mineral salts.
·060 ,,	.. .. ..	sulphuric anhydride.
·008 ,,	.. .. ..	chlorine.
·002 ,,	.. .. ..	nitric anhydride.
·200 ,,	.. .. ..	alkaline earths.
·030 ,,	.. .. ..	silica.
·003 ,,	.. .. ..	iron.

In the Municipal Laboratory of Paris, the following standards for potable waters are employed. One litre must not contain more than :—

0·5 to 0·6 gramme	.. ..	total mineral residue.
0·25 ,, ,,	.. ..	calcium sulphate.
0·015 ,, ,,	.. ..	chlorine.
0·005 ,, ,,	.. ..	organic matter (calculated as oxalic acid).
0·001 ,, ,,	..	albuminoid ammonia.
0·001 ,, ,,	..	metals precipitated by sulphuretted hydrogen.
0·003 ,, ,,	..	iron.
		No sulphuretted hydrogen.

100 c.c. should contain 3·25 c.c. of gas, 10 per cent. of which should be carbonic acid and 33⅓ per cent. oxygen.

Professor J. W. Mallet[*] suggests the idea, that the noxious character of potable waters containing nitrates and nitrites, with but small proportions of organic matter, may be due to the presence of a special nitrifying ferment belonging to the lower organisms, which are capable of propagating disease.

In regard to the degree of importance that should attach to definite and arbitrary standards of purity, it appears to be accepted that, although the data afforded as the result of chemical tests are often of value in discriminating

[*] 'Annual Report of the National Board of Health,' 1882, p. 207.

between pure and impure waters, but little reliance should be placed upon such criteria alone.

Professor Mallet, who has devoted much attention to the investigation of potable waters, and whose opinion on this subject is entitled to the highest consideration, arrived at the following conclusions concerning the more vital points at issue in the determination of the hygienic character of water :—

" 1. It is not possible to decide absolutely upon the wholesomeness or unwholesomeness of a drinking water by the mere use of any of the processes examined for the estimation of organic matter or its constituents.

" 2. I would even go further, and say that in judging the sanitary character of the water, not only must such processes be used in conjunction with the investigation of other evidence of a more general sort, as to the source and history of the water, but should even be deemed of secondary importance in weighing the reasons for accepting or rejecting a water not manifestly unfit for drinking on other grounds.

" 3. There are no sound grounds on which to establish such general 'standards of purity' as have been proposed, looking to exact amounts of 'organic carbon' or 'nitrogen,' 'albuminoid-ammonia,' 'oxygen of permanganate consumed,' etc., as permissible or not.

" 4. Two entirely legitimate directions seem to be open for the useful examination by chemical means of the organic constituents of drinking water, namely ; first, the detection of *very gross* pollution,   *   *   *   *   and, secondly, the periodical examination of a water supply, as of a great city, in order that the normal or usual character of the water having been previously ascertained, any suspicious changes, which from time to time may occur, shall be promptly detected and their cause investigated."

The microscopic and biological investigations of water are useful adjuncts to the chemical examination. The former is made by allowing a litre or more of the sample to remain at rest for several hours, collecting the deposit formed and inspecting it by means of the microscope, using low magnifying power at first. It will be found advantageous to stain portions of the sediment obtained with aniline violet, which, by a sort of predilection, attaches itself to particular forms of vegetable and animal life, thereby rendering them more distinct. The matters most usually observed in the microscopic examination of the deposit are :—

1st. Numerous lifeless substances, such as mineral matters, vegetable *debris*, muscular and cellular tissues, hairs, hemp, wool, cotton, silk, starch cells, insect remains, and pollen grains.

2nd. Living vegetable forms, such as confervæ, various algæ, oscillatoria, desmids, diatoms, and bacteria.

3rd. Living animal forms, including many varieties of infusoria and animalcula. Of the latter, those known as "saprophytes" are regarded as specially indicating the presence of sewage contamination.

Certain varieties of bacteria have been found associated with some forms of disease, and particular attention has been bestowed upon the study of these germs. The biological examination of water consists of pathological experiments on living animals, made by injecting a solution of the water-residue beneath the skins of rabbits, etc., and of experiments made by inoculating culture gelatine with the water. Of the latter methods of examination, that originally suggested by Dr. Koch, of Berlin, and described by Dr. Percy F. Frankland,* is well worthy of mention. In this process, the lower forms of life are cultivated in a solid medium, by means of which the growth of each colony is localised and rendered suitable for microscopic inspection.

The medium employed by Dr. Frankland has the following composition :

* Jour. Soc. Chem. Indus., Dec. 1885.

Lean meat	..	..	..	..	..	..	1 lb.
Gelatine	..	..	..	..	..	..	150 grammes.
Solid peptone	..	..	..	..	..	10	„
Sodium chloride	..	..	..	..	..	1	„
Distilled water	..	..	..	..	..	1 litre.	

The finely-cut meat is first infused in half a litre of cold water for two hours and strained; the gelatine is digested in the other half-litre of water, then mixed with the meat-extract, and the whole heated until the gelatine is completely dissolved, when the peptone and salt are added.

The liquid is now cautiously neutralised with sodium carbonate, and clarified by beating it together with two or three eggs, boiling, straining through cloth, and filtering hot through bibulous paper; upon cooling it sets to a transparent jelly. Before setting, 7 c.c. of the liquid are introduced into a series of clean test-tubes, which are tightly plugged with cotton-wool and then sterilised by steaming them half-an-hour for three or four consecutive days. It is necessary to observe special precautions in the collection of the sample of water to be examined. Glass-stoppered bottles are well adapted for this purpose. These are to be very thoroughly washed with distilled water, then dried and finally sterilised by heating in an air-bath for three or four hours at a temperature of from 150° to 180°.

The actual examination of the water is executed by first heating one of the test-tubes containing the sterilised gelatin medium in a water-bath to 30°, by which it is fused. The external portion of the cotton-wool is next burned, the tube opened, and a certain number of drops of the water to be tested (previously well shaken) are introduced by means of a sterilised pipette. The mixture is immediately poured out upon a clean and sterilised glass plate which rests in a perfectly horizontal position, and is covered by a glass shade. The plate is supported by a glass tripod which dips into a dish containing a two per cent. solution of mercuric chloride—thus forming an antiseptic protection from the external air. The tripods, dishes, etc., are sterilised by washing them with the mercuric chloride solution. As soon as the gelatine mixture has set, the glass plate (together with the cover) is introduced into an air-bath kept at a temperature of from 20°–25°, where it is allowed to remain for two to five days for incubation. The individual organisms and the progress of the formation of colonies are observed from time to time by inspecting the plate, which can be done without removing the glass cover. As soon as they have become easily visible to the naked eye, the plate is removed from the bath, and placed upon another glass plate, which is ruled in squares, and put over a black paper. The colonies are then counted by aid of a lens, or, if they are too numerous to admit of this, the number contained in a few of the squares is determined and multiplied accordingly.

Dr. Frankland has applied the foregoing method to the examination of the London water supply (1885), with the following results :—

MICRO-ORGANISMS IN 1 C.C.

	Jan.	Feb.	March.	May.	June.		Sept.	Oct.	Nov.
River Thames at Hampton	..	..	..	..	155	..	1644	714	1866
Chelsea	8	23	10	14	22	81	13	34	3
West Middlesex	2	16	7	3	..	26	2	2	5
Southwark ..	13	26	246	24	..	47	18	24	32
Grand Junction	382	57	28	3	21	18	43	40	40
Lambeth	10	5	69	30	..	38	103	26	26
RIVER LEA.									
River Lea at Chingford Mill	..	..	..	..	..	..	..	..	954
New River ..	7	7	95	3	..	27	3	2	11
East London ..	25	39	17	121	..	22	29	53	14
DEEP WELLS.									
Kent (well at Deptford)	..	..	..	..	6	..	..	6	8
Kent (supply) ..	10	41	9	20	26	..	14	18	

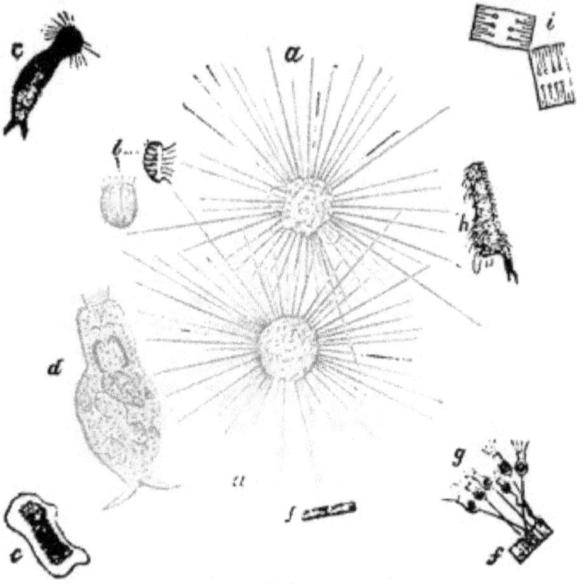

PLATE XI.

FIG. 2.

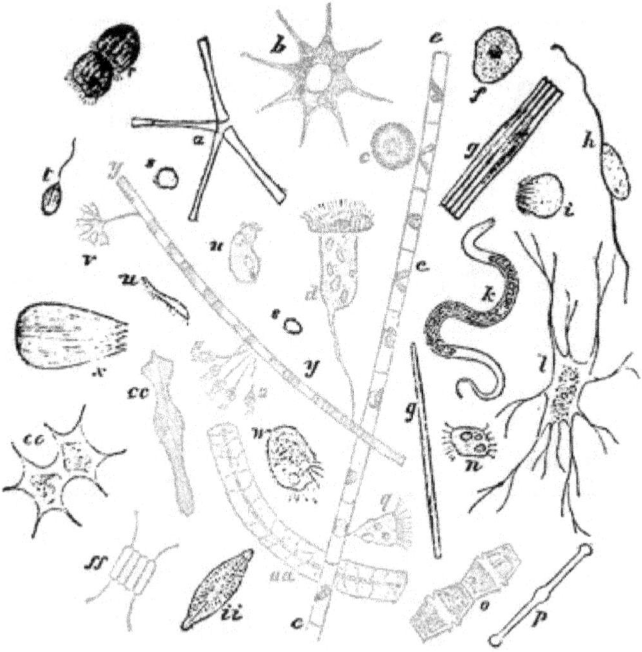

FIG. 1

In Plate XI., Fig. 1 exhibits the animal and vegetable living forms contained in Croton water. They have been catalogued as follows :—

(*a*) Asterionella formosa, vegetable ; a diatom, × 312.
(*b*) Pediastrum simplex, vegetable ; a desmid, × 200.
(*c*) Cyclotella astræa, vegetable ; a diatom, × 200.
(*d*) Vorticella ; an animalcule, × 312.
(*e*) Conferva, vegetable ; "green scum," × 40.
(*f*) Epithelial cell ; × 200.
(*g*) Fragillaria cupucina, vegetable ; a diatom, × 200.
(*h*) Heteromita ovata ; an animalcule, × 500.
(*i*) Halteria grandinella (?); an animalcule, × 200.
(*k*) Anguillula fluviatilis ; a water-worm, × 312.
(*l*) Amœba porrecta ; an animalcule, × 200.
(*n*) Dinophrys ; an animalcule, × 200.
(*o*) Didymoprium borreri, vegetable ; a desmid, × 200.
(*p*) Tabellaria fenestrata, vegetable; a diatom, × 312.
(*q*) Free vorticella ; an animalcule, × 200.
(*r*) Coccudina costata, dividing ; an animalcule, × 312.
(*s*) Monas umbra ; an animalcule, × 312.
(*t*) Cyclidium obscissum ; an animalcule, × 312.
(*u*) Chilodon cucullulus ; an animalcule, × 200.
(*v*) Epistylis nutans ; young animalcules, × 200.
(*w*) Paramecium ; an animalcule, × 200.
(*x*) Difflugia striolata, the lorica or case ; an animalcule, × 200.
(*y*) Conferva ; vegetable "green scum," 312.
(*z*) Vorticella microstoma ; an animalcule, × 200.
(*a a*) Fragments of dyed wood, × 200.
(*c c*) Gomphonema acuminatum, vegetable ; a diatom, × 200.
(*e e*) Arthrodesmus octocornis, vegetable ; a desmid, × 312.
(*f f*) Scenodesmus quadricauda, vegetable; a desmid, × 200.
(*i i*) Navicula rhynchocephala (?), vegetable ; a diatom, × 200.

Fig. 2 represents the organisms found in the Brooklyn (Ridgwood) water supply :—

(*a*) Actinophrys sol ; an animalcule, × 200.
(*b*) Coccudina costata ; an animalcule, × 200.
(*c*) Chætonotus squamatus ; hairy-backed animalcule, × 200.
(*d*) Notommata; a rotiferous animalcule, × 200.
(*e*) Amœba guttula ; an animalcule, × 200.
(*f*) Melosira orichalaea, vegetable ; a diatom, × 200.

(*g*) Vorticella microstoma ; animalcules, × 200.

(*h*) Chætonotus larus ; hairy-backed animalcule, × 200.

(*i*) Tabellaria flocculosa, vegetable ; a diatom, × 200.

The original drawings from which Plate XI. is taken were prepared by Mr. William B. Lewis, for the Metropolitan Board of Health.

The presence of these organisms, however startling some of them may be in appearance, is usually not objectionable ; indeed, microscopic vegetable growths are frequently of service in the purification of potable water. The more important forms of bacteria (bacilli, etc.), present minute rod-like shapes, far less impressive in appearance.

Considerable difference of opinion exists in regard to the sanitary value of the results afforded by the biological examination of water. While the number of bacteria found in a given quantity of water may be of aid in the formation of an opinion as to its relative safety for domestic purposes, it should be borne in mind that these micro-organisms are almost omnipresent, being contained in the air, and in soils, and articles of food.

The following tabulation shows the relative purity of the water supply of several American cities, as determined by Prof. A. R. Leeds, in June, 1881 :—

Parts in 100,000	New York.	Brooklyn.	Jersey City.	Philadelphia.	Boston.	Washington.	Rochester.	Cincinnati.
Free ammonia..	0·0027	0·00075	0·00475	0·001	0·01325	0·006	0·0114	0·0115
Albuminoid ammonia.	0·027	0·00825	0·0427	0·018	0·0605	0·027	0·023	0·024
Oxygen required	0·81	0·413	0·95	0·46	1·77	0·600	0·790	0·860
Nitrites	None	None	None	None	None	None	None	None
Nitrates	0·8325	1·2025	0·9065	0·6845	1·2395	0·8325	0·629	0·740
Chlorine	0·350	0·550	0·235	0·3000	0·315	0·270	0·195	0·805
Total hardness..	3·300	2·270	3·200	4·400	2·100	4·800	5·500	6·400
Total solids ..	11·800	6·000	9·300	14·300	8·500	11·500	10·000	16·200
Mineral matter	5·000	5·000	3·400	6·000	2·000	5·500	4·000	9·000
Organic and volatile matter.	6·800	1·000	5·900	8·300	6·500	6·000	6·000	7·200

Parts per 100,000.	April.	May.	May.	June.	June.	July.	July.	August.	August.	September.	September.	October.	October.	November.	December.
	3rd.	6th.	26th.	13th.	30th.	15th.	30th.	19th.	31st.	13th.	29th.	14th.	30th.	13th.	1st.
Appearance, &c...	Cl.	Sl. Tb.	Tb.	Cl.	Cl.	Cl.	Cl.	Cl.	Cl.	Cl.	Cl.	Cl.	Cl.	Cl.	Cl.
Odour (heated to 100° Fahr.)	None	None	None	None	None	None	None	None	None	None	None	None	None	None	None
Chlorine in chlorides	0·278	0·348	0·244	0·348	0·226	0·279	0·226	0·278	0·313	0·209	0·208	0·272	0·243	0·312	0·295
Equivalent to sodium chloride	0·459	0·575	0·400	0·574	0·374	0·459	0·374	0·459	0·517	0·344	0·343	0·456	0·400	0·515	0·486
Phosphates	None	None	None	None	None	None	None	None	None	None	None	None	None	None	None
Nitrites	None	None	None	None	None	None	None	None	None	None	None	None	None	None	None
Nitrogen in nitrates and nitrites	0·0403	0·0494	0·034	0·0469	0·0371	0·0395	0·0387	0·0469	0·0486	0·037	0·0477	0·041	0·047	0·048	..
Free ammonia	0·001	0	0·002	0·003	0·0005	0·002	0·003	0·003	0·001	0·004	0·002	0	0·003	0·001	0·032
Albuminoid ammonia	0·009	0·0166	0·0086	0·007	0·014	0·008	0·011	0·014	0·009	0·016	0·0094	0·013	0·015	0·014	..
"Hardness" equivalent to carbonate of lime—Before boiling	4·73	4·082	4·280	3·860	4·968	4·268	4·332	4·586	4·332	5·096	3·949	4·520	4·512	3·840	3·729
After boiling	4·31	3·787	3·510	3·500	4·586	4·268	4·332	3·949	4·332	4·459	3·822	4·294	4·512	3·390	3·164
Organic and volatile (loss on ignition).	6·00	1·500	3·00	2·50	2·00	0·50	2·50	3·00	2·00	2·50	2·50	2·50	3·00	3·00	..
Mineral matter (non volatile).	5·00	4·000	4·50	4·50	5·50	5·00	5·00	5·00	4·50	4·00	4·00	4·00	4·50	4·00	..
Total solids (by evaporation).	11·00	5·50	7·50	7·00	7·50	5·50	7·50	8·00	6·50	6·50	6·50	6·50	7·50	7·00	..

Cl. signifies *clear.* Sl. *slightly turbid.* Tb, *slightly turbid.* Tb, *turbidity somewhat more marked.*

PARTS PER 100,000.

Description of Sample.	Date when taken.	Time when drawn.	Appearance in two-foot tube.	Odour when heated to 38°.	Chlorine in Chlorides.	Equivalent to Sodium Chloride.
	1884.					
Mohawk River, above Diamond Woollen Mills	Dec. 5	..	Turbid, greenish yellow	Faint, aromatic	0·233	0·371
Hudson River, above Lansingburg	Nov. 12	..	Faintly turbid, light greenish yellow	Faint, vegetable	0·233	0·371
Troy hydrant	,, 12	..	Faintly turbid, light greenish yellow	Faint, vegetable	0·233	0·371
Hudson River, at Maple Island	Dec. 6	..	Faintly turbid, greenish yellow	Faint, marshy	0·167	0·265
Hudson River, at inlet	Nov. 1	High tide	Clear, light yellow	Faint	0·333	0·530
Hudson River, at inlet	,, 1	,,	Faintly turbid, light yellow	Faint, stale	0·333	0·530
Hudson River, at inlet	,, 1	Low tide	Clear, brownish yellow	Faint	0·366	0·583
Hudson River, at inlet	,, 1	,,	Turbid, brownish yellow	Faint	0·366	0·583
Hudson River, 50 ft. south of inlet	Dec. 4	High tide	Slightly turbid, brownish yellow	Oily	0·233	0·371
Hudson River, at inlet	,, 4	Low tide	Turbid, brownish yellow	Oily	0·183	0·291
Bleecker Reservoir ..	Nov. 1	..	Clear, faint yellow	..	0·340	0·541
Bleecker Reservoir ..	,, 1	..	Turbid, faint yellow	Faint, stale	0·340	0·541
Tivoli Lake	,, 6	..	Faint milkiness	Faint, stale	0·833	1·325
Tivoli Lake	,, 6	..	Whitish, milky	Faint, stale	0·833	1·325
Tivoli Lake	Dec. 4	..	Turbid, greenish	Faint, marshy	0·966	1·537

PARTS PER 100,000.

Phosphates.	Nitrites.	Nitrogen in Nitrates and Nitrites.	Free Ammonia.	Albuminoid Ammonia.	Oxygen absorbed at 80° Fahr.		Hardness equivalent to Carbonate of lime.		Organic and Volatile Matter.	Mineral Matter.	Total Solids dried at 110°.
					In 15 Minutes.	In 4 hours.	Before Boiling.	After Boiling.			
..	..	0·0705	0·0044	0·0074	0·2071	0·3704	6·838	6·838	1·70	9·00	10·70
..	..	0·0247	..	0·0150	0·2691	0·4150	3·818	3·818	2·20	5·80	8·00
..	..	0·0284	0·0015	0·0151	0·2750	0·4000	4·498	4·498	2·60	6·50	9·00
..	..	0·0614	0·0014	0·0082	0·2827	0·4100	5·049	4·839	2·40	5·30	7·70
..	..	0·0277	0·0064	0·0002	0·1670	0·3111	5·897	5·897	1·40	9·80	11·20
..	..	0·0265	0·0038	0·0142	0·1890	0·3422	6·237	6·237	5·00	7·20	12·20
..	..	0·0471	0·0028	0·0134	0·2180	0·3180	6·237	6·086	1·80	9·20	11·00
..	..	0·0288	0·0050	0·0124	0·2200	0·3470	6·048	6·048	4·80	8·20	13·00
..	..	0·0647	0·0054	0·0114	0·2509	0·4340	5·470	5·470	3·50	4·50	8·00
..	..	0·0606	0·0064	0·0090	0·2230	0·4420	5·838	5·838	1·50	7·50	9·00
..	..	0·0484	0·0052	0·0068	0·1511	0·2578	5·330	3·893	2·50	8·80	11·30
..	..	0·0489	0·0046	0·0102	0·1755	0·3020	6·577	6·577	5·70	6·80	12·50
Faint trace	Faint trace	0·0507	0·0184	0·0080	0·0780	0·2030	7·069	4·309	2·00	12.00	14·00
Faint trace	Faint trace	0·0611	0·0198	0·0280	0·1200	0·1852	7·409	5·481	6·00	11·00	17·00
Faint trace	Faint trace	0·1334	0·0380	0·0118	0·1075	0·1762	8·468	8·468	3·20	10·40	13·60

The variation in the composition of Croton water, at different seasons of the year, is exhibited by the table on p. 221, which gives the results of the semi-monthly examinations made by Dr. Elwyn Waller during the year 1885.*

For the results of the analyses of the water of the Hudson River, recently made by Dr. C. F. Chandler, see table, pp. 222, 223.

The rather common belief that freezing purifies water is incorrect. It is said, that the greater part of the ice supply of New York City (three millions of tons) is gathered from the Hudson River between Albany and Poughkeepsie, most being drawn within thirty miles of the former city, and therefore liable to be polluted with sewage. The average number of bacteria in one c.c. of ordinary ice is stated to approximate 400, but Hudson River ice has been found to contain nearly 2000 bacteria per c.c.† The number of bacteria in one c.c. of snow is usually about 9000; Hudson River snow-ice contains 20,000 per c.c.; and, although the great majority of these organisms are perfectly harmless, cases are on record where epidemics (as of gastro-enteritis) have been directly traced to the use of impure ice.

* Jour. Am. Chem. Soc., viii. p. 6.
† See paper read by Dr. T. M. Prudden before the New York Academy of Medicine, March 18th, 1887.

VINEGAR.

VINEGAR is a dilute aqueous solution of acetic acid, containing inconsiderable proportions of alcohol, aldehyde, acetic ether, and extractive matters, which, to some extent, impart a characteristic flavour and aroma. The process most frequently involved in the preparation of vinegar is known as the acetous fermentation, and may be induced in various saccharine juices and infusions, such as those of apples, wine, malted grain, etc., when, in presence of a ferment, they are exposed to the action of the air, at a temperature between 24° and 32°. In the oxidation of alcohol, an intermediate compound (aldehyde) is at first formed, which, by the continued action of oxygen, is ultimately converted into acetic acid. A dilute solution of alcohol is, however, not oxidised to acetic acid by simple exposure to the air ; it is usually necessary that a peculiar microscopic plant (*mycoderma aceti*) should be present. This fungus includes two varieties, viz., minute globules (*micrococci*) and rod-like forms (*bacilli*) varying in size ; and is often developed in old casks that have been long employed for making vinegar. It constitutes a gelatinous mass ("mother of vinegar") having the appearance of glue that has been soaked in cold water ; the surface quickly becomes coated with a bluish mould (*Penicillium glaucum*).

Pasteur regards acetification as a product of the development of the *mycoderma aceti*, i.e., as a physiological fermentation—but it appears probable that the process is rather one of oxidation, and that the fungus accelerates the change by condensing the oxygen upon its surface and delivering it to the alcohol, possibly in the form of ozone. Indeed,

Q

the process of vinegar making may take place in the entire
absence of the *mycoderma*, as when spongy platinum is
brought into contact with alcoholic solutions ; and Buchner
has examined shavings which had been used in a vinegar
factory for over twenty-five years, and found them to be
absolutely free from the fungoid plant.   In the United
States, the best known and most esteemed kind of vinegar
is that obtained by the acetification of apple cider ; but by
far the largest quantity is manufactured from alcohol and
spirituous liquors. Cider vinegar is free from aldehyde but
contains malic acid.   The usual source of vinegar in Great
Britain is a wort prepared from mixtures of malt with other
grain ; while, in Continental Europe, inferior sorts of new
wine (especially white wine) are extensively employed for
its production.

Malt vinegar possesses a brown colour and a density
ranging from 1·006 to 1·019; that known as proof vinegar
contains from 4·6 to 5 per cent. of acetic acid.   In Great
Britain the manufacturer is allowed by law to add 0·1 per
cent. of sulphuric acid to vinegar, on account of its supposed preservative action, and, although the practice is now
known to be unnecessary, it is still sometimes resorted to.
The specific gravity of wine vinegar varies from 1·014 to
1·022.   100 c.c. should neutralise from 0·6 to 0·7 grains of
sodium carbonate, and the solids obtained upon evaporation
to dryness should approximate two per cent.   According
to the United States Pharmacopœia, one fluid ounce of
vinegar should require for saturation not less than 35 grains
of potassium bicarbonate.

In 500 samples of imported wine and malt vinegar tested
by the author, the minimum and maximum strength ranged
from 3 to 10·6 per cent. of acetic acid, the specific gravity
from 1·0074 to 1·0150, and the number of grains of potassium bicarbonate required to neutralise one troy ounce
from 22 to 84.   Of 273 samples of vinegar tested in 1884
by the Massachusetts State Board of Health, 52 were above

the then legal standard of 5 per cent. of acetic acid, and 221 below ; 109 of the latter contained more than 4 per cent. ; the strongest sample showed 8·86 per cent., and the weakest contained but 0·66 per cent. of acetic acid. In the year 1885, 114 samples were examined, of which 45 were above and 69 below the standard of 4½ per cent. acetic acid.

In the State of New York, the legal standard for vinegar is 4·5 of absolute acetic acid, and, in the case of cider vinegar, the proportion of total solids must not fall below 2 per cent. In Massachusetts, also, the acidity must be equivalent to 4½ per cent. of acetic acid, and cider vinegar must contain, at least, 2 per cent. of solid matter. The English standard of strength is 3 per cent. of acetic acid.

Analysis.—For the requirements of the United States Customs Service, the only estimations ordinarily made are the specific gravity, and a determination of the acidity. The former is accomplished by means of the specific gravity bottle ; the latter, by placing 10 c.c. of the sample in a beaker, adding about 30 c.c. of water, then a few drops of an alcoholic solution of phenol-phthalein (to serve as the indicator), and titrating with a normal alkali-solution ; the number of c.c. used divided by 10 and multiplied by 48, gives the amount, in grains, of potassium bicarbonate required to neutralise one troy ounce of the vinegar. In the presence of sulphuric acid, it is necessary to distil a measured quantity of the sample almost to dryness and titrate the distillate, it being assumed that 80 per cent. of the total acetic acid present passes over.

The determination of the extract or solid residue in vinegar is executed in the same manner as described under beer and wine. Several tests have been suggested for the detection of the presence of free sulphuric acid. The usual reagent—barium chloride—is not well adapted to the direct determination of this acid, since sulphates, which are as readily precipitated as the free acid, may also be present. The following methods may be employed :—

1. A piece of cane sugar is moistened with a small quantity of the sample and exposed to the heat of the water-bath for some time, when, in presence of free sulphuric acid, the residue will become more or less carbonised, according to the proportion of acid present.

2. Five centigrammes of pulverised starch are dissolved in a decilitre of the sample by boiling, and after the liquid has become completely cooled, a few drops of iodine solution are added.   Dilute acetic acid does not affect starch, and if the sample is pure, a blue coloration will be produced ; if, however, but a minute quantity of sulphuric or other mineral acid is present, the starch is converted into dextrine, and the addition of iodine fails to cause the blue coloration.

3. According to Hilger,* if two drops of a very dilute solution of methyl aniline violet (0·1 to 100) are added to about 25 c.c. of pure vinegar no change of colour takes place ; whereas, in the presence of 0·2 per cent. of mineral acid, a bluish coloration is produced ; in case the proportion of acid reaches 1 per cent. the liquid acquires a greenish tint.

4. A recent test for mineral acids has been suggested by Hager.†   It consists in warming together two drops of East Indian copaiba balsam, and 30 drops of pure acetic acid, and subsequently adding to the mixture two or three drops of the vinegar under examination ; if either sulphuric or hydrochloric acid be present, a blue-violet colour is produced.

The free mineral acids in vinegar may be quantitatively estimated by saturating a weighed quantity of the sample with quinine, evaporating the mixture to dryness over the water-bath, and dissolving the quinine salts formed in alcohol, which is then removed by distillation.   The second residue is next dissolved in water, and the quinine precipitated by addition of ammonia, and separated by filtration.

* Archiv. der Pharm., 1876, p. 193.
† Pharm. Centralb., N.F. 7, p. 292.

The filtrate will contain the mineral acids present, and their amount is determined by the ordinary methods.

The free sulphuric acid in vinegar can also be quantitatively estimated, according to Kohnstein,* as follows: 100 c.c. of the sample are shaken with pure and freshly calcined magnesia until completely neutralised. The mixture is filtered, the filtrate evaporated to dryness in a platinum dish and the residue ignited at a moderate temperature. By this treatment magnesium acetate is converted into the corresponding carbonate, while any magnesium sulphate present will remain unaltered. The ignited residue is moistened and evaporated with a little carbonic acid water, then digested with hot water, and the solution filtered; the insoluble magnesium carbonate remains upon the filter, the sulphate going in solution; the precipitate is thoroughly washed. After removing the traces of lime possibly present, the amount of magnesia contained in the filtrate is determined as pyrophosphate, from the weight of which the proportion of free sulphuric acid originally contained is calculated. The presence of metallic impurities in vinegar is detected by means of the usual reagents, such as hydrosulphuric acid and ammonium sulphide. In addition to water and sulphuric acid, the most common adulterants of vinegar are capsicum, sulphurous acid and various colouring matters. The presence of capsicum and other acrid substances is usually revealed by the pungent odour produced upon burning the solid residue obtained by the evaporation of the sample to dryness, and by the peculiar taste of the residue. Sulphurous acid is sometimes detected by its characteristic odour; its determination is described on p. 177.

Caramel is recognised by extracting the solid residue with alcohol, and evaporating the solution to dryness; in its presence, the residue now obtained will possess a decidedly dark colour, and a bitter taste. Fuchsine, which

* Dingl. Poly. Journ., 256, p. 129.

is said to have been employed for colouring vinegar, is detected by the tests mentioned under Wine.

As already stated, a very large proportion of vinegar is made in the United States from spirituous liquors. It is probable that fully 90 per cent. of the total production is obtained by the acetification of whisky. Much of this product is mixed with cider vinegar, or simply coloured with caramel, and then put on the market as apple vinegar. It is certain that the manufacturers of whisky vinegar, who are permitted by law to make "low wines" on their premises, without being subjected to the usual Internal Revenue Tax, are frequently enabled to perpetrate a fraud on the Government by disposing of the spirits so produced to the whisky trade, instead of converting it wholly into vinegar. To so great an extent is this practice carried on, that many of the cider vinegar producers have found it impossible to successfully compete with the less scrupulous manufacturers. Whisky vinegar is nearly colourless, usually possesses a greater strength than cider vinegar, and is free from malic acid. Cider vinegar exhibits a light-brownish colour and a characteristic odour. Some of the differences between these two varieties are shown by the following results, obtained by the author by the examination of samples of pure apple and whisky vinegar, fresh from the factories :—

	Cider Vinegar.	Whisky Vinegar.
Specific gravity	1·0168	1·0107
Specific gravity of distillate from neutralised sample ..	0·9985	0·9973
Acetic acid	4·66 p. c.	7·36 p. c.
Total solids	2·70 ,,	0·15 ,,
Mineral ash	0·20 ,,	0·038 ,,
Potassa in ash	Considerable	None
Phosphoric acid in ash ..	Considerable	None
Heated with Fehling's solution	Copious reduction	No reduction
Treated with basic lead acetate	Flocculent precipitate	No precipitate

Naturally the addition of caramel or cider vinegar to whisky vinegar would greatly affect the above tests.

Attempts made to differentiate between the two samples by means of qualitative reactions for aldehyde and malic acid were not sufficiently distinctive in their results to be of much value.

It has been suggested that the presence of *nitrates* in vinegar would point to its origin from spirits. The apple vinegar manufacturer, however, frequently finds his product above the standard, in which case he reduces its strength by adding water, thus rendering this test of little or no avail.

Regarding the addition of mineral acids to vinegar in the United States, it is satisfactory to note that, of a large number of samples tested by the New York City Vinegar Inspector during the past year, not a single sample was found to contain these adulterants.

Fermented infusions of molasses, "black strap," etc., are occasionally employed in the manufacture of vinegar. The product obtained from these sources has been found in some instances to contain acrid and probably noxious ingredients.

PICKLES.

THE examination of pickles naturally includes a determination of the character of the vinegar used in their preparation.   This is made by the methods just described. The practice of imparting a bright green colour to pickles which have become bleached by long preservation in brine or by other means, is doubtless still prevalent, and calls for a brief notice.   The greening of pickles is effected either by the direct addition of cupric sulphate to the water in which they are heated, or by introducing some form of metallic copper into the bath.   Alum is stated to be also occasionally employed for the same purpose.   The presence of copper is readily detected by incinerating a rather considerable quantity of the pickles, treating the ash with a little nitric acid and adding an excess of ammonium hydroxide to the solution, when, in presence of the metal, a blue coloration will be produced.   The quantitative estimation of copper is made by boiling the residue, obtained by the evaporation of the vinegar or the incineration of the pickles, with dilute nitric acid, adding a small quantity of sulphuric acid and expelling the excess of nitric acid by evaporating nearly to dryness.   The solution is next diluted with water, filtered, and the filtrate placed in a platinum capsule.   The copper is then deposited by electrolysis.   In the Report of the Brooklyn Board of Health for the year 1885, a case is recorded where a child ate a portion of a pickle coloured with cupric sulphate (containing an estimated quantity of $2\frac{1}{2}$ grains of the salt), with fatal results.

OLIVE OIL.

OLIVE OIL is extracted from the pericarp of the fruit of the *Olea Europea*. When pure, it exhibits a pale yellow or greenish colour, has a specific gravity of 0·9176, and possesses a faint, pleasant odour and a bland and agreeable taste. It is insoluble in water, very slightly in alcohol, but dissolves in about 1½ parts of ether. Olive oil boils at 315°, and begins to deposit white granules at 10°; at 0°, it solidifies to a solid mass which, by pressure, may be separated into tripalmetine and trioleine. Upon saponification, it is decomposed into oleic, palmetic, and stearic acids and glycerine. The best-known varieties of olive oil met with in commerce, in the order of their quality, are— Provence, Florence, Lucca, Genoa, Gallipoli, Sicily, and Spanish.*

Owing to the high price of the pure article, and perhaps to the difficulty experienced in detecting foreign admixtures, olive oil is probably more extensively adulterated than any substance of general consumption. The oils most employed as adulterants are those of cotton-seed, poppy, pea-nut, sesamé, rape-seed, arachis, and lard. Although the subject of the adulteration of olive oil has received the attention of numerous chemists, including several of exceptionally high standing, the results obtained, while of service in indicating the presence of some foreign oil, are unfortunately often of but little use in the positive identification of the particular adulterant used. Of the

* It has been stated that American olive oil of superior excellence is made in the States of N.C., Miss. and Cal. ; but this product does not, as yet, appear to be generally known on the New York market.

many methods of examination that have been suggested, the following are the most satisfactory :—

1. *Specific gravity.*—The density of olive oil is lower than that of the majority of the oils with which it is mixed, and it is sometimes possible to detect the presence of the latter by means of this property, especially when they are contained in a considerable proportion. Cotton-seed oil differs more in specific gravity than the other oils generally employed as adulterants. Donny[*] applies the test by placing in the suspected sample a drop of olive oil of known purity which has been dyed with ground alkanet root, and observing whether it remains stationary. A more satisfactory method is to determine the density by the gravity bottle. The following tabulation gives the densities (at 15°) of olive and several other oils liable to be met with as admixtures :—

Olive oil	..	..	..	·914 to ·917
Poppy oil	..	..	..	·924 ,, ·927
Cotton-seed oil	..	..		·922 ,, ·930
Sweet almond oil..	..			·914 ,, ·920
Arachis oil	..	..	..	·916 ,, ·920
Colza oil	..	..	..	·914 ,, ·916
Sesamé oil	..	..	..	·921 ,, ·924
Rape-seed oil		..	..	·914 ,, ·916
Lard oil..	..	..	..	·915

2. *Solidifying point.*—Attempts have been made to utilise the fact that some of the oils added to olive congeal at a lower temperature than the pure oil. Thus, cotton-seed oil solidifies at −22°, ground-nut oil at −33°, poppy at −18°.

3. *Elaïdin and colour tests.*—Pure olive oil is converted into a solid mass when treated with various oxidising agents, the change being retarded by the presence of some of its adulterants. The test may be made in several ways :—

* Frens. Zeitsch. 3, 1864, p. 513.

(*a*) Ten grms. of the sample are shaken with 5 grms. of nitric acid (sp. gr. 1·40) and 1 grm. of mercury, and the colour produced and time required for solidification noticed. In this manner the following results have been obtained :—

Oil.	Coloration.	Minutes for Solidification.
Olive	Pale yellowish green	60
Almond	White	90
Arachis	Pale reddish	105
Rape	Orange	200
Cotton-seed	Orange red	105
Sesamé	Yellowish orange	150
Beech-nut	Reddish orange	360
Poppy	Red	Remains fluid.

(*b*) Or a few pieces of copper foil are added to a mixture of equal parts of the oil and nitric acid, the liquor occasionally stirred, and then set aside. If the oil be pure, it will be converted into a nearly white buttery mass in from three to six hours ; sesamé oil yields a red, cotton and rape-seed a brown, and beech-nut a reddish-yellow colour, the solidification being delayed from 10 to 20 hours, while poppy oil fails to solidify at all.

(*c*) Nine parts of the sample are oxidised by heating with one part of concentrated nitric acid, the mixture being well stirred ; pure olive oil forms a hard, pale-yellow mass in the course of two hours ; seed oils (including cotton-seed) turn orange-red in colour and do not become solid in the same time or manner.

(*d*) A portion of the sample is well mixed with one-fourth of its weight of chromic acid ; if pure, the oil will be converted into an opaque mass.

(*e*) Introduce 2 c.c. of the sample into a narrow graduated glass cylinder, add 0·1 gramme potassium dichromate, next 2 c.c. of a mixture of sulphuric and nitric acids, shake well, and then add 1 c.c. of ether ; shake again and allow the mixture to stand at rest. Lively effervescence and evolution of nitrous fumes soon take place, and the oil rises to the surface, showing a characteristic coloration. Olive oil exhibits a green colour, whereas in presence of 5 per cent. of sesamé, arachis, cotton-seed, or poppy oil, the colours will vary from greenish-yellow to yellow or yellowish red. The coloration is more readily observed upon agitating the mixture with water and setting it aside for a short time.

(*f*) Several portions of the oil are placed upon a porcelain slab and separately treated with a few drops of concentrated sulphuric acid, nitric acid, and a solution of potassium dichromate in sulphuric acid, and notice taken of the colours produced, comparative tests being simultaneously made with olive oil of undoubted purity.

(*g*) The presence of sesamé oil is readily detected by the formation of a deep green colour when the oil is agitated with a mixture of equal parts of nitric and sulphuric acid.

(*h*) Upon mixing samples containing cotton-seed oil with an equal volume of nitric acid (40° B.) a coffee-like colour is produced. Olive oil gives a pale green, rape and nut, a pale rose, and sesamé oil a white-coloured mixture.

The presence of rape- and cotton-seed oils may also be detected as follows :—Dissolve 0·1 gramme silver nitrate in a very little water, and add about 4 c.c. of absolute alcohol. This solution is added to the sample of olive oil to be tested, the mixture well shaken and put aside for one or two hours ; it is then to be heated for a few minutes. If cotton-seed or rape-seed oil is present, the oily stratum which separates on standing will exhibit a brownish-red or blackish colour, due to the reduction of silver. Olive oil fails to cause an appreciable coloration. Experiments made by the author with samples of olive oil containing 10 per cent. of cotton-seed and rape-seed oils furnished the following results:—On standing one hour, without heating, the mixture containing cotton-seed oil showed a slightly dark colour, that adulterated with rape-seed oil a decidedly dark colour; upon the application of heat, the former exhibited a dark-red colour, while the latter turned quite black.

Maumené's test.—This test is founded upon the fact that the elevation of temperature caused by mixing olive oil with strong sulphuric acid is considerably less than that produced with the oils commonly employed as its adulterants. With these latter an evolution of sulphurous acid generally takes place, which is not the case with pure olive oil. The best method of procedure is as follows:—10 c.c. of sulphuric acid (sp. gr. 1·844) are gradually added to 50 grammes of the sample, the mixture being constantly stirred with a small thermometer, and observations made of the maximum increase of temperature produced, as well as of the evolution of gas. When treated in this manner, genuine olive oil causes an elevation of about 42°; that given by various other oils, often added to it, ranges from 52° to 103°, and it is frequently possible to recognise their presence in admixtures by the high temperature produced. The following are the increases of temperature observed by L. Archbutt:—olive, 41–45; rape, 55–64; arachis, 47–60; sesamé, 65; cotton-seed (crude) 70; (refined), 75–76; poppy-seed, 86–88; menhaden, 123–128. In the Paris Municipal Laboratory an acid of 1·834 sp. gr. is used, and the following heating powers are regarded as standards:—For olive oil, 55·5°; for cotton-seed, 69·5° for nut, 62°; for sesamé, 66°; for poppy oil, 73°.

The application of Hubl's test for butter (see p. 75) is one of the most useful means for the detection of foreign oils in olive oil. The iodine absorption number of the pure oil is considerably below that of its most common adulterants.

The prevalence of the adulteration of olive oil has been abundantly demonstrated. Of 232 samples examined by the New York and Massachusetts State Boards of Health, 165 (71 per cent.) were spurious. It is a notorious fact that large quantities of cotton-seed oil are exported from the United States to France and Italy, much of which returns home under the guise of the genuine product of the olive.

MUSTARD.

MUSTARD is the product obtained by crushing and sifting the seeds of *Sinapis nigra* and *Sinapis alba*, of the genus Brassicaceæ. In the manufacture of the condiment, both the black and white seeds are used. According to analyses made by Piesse and Stansell,* fine grades of the two varieties of mustard possess the following composition :—

	Black Mustard.	White Mustard.
	per cent.	per cent.
Moisture	4·52	5·78
Fixed oil or fat	38·02	35·74
Cellulose	2·06	4·15
Sulphur	1·48	1·22
Nitrogen	5·01	4·89
Albuminoids	30·25	30·56
Myrosin and albumen	6·78	6·67
Soluble matter	32·78	36·60
Volatile oil	1·50	0·04
Potassium myronate	5·36	..
Ash	4.84	4.31
Soluble ash	0·98	0·55

Clifford Richardson regards the following proportions of the more prominent constituents of pure mustard flour as a basis for detecting adulterations :—

		Per cent.	
Water	5·00 to	10·00
Ash	4·00 „	6·00
Fixed oil	33·00 „	37·00
Volatile oil	0·25 „	1·00
Crude fibre	0·50 „	2·00
Nitrogen	4·50 „	6·00

The following results were obtained by Messrs. Waller

* 'Analyst,' 1880, p. 161.

and Martin from the examination of 14 samples of very low
grade dry mustard, as found on the New York market : *—

			Per cent.
Moisture, ranged from	..	.. ..	5·43 to 9·86
Fixed oil	,,	,, ...	6·81 ,, 22·56
Total ash	,,	,, ...	2·05 ,, 16·05
Soluble ash	,,	,, ...	0·15 ,, 2·90
Insoluble ash	,,	,, ...	1·69 ,, 13·15

Eight samples were coloured with turmeric, 4 with
Martius' yellow, 12 contained starch, and 5 showed the
presence of calcium sulphate.

The article usually sold as mustard is a mixture of
mustard farina, prepared from different varieties of the
seed, with wheaten flour or starch, and turmeric. It is
claimed by the manufacturers that pure mustard possesses
too acrid a taste to be suitable for use as a condiment;
and its admixture with the foregoing substances is so
generally resorted to and recognised, that the New York
State Board of Health, in 1883, legally sanctioned the
practice, provided the fact is distinctly stated upon the
label of the packages. Other prevalent forms of sophistication consist in the partial extraction of the fixed
oil from the mustard before its introduction on the market,
and in the addition of cocoa-nut shells, *terra alba*, and
"Martius' yellow" (potassium dinitronaphthalate). The
latter colouring matter is specially objectionable, being
poisonous in its action. The presence of organic admixtures is usually recognised upon a microscopic examination of the sample. The anatomical structure of mustard
seed is described by Fluckigen and Hamburg in 'Pharma-
cographia.' Wheaten flour or starch is readily identified
by the iodine test. The following methods are employed
for the detection of turmeric :—

1. A portion of the sample is agitated with castor oil
and filtered. In case turmeric is present, the filtrate will
exhibit a marked greenish fluorescence.

* ' Analyst,' ix. p. 166.

2. Upon treating the suspected sample with ammonium hydroxide, an orange-red colour is produced in presence of turmeric. Or, the mustard is boiled with methylic alcohol, the extract filtered, evaporated to dryness, and the residue treated with hydrochloric acid ; if turmeric be present, an orange-red coloration takes place, which changes to a bluish-green upon adding an excess of sodium hydroxide. In addition to the above qualitative tests, valuable indications regarding the purity of mustard are to be obtained by the determination of the proportions of fixed oil, sulphur, and ash contained in the sample under examination.

Fixed Oil.—The amount of fixed oil is estimated by digesting a weighed portion of the mustard with ether in a closed vessel, filtering, and determining the weight of the residue left upon evaporating the ethereal solution to dryness over the water-bath. The oil possesses a specific gravity ranging from 0·915 to 0·920. The percentage of fixed oil in pure mustard is very considerable (usually over 34 per cent.), whereas the substances commonly added contain but a very small quantity. In case wheaten flour has been employed as an adulterant, the proportion of pure mustard (x) in a mixed sample, can be approximately calculated by the following formulæ, in which y is the fixed amount of oil contained.[*]

$$\frac{33\cdot9x}{100} + \frac{1\cdot2(100-x)}{100} = y,$$
$$\frac{36\cdot7x}{100} + \frac{2\cdot(100-x)}{100} = y.$$

In the absence of flour, a low percentage of fixed oil indicates the presence of exhausted mustard cake.

Sulphur.—Blyth determines the total sulphur by oxidation with fuming nitric acid, diluting the liquid considerably with water, filtering and precipitating the sulphates formed by means of barium chloride. The proportion of sulphates

[*] Blyth, op. cit.

R

(in terms of barium sulphate) found in the ash is to be
deducted from the weight of the precipitate obtained; the
remainder, multiplied by 0·1373, gives the amount of sulphur present in organic combination, and, as the quantity
contained in this form in mustard is far greater than in any
of the substances employed for its adulteration, the estimation is frequently very useful.

Ash.—The amount of ash is determined in the usual
manner, *i.e.* by the incineration of a weighed portion in
a platinum capsule. Genuine mustard contains about 5 per
cent. of ash, of which nearly 1 per cent. is soluble in water.
In presence of inorganic impurities, the quantity of ash is
naturally increased, while a proportion under 4 per cent. is
usually considered an indication of organic admixture.

The composition of the ash of mustard seed is given
below :—

						Per cent.
Potassa	..	..	..	..	..	16·15
Lime ..	..	..	..	..	..	19·24
Magnesia ..		..	..	..	..	10·51
Ferric oxide	..	..	..	..	..	0·99
Phosphoric acid		..	..	..	..	39·92
Sulphuric acid ..		..	..	..	..	4·92
Chlorine	..	..	..	..	..	0·53
Silica ..	..	..	..	..	..	2·48

The adulteration of mustard is very extensively practised.
Of 18 samples bought at random in the shops and tested for
the New York State Board of Health, 12 were found to be
impure ; of 88 samples, examined in the year 1884 by the
Massachusetts State Board, 20 were compounds (labelled
as such, but in a manner designed to deceive the purchaser).
37 were adulterated with flour, turmeric, and, in some cases,
with cayenne, and 31 were found to be pure ; in 1885, 211
samples were tested, of which 124 were sophisticated ; of
27 samples tested by the National Board of Health, 21
contained foreign admixtures, consisting chiefly of wheat
or flour and turmeric, but also including corn-starch, rice,
cayenne, and plaster of Paris.

PEPPER.

BLACK PEPPER is the dried unripe berry of *Piper nigrum ;* white pepper, which is much less in use, being the same fruit deprived of its outer skin by maceration in water and friction. The more important constituents of pepper are an alkaloid (piperin), the volatile oil, and the resin, and upon these ingredients its value as a condiment depends. The partial composition of genuine pepper, as given by Blyth, is shown below :—

Variety.	Moisture.	Piperin.	Resin.	Aqueous Extract.	Ash.	
					Soluble.	Total.
	per cent.	per cent.	per cent.	per cent.	per cent.	per cent.
Penang	9·53	5·57	2·08	18·33	2·21	4·18
Tellicherry	12·90	4·67	1·70	16·50	3·38	5·77
Sumatra	10·10	4·70	1·74	17·59	2·62	4·31
Malabar	10·54	4·63	1·74	20·37	3·45	5·19

The percentages of piperin, resin, extract, and ash are calculated on the sample dried at 100°. König's analysis of pepper is as follows :—

	Per cent.
Water	17·01
Nitrogenous substances	11·99
Volatile oil	1·12
Fat	8·82
Other non-nitrogenous substances	42·02
Cellulose	14·49
Ash	4·57 to 5·00

Heisch * has analysed several varieties of pure and commercial pepper, with the following results:—

	Water.	Total Ash.	Ash Soluble in Water.	Ash Soluble in Acid.	Ash Insoluble.	Alkalinity as K_2O.	Starch.	Alcoholic Extract.	Piperin.
	per cent.	per cent.	per cent.	per cent.	per cent.	per cent.	per cent.	per cent.	per cent.
Black berry .. .. {	9·22 to 14·36	4·35 to 8·99	1·54 to 3·34	1·51 to 3·83	0·36 to 4·38	0·72 to 1·57	48·53 to 56·67	10·47 to 16·20	4·05 to 9·38
White berry.. .. {	13·67 to 17·32	1·28 to 8·78	0·217 to 0·618	0·84 to 2·80	0·22 to 0·69	0· to 0·22	76·27 to 77·68	9·23 to 9·73	5·13 to 6·14
Fine ground (white)	13·90	1·58	0·16	0·90	0·52	0·0	75·31	10·66	4·51
Long pepper ..	12·15	13·48	2·28	5·52	5·68	0·53	58·78	8·29	1·71
Adulterated ground	11·12	14·70	2·02	4·07	8·61	0·78	35·85	11·57	2·02

The same authority regards 50 per cent. of starch as the minimum standard for unadulterated pepper. The granules of pepper-starch are characterised by their exceedingly small size, being only about ·008 mm. in diameter.

The proportion of ash in genuine pepper seldom exceeds 7 per cent., of which not over $\frac{1}{10}$th should consist of sand; but in the commercial article, the total ash often approximates 10 or 12 per cent., 40 or 50 per cent. of which is sand and other insoluble substances.

COMPOSITION OF PEPPER ASH.

Potassa	31·36
Soda	4·56
Magnesia	16·34
Lime	14·59
Ferric oxide	0·38
Phosphoric acid	10·85
Sulphuric acid	12·09
Chlorine	9·52

The list of adulterations used as admixtures to pepper, as well as to most other ground condiments and spices, is quite extensive, and includes such cheap and neutral substances

* 'Analyst,' 1886, p. 186.

as ship-bread, corn, ground cocoanut shells, beans, peas, hulls of mustard seed, sand, etc., etc. It is stated that in England large quantities of preparations consisting of linseed-meal, mustard husks and rice-meal, known to the trade respectively as P.D., H.P.D., and W.P.D., are very generally employed in the adulteration of pepper. P.D. (pepper-dust), would appear to also signify the sweepings collected from pepper factories, and sometimes fortified with cayenne, the manufacture of which article has given rise to a special industry. It is utilised as a diluent of the various spices, the sophisticated products being sold as "P.D. pepper," "P.D. cloves," "P.D. cinnamon," etc. Unfortunately the character of most of the adulterants of pepper, as of other spices, is such, that little assistance is afforded the analyst by chemical tests. A microscopic examination of the suspected sample furnishes far more trustworthy information and should in all instances be employed, comparative observations being made with an article of known purity.

The appearance of several of the starch granules of various flours often found in adulterated condiments and spices is represented in Plate IX.

In the special case of pepper, it is of advantage to make chemical determinations of the moisture, ash, piperin and resin.

Moisture.—The proportion of moisture is estimated by the ordinary method of drying a weighed portion of the pepper in a platinum capsule at 100°, and noting the loss in weight sustained.

Ash.—The dry sample is incinerated, and the amount of mineral residue determined. As already intimated, the proportion of sand present is of especial import.

Piperin and Resin.—The pepper is repeatedly digested with absolute alcohol, the mixture filtered and the filtrate evaporated to dryness over a water-bath. The extract is weighed and then treated with sodium hydroxide solution, in which the resin is soluble. The alkaline liquid is then removed, and the remaining piperin dissolved in alcohol, the solution filtered, evaporated to dryness, and the weight of the residue determined. The proportion of piperin in unadulterated pepper ranges from 4·5 to 5·5 per cent., that of resin from 1·7 to 2 per cent.

Niederstadt,[*] from the results of his investigations, concludes, that genuine pepper should yield as much as 7·66 per cent. of piperin, and employs this factor for estimating the purity of mixtures; thus, a sample adulterated with palm kernels and husks, to the extent of about 80 per cent., contained but 1·62 per cent. of piperin.

Pepper contains a greater proportion of starch than some of the substances employed in its adulteration. The following method, suggested by Lenz,[†] may be used for the determination of this constituent :—4 grammes of the sample are digested for several hours in a flask with 250 c.c. of water, with occasional shaking, and the decoction decanted upon a filter. The residue is washed and returned to the flask, which is filled with water to a volume of 200 c.c., 20 c.c. of hydrochloric acid (sp. gr. 1·121) are added, the flask connected with an ascending Liebig's condenser, and heated on the water-bath for three hours. After cooling, the contents of the flask are filtered into a half-litre flask, and the filtrate carefully neutralised with sodium hydroxide and diluted up to the 500 c.c. mark. It is finally tested by Fehling's solution. The clarification of the hot solution is assisted by the addition of a few drops of zinc chloride. Lenz obtained by this process the following percentages of sugar, calculated on the ash-free substances :—

Black pepper	..	..	..	..	..	52
White pepper	..	..	..	..	..	60
Palm-nut meal	..	..	..	..	..	22·6
Pepper husks	..	..	..	..	..	16·3

---

* Rép. anal. Chem., iii. p. 68.
† Zeit. f. anal. Chem., 1884, p. 501.

The application of this method to the examination of commercial American peppers, when they contain as adulterants substances rich in starch, is obviously of little value. A sample of German pepper, sold as "*Pfefferbruch*," recently analysed by Hilger,[*] had the following composition :—

				Per cent.
Pepper husks ..	..	..	..	50
Palm nut meal	..	..	..	30
Pepper dust ..	..	..	..	15
Paprika	..	..	..	1
Brick-dust ..	..	..	..	4

Cayenne Pepper.—Cayenne pepper is the ground berry and pods of *Capsicum annuum*. Its well-known active properties, which were formerly ascribed to an acrid oil termed *capsicin*, have lately been shown to be due to the presence of the crystalline compound *capsaicin* ($C_9H_{14}O_3$), fusing at 55°, and capable of volatilisation at 115° without decomposition. The proportion of moisture in cayenne pepper is about 12 per cent.; the alcoholic and ethereal extracts should approximate, respectively, 25 and 9 per cent. The ash ranges from 5·5 to 6 per cent., of which nearly one-half should be soluble in water. Strohmer [†] has analysed Hungarian cayenne, known as "Paprika"; his results were as follows :—

	Seeds.	Husks.	Entire Fruit.
	per cent.	per cent.	per cent.
Water and volatile matter at 100°	8·12	14·75	11·94
Nitrogenous substances, as protein	18·31	10·69	13·88
Fat	28·54	5·48	15·26
Ethereal extract (free of nitrogen)	24·33	38·73	32·63
Fibre	17·50	23·73	21·09
Ash	3·20	6·62	5·20
Nitrogen	2·93	1·71	2·22

[*] Archiv. der Pharm., 233, p. 825.
[†] Chem. Centralb., 1884, p. 577.

A commercial brand of the same article had the following composition :—

	Per cent.
Volatile at 100°	12·69
Nitrogenous substances, as protein	13·19
Ethereal extract	13·35
Ash	7·14

The organic adulterants sometimes met with in cayenne (flour, mustard seed, husks, etc.), are detected by means of the microscope. Among the mineral substances said to be employed as colouring agents, such as iron ochre, brick-dust, red lead, and vermilion, the two former are of more frequent occurrence, and may be recognised upon an examination of the ash obtained by the incineration of the sample.

An adulterant of pepper, known in the trade as "Poiv-rette" or "Pepperette," has recently made its appearance in England. It forms a cream-coloured powder, much resembling the inner layer of the pepper-berry in bulk and cellular structure, is exported from Italy, and evidently consists of ground olive-stones, as is indicated by the following analyses, made by J. Campbell Brown : *—

	Ash.	Matters Soluble by boiling in Dilute Acid.	Albuminous and other matters Soluble in Alkali.	Woody Fibre Insoluble in Acid and Alkali.	Starch.
White pepperette	1·33	38·32	14·08	48·48	None
Black pepperette.. ..	2·47	34·55	17·66	47·69	,,
Ground almond shells ..	2·05	23·53	24·79	51·68	,,
Ground olive stones	1·61	39·08	15·04	45·38	,,

The extent to which the various forms of pepper are fraudulently contaminated in the United States is illustrated by the fact that, out of 386 samples of the condiment examined by the chemists of the New York, Massachusetts and National State Boards of Health, 236 (or about 61 per cent.) were found to be adulterated.

* 'Analyst,' Feb. 1887, p. 23 ; Mar. p. 47.

SPICES.

As is the case with mustard and pepper, the adulteration of the ordinary spices is exceedingly prevalent in the United States. Probably those most subject to admixture, are cloves, mace, cinnamon, allspice, and ginger. The fact that these condiments are frequently offered for sale in a ground state furnishes an opportunity to incorporate with them various cheaper vegetable substances, of which the manufacturer too often makes use. For the detection of these additions the use of the microscope is of pre-eminent importance ; and, in this regard, no more useful information could be afforded than by quoting the following remarks, furnished to the author by Clifford Richardson, Assistant Chemist of the United States Department of Agriculture, who has lately made a valuable contribution to the literature of spice adulteration.*

" Spices consist of certain selected parts of aromatic or pungent plants possessing a characteristic anatomical structure and proximate composition which, when they have been carefully studied and recorded, serve as a means of recognising the pure substances when under examination, and distinguishing them from the different structure and composition of the adulterants which have been added to them.

" To carry on an investigation of this description a limited knowledge of botanical physiology (as well as of proximate chemical analysis) is therefore necessary. For the physiological part, the use of the microscope, as a means of determining structure, is necessary.

" The structure of the plant parts which constitute the spices and their adulterants as well, is characterised by the

* Bulletin No. 13, Part 2, Chemical Division ; United States Department of Agriculture.

presence or absence of different forms of cells and of starch, and their relative arrangement. At least, this is as far as it is necessary to go from the analyst's point of view. By studies of sections of pure whole spices one must become familiar with the forms usually met with in the spices and those which are prominent in adulterants and be able to recognise the presence of starch and by the character of the granules to determine their source.

" The common forms of cells which are met with in the spices, and with which one should be familiar, are known as parenchyma cells, sclerenchyma cells, those of fibro-vascular bundles, spiral and dotted cells, and those of peculiar form in the cortex and epidermis.

" *Parenchyma* consists of thin-walled cells, such as are well illustrated in the interior of a corn-stalk and are found in the centre of the pepper kernel. They are often filled with starch, as in the cereals and pepper, but at times are without it, as in the mustard seed.

" *Sclerenchyma*, or stone cells, are of a ligneous character, their walls being greatly thickened. They are commoner in the adulterants than in the spices, and are well illustrated in the shell of the cocoa-nut, in clove stems, and a few are seen in pepper hulls.

" *Spiral and Dotted Cells* are found in woody tissue, and their characteristics are denoted by their names. They are more commonly found in adulterants, and their presence in large amounts is conclusive, in many instances, of impurity. They may be seen in sections of cedar-wood and in cocoa-nut shells, and to a small extent in pepper husks.

" *The Fibro-vascular Bundles*, as their name implies, are aggregations which appear to the eye, in some instances, as threads running through the tissue of the plant. They are easily seen in the cross-section of the corn-stalk, and are common in ground ginger, having resisted comminution from their fibrous nature. They are made up of cells of various forms.

" *The Cells of the Cortex and Epidermis* are in many cases extremely characteristic in form, and of great value for distinguishing the origin of the substances under examination. They are too numerous in shape to be particularly described, and are well illustrated in the husk of mustard, and the pod of *Capsicum* or cayenne.

"Other forms of tissue are also met with, but not so prominently as to render it advisable to burden the memory with them at first, or to seek them before they are met.

"These forms of cells and their combinations which have been described, present in addition some peculiarities, aside from their structure, which assist in distinguishing them.

" Parenchyma is optically inactive, and is not stained by iodine solution, except in so far as its contents are concerned. Sclerenchyma, the stone cell, is optically active, and in the dark field of the microscope, with crossed Nicols, appears as shining silvery cells, displaying their real structure. The fibro-vascular bundles are stained yellowish brown by iodine, and are thus differentiated from the surrounding tissue.

"Starch is stained a deep blue, or blue black, by iodine solution, and since the contents of the parenchyma cells often consist of much starch, the parenchyma in these cases seems to assume this colour.

"To distinguish some of the peculiarities of structure which have been mentioned requires some little practice and skill, but not more than is readily acquired with a short experience. There are however some aids which should not be neglected.

" In the ground spices it will be found more difficult to recognise the anatomy of the parts than in a carefully prepared section. The hardest parts are often the largest particles, and scarcely at all transparent. The mounting of the material in water or glycerine will render them more so, but it is necessary to employ some other means of which two are available. A solution of chloral hydrate in water, 8 to 5, serves after 24 hours to make the particles less

obscure.   In many instances also, it has been found
advisable to bleach the deep colour by Schulze's method,
using nitric acid of 1·1 sp. gr. and chlorate of potash.
When this is done, hard tissue is broken down and rendered
transparent where otherwise nothing could be seen.   As
examples, olive stones and cocoa-nut shells will serve.
Without treatment little can be made out of their structure.

"Of course, it is plain that the detection of starch must be
in a portion of the material which has received no treatment, and that progress must be made from the least to
the most violent reagents.

"For this work an elaborate microscope is unnecessary.
It should, for work with starches, have objectives of ½ and
⅕ inch equivalent focus, arrangements for polarising light,
and if possible, a condenser system.   Many good stands are
to-day made at reasonable prices which will serve the
purpose."

The microscopical appearance of various starches in
polarised light is shown in Plate IX.   Plate XII. exhibits
several spices, under polarised light, in a pure and adulterated state.   Those represented are :—

Ginger, pure, and adulterated with foreign starch.

Cinnamon and Cassia ; the pure barks, ground, showing
the relative greater frequency of fibro-vascular bundles in
the former.

Cayenne, pure, and adulterated with rice starch.

The chemical analysis of spices, although usually of
minor importance, often serves to confirm the results
secured by aid of the microscope.   The principal determinations required are the ash, oil, starch, and sugar.   The
more common forms of spice adulteration are the following :—

Cloves.—This spice is said to be sometimes deprived of
its volatile oil before being put on the market.   In the
genuine article the proportion of oil seldom falls below
17 per cent. The oil is readily estimated by distilling the sus-

PLATE XII

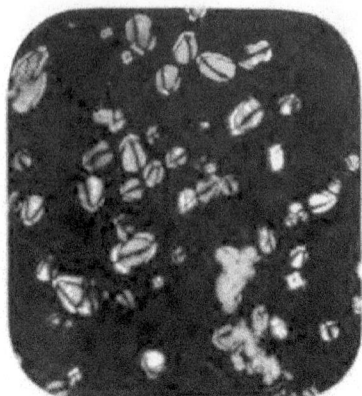

Ginger Starch.

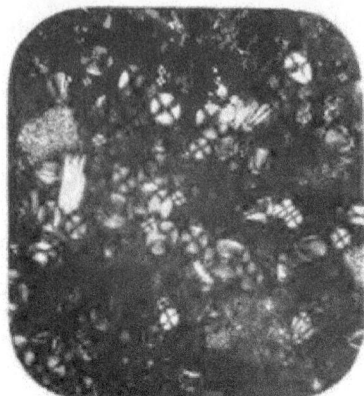

Ginger Adulterated.

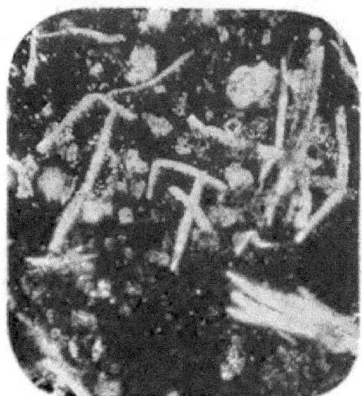

Cinnamon.

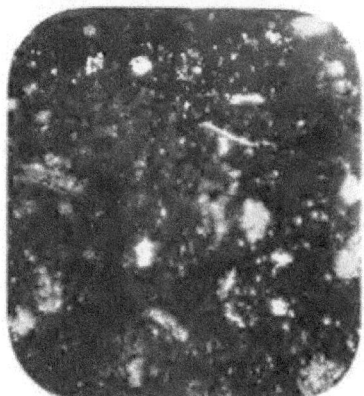

Cassia.

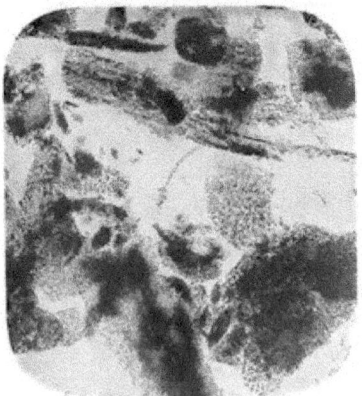

Cayenne.

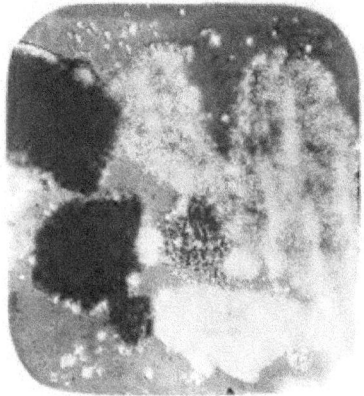

Cayenne Adulterated.

SPICES.

pected sample with water. The usual adulterants of ground cloves consist of clove-stems, allspice, flour and burnt shells.

Mace.—True mace is frequently mixed with the false spice, the presence of which is indicated by its dark-red colour. The other foreign substances most commonly used are turmeric, wheaten flour, rice, corn meal, and roasted beans.

Cinnamon.—The chief admixtures to be sought for are cassia, ground shells, crackers, etc.

Allspice.—Owing to its cheapness, allspice is probably less adulterated than the preceding spices. The addition of mustard-husks, ground shells, and clove stems, and the removal of the volatile oil, are, however, sometimes practised. The oil in genuine allspice should amount to about 5 per cent.

Ginger.—Ginger is likewise comparatively little exposed to sophistication, although it has occasionally been found coloured with turmeric, and admixed with corn meal, mustard-husks, cayenne, and clove stems. It is stated that the manufacturers of ginger extract dispose of the exhausted article to spice dealers who utilise the impoverished product for the adulteration of other spices.

Mixed Spices.—These consist of mixtures of the foregoing, and are liable to the sophistications practised upon their ingredients, the addition of the cheaper flours and starches being especially prevalent.

The following table shows the results of the examination of various spices, lately officially made in the States of New York and Massachusetts, and by the National Board of Health in Washington :—

	Number Examined.	Number Adulterated.	Percentage Adulterated.
Cloves	132	60	45·5
Mace	79	50	66·3
Cinnamon	149	78	52·4
Allspice	90	39	43·3
Ginger	157	40	25·4

MISCELLANEOUS.

A VARIETY of articles of food, which do not properly come
under any of the heads previously treated, have, during
the past few years, been found on our markets in an adulterated state.   Prominent among these, are the various
kinds of canned meats, fruits, and vegetables, which have
not unfrequently been the cause of serious cases of illness.
This result may be owing to the original bad condition of
the goods, or to fermentation having taken place ; but, in
many instances, the trouble has been traced to the improper
methods of canning used, resulting in the contamination of
the preserved articles with metallic poisons.   The fact that
fermentation has occurred is frequently indicated by the
external appearance of the head of the can, which, in this
case, will be slightly convex, instead of being, as it should
be, concave.   The metals most often detected in canned
goods are lead, tin, and copper.   The presence of lead is
usually due to the use of an impure grade of tin, known as
"terne-plate," in the manufacture of the cans, or to care-
lessness in the soldering process.   The origin of copper is
probably to be found in the methods sometimes practised
of heating the goods in vessels made of this metal previous
to canning them.   The presence of tin results from the
action of partially decomposed fruits and vegetables upon
the can.   Preserved fruits and jellies are sometimes put up
in unsealed tin pails or cans, when they almost invariably
contain notable amounts of this metal.

Asparagus seems to be especially liable to contamination
with metals, doubtless owing to the formation of aspartic
acid.   As much as half a gramme of tin has been found in

a quart can of this vegetable. The use of zinc chloride as a flux in soldering, has, to the writer's knowledge, occasioned the presence of an appreciable proportion of the salt in canned goods.

Of 109 samples of canned food lately examined by our health officials, 97 contained tin; 39, copper; 4, zinc; and 2 lead. In the analysis of food of this description, the organic matters are first destroyed by heating with oxidising agents, such as a mixture of potassium chlorate and hydrochloric acid. The solution is then evaporated to a small volume. It is next diluted with water, and tested with sulphuretted hydrogen, ammonium sulphide, and the usual reagents.

Messrs. Waller and Martin have made an investigation in regard to the proportion of copper which may be present in various natural grains and vegetables. Their results show that these plants frequently take up a minute quantity of this metal from the soil. The amounts of copper found were as follows :—

	Parts of copper per million.
Raw wheat and other grains, from	4· to 10·8
Green cucumbers	2·5
„ peas	3·1
„ pea pods	1·0

The following proportions were detected in canned vegetables :—

Pickles	29 to 91
Peas	79 „ 190
Beans	87 „ 100

Meat extracts, while not subjected to adulteration, have acquired a popular reputation as articles of food which is not always deserved. As stimulants and useful adjuncts to food proper for invalids, the value of these preparations is undoubted. The chemical composition of several of the best known brands, as determined by American and English health officials, is given below :—

Brand.	Water.	Organic Substance.	Ash.	Soluble Albumin.	Alcoholic Extract.	Phosphoric Acid.	Potassa.
	per cent.	per cent.	per cent.	per cent.	per cent.	per cent.	per cent.
Liebig's extract	18·27	58·40	23·25	0·05	44·11	7·83	10·18
Berger's extract of beef ..	40·65	39·85	19·50	1·11	13·18	..	..
Starr's extract of beef ..	37·00	55·65	7·35	1·10	10·13	..	..
Johnson's fluid beef	41·20	50·40	8·40	1·17	15·93	1·91	1·72
Gaunt's beef peptone ..	37·15	54·92	7·43	0·00	20·14	..	..
London Co.'s extract of beef	81·90	16·80	1·30	..	..	..	..
London Co.'s extract of mutton	78·00	19·50	2·50	..		..	
London Co.'s extract of chicken	71·60	27·10	1·30	..	..	..	..
Brand's essence of beef ..	89·19	9·50	1·31	..	..	0·19	0·20
Carnrick's beef peptonoids	6·75	87·75	5·50	..	..	1·27	1·33
Kemmerick's extract of beef	20·95	60·81	18·24	..	..	6·56	8·30
Murdoch's liquid food ..	83·61	15·83	0·56	..		0·10	4·17
Savory and Moore's fluid meat	27·01	60·89	12·10	..		1·49	4·20
Valentine's meat juice ..	50·67	29·41	11·52	..	..	3·76	5·11

The factitious manufacture of jellies has lately excited considerable attention. Many of the more expensive kinds of this article are imitated by mixtures consisting largely of apple jelly.

A brand of spurious currant jelly, which is manufactured in France, and has recently made its appearance on the American market, is prepared from a gelatinous seaweed found in Japan (*Arachnoidiscus Japonicus*), to which glucose, tartaric acid, and an artificial essence of currants are added, the desired colour being obtained by means of cochineal and *Althea roseata*. The product is offered for sale at five cents a pound.

The flour employed in the manufacture of the maccaroni and vermicelli commonly met with in our larger cities, is not always of good quality. A more serious form of adulteration consists in the artificial colouring of these preparations. The substances used for this purpose, which have been detected by the public authorities, are turmeric, saffron, and chrome yellow. Meat has been found tinted with aniline red, and Bologna sausages, coated with iron pigments, have occasionally been encountered.

The flavouring syrups used in connection with the popular American beverage, "soda water," frequently consist almost wholly of glucose and artificial compound ethers. Dr. Cyrus Edson, of the New York City Board of Health, has lately directed public notice to the fact that many manufacturers of soda water use water obtained from artesian wells, which are driven on their premises, and which, from the nature of the geological formation of Manhattan Island, are very liable to contain sewage contamination.

APPENDIX.

BIBLIOGRAPHY.

THE literature of Food Adulteration has acquired such extensive proportions during the past few years, that a complete list of the memoirs which have been contributed to scientific journals would alone form a moderately sized volume. In the following pages the more important periodicals, official reports, etc., are mentioned, together with a chronological catalogue of the works on Adulteration and allied subjects.

Periodicals.

Zeitschrift für Untersuchung von Lebensmittel. Eichstatt.
Zeitschrift gegen Verfälschung der Lebensmittel. Leipzig.
The Analyst. London, from 1877 to date.
The Food Journal. London, 1870 to 1874.
The Sanitary Engineer. New York, 1877 to date.
Food, Water, and Air in relation to the Public Health. London, 1872.
Jacobson's Chemisch-techniches Repertorium. 1862 to date.
Repertorium der Analytischen Chemie. 1881.
Schäfer's Wieder die Nahrungsfälscher. Hanover, 1878.
Biederman's Centralblatt. 1880 to date.
Zeitschrift für Analytische Chemie. 1862 to date.
Wagner's Jahresberichte. 1880 to date.
American Analyst. New York, 1884 to date.
Vierteljahresschrift der Chemie der Nahrungs- und Genussmittel. Berlin, 1887.

Reports.

Reports of the Select Committee on Adulteration of Food. London, 1855, 1856, 1872, 1874.
Canadian Reports on the Adulteration of Food. Ottawa, 1876 to date.
First and Second Reports of the Municipal Laboratory of Paris.

Annual Reports of the National Academy of Sciences. Washington, 1882 to date.
Annual Reports of the National Board of Health. Washington, 1881 to date.
Annual Reports of the State Boards of Health of New York, New Jersey, Massachusetts, and Michigan. 1882 to date.
Annual Reports of the New York State Dairy Commissioner. 1885-1886.
Annual Reports of the Inspector of Wines and Liquors to the Commonwealth of Massachusetts. 1876 to date.
Annual Reports of the New York City Board of Health. 1871, 1873.
Annual Reports of the Brooklyn Board of Health.
Bulletins of the Chem. Div., U.S. Dept. of Agriculture.

Special Technical Journals.

Milk Journal. London.
Milch-Zeitung.
La Sucrerie Indigène. Compiègne.
Jahresbericht über die Untersuchungen und Fortschritte auf dem Gesammtgebiete der Zuckerfabrikation.
Wochenschrift für die Zuckerfabrikanten. Braunschweig.
Zeitschrift für Zuckerindustrie. Prag.
The Sugar Cane. Manchester.
Der Bierbrauer. Leipzig.
Der Amerikanische Bierbrauer. New York.
Le Brasseur. La Sedan.
Bayerischer Bierbrauer. München.
Norddeutsche Brauer-Zeitung. Berlin.
The Western Brewer. Chicago and New York.
The Brewer's Gazette. New York.
The Brewer's Journal. London.
Le Moniteur de la Brasserie. Bruxelles.

Important articles on Food Adulteration and Analysis are contained in the following general works of reference :—

Watts' Dictionary of Chemistry.
Spons' Encyclopædia of Arts, Manufactures, etc.
Muspratt's Encyclopædia of Chemistry.
Lippincott's Encyclopædia of Chemistry.
Ure's Dictionary of Chemistry.
Gmelin's Handbook of Chemistry.
Cooley's Practical Receipts.
Wurtz's Dictionnaire de Chimie.

General Works, chronologically arranged.

Boyle, Medicina Hydrostatica. London, 1690.

Sande, Les falsifications des médicaments dévoilées. La Haye, 1784.

Fraise, Alimentation publique. Anvers, 1803.

Favre, De la sophistication des substances médicamenteuses et des moyens de la reconnaître. Paris, 1812.

Accum, A Treatise on Adulteration of Foods and Culinary Poisons. London, 1820.

Ebermayer, Manuel des pharmaciens et des droguistes. Paris, 1821.

Culbrush, Lectures on the Adulteration of Food and Culinary Poisons. Newbury, 1823.

Branchi, Sulla falsificazione delle sostanze specialmente medicinali e sui mezzi atti ad scoprirli. Pisa, 1823.

Desmarest, Traité des falsifications. Paris, 1827.

Bussy et Boutron-Charlard, Traité des moyens de reconnaître les falsifications des drogues. Paris, 1829.

Walchner, Darstellung der wichtigsten im bürgerlichen Leben vorkommenden Verfälschungen der Nahrungsmittel und Getränke. Karlsruhe, 1840.

——, Darstellung der wichtigsten, bis jetzt erkannten Verfälschungen der Arzneimittel und Droguen. Karlsruhe, 1841.

Brum, Hilfsbuch bei Untersuchungen der Nahrungsmittel und Getränke. Wien, 1842.

Pereira, A Treatise on Food and Diet. London, 1843.

Richter, Die Verfälschung der Nahrungsmittel und anderer Lebensbedürfnisse. Gotha, 1843.

Garnier, Des falsifications des substances alimentaires, et des moyens de les reconnaître. Paris, 1844.

Trebuschet, Exposé des recherches du Conseil de Salubrité de Paris. Paris, 1845.

Bertin, Sophistication des substances alimentaires, et moyens de les reconnaître. Nantes, 1846.

Beck, Adulterations of various substances used in Medicine and in the Arts. New York, 1846.

Friederich, Handbuch der Gesundheitspolizei. Ansbach, 1846.

Duflos, Die wichtigsten Lebensbedürfnisse, ihre Aechtheit, Güte, und Verunreinigungen, etc. Breslau, 1846.

Acam, Traité des falsifications des substances médicamenteuses, &c. Anvers, 1848.

Batilliat, Traité sur les Vins de France. Paris, 1848.

Mitchell, Treatise on the Adulteration of Food. London, 1848.

Pedroni, Manuel complet des falsifications des drogues, simples et composées. Paris, 1848.

Normandy, Commercial Handbook of Chemical Analysis. London, 1850.

Cottereau, Des altérations et des falsifications du vin et des moyens physiques et chimiques employés pour les reconnaître. Paris, 1850.

Dungerville, Traité des falsifications des substances alimentaires, etc. Paris, 1850.

Marcet, Composition, Adulteration, and Analysis of Foods. London, 1850.

Tauber, Verfälschung der Nahrungstoffe und Arzneimittel. Wien, 1851.

Chevallier et Baudrimont, Dictionnaire des altérations et falsifications des substances alimentaires, etc., avec l'indication des moyens pour les reconnaître. Paris, 1851.

Büchner, Die Baierische Bierbrauerei und ihre Geheimnisse. Leipzig, 1852.

McMullen, Handbook of Wines. New York, 1852.

Pierce, Examination of Drugs, Medicines, Chemicals, etc., as to their Purity and Adulterations. Cambridge, U.S., 1852.

Fop, Adulteration of Food. London, 1853.

Moleschott, Lehre der Nahrungsmittel für das Volk. Erlangen, 1853.

Gille, Falsifications des substances alimentaires. Paris, 1853.

Babo, Von dem Weinbau. 1855.

Bureaux, Histoire des falsifications des substances alimentaires. Paris, 1855.

Hassall, Food and its Adulteration. 1855 (there are several later editions).

How, Adulteration of Food and Drink. London, 1855.

Klencke, Die Nahrungsmittelfrage in Deutschland. Leipzig, 1855.

Fresenius, Auffindung unorganischer Gifte in Speisen. Braunschweig, 1856.

Ganeau, Altérations et falsifications des farines. Lille, 1856.

Dodd, The Food of London. London, 1856.

Gall, Praktische Anweisung sehr gute Mittelweine aus unreifen Trauben zu erzeugen. Trier, 1856.

Payen, Des substances alimentaires. Paris, 1856.

Trommer, Die Kuhmilch in Bezug auf ihre Verdünnung und Verfälschungen. Berlin, 1857.

Dalton, Adulteration of Food. London, 1857.

Bouchardet et Quevenne, Du Lait. Paris, 1857.

Müller, Die Chemie des Bieres. Leipzig, 1858.

Klencke, Die Verfälschung der Nahrungsmittel und Getränke. Leipzig, 1858.

Vernois, Du Lait, chez la femme dans l'état de santé et dans l'état de maladie. Paris, 1858.

Petit, Instructions simplifiées pour la constatation des propriétés des principales denrées alimentaires. Bordeaux, 1858.

Müller, Anleitung zur Prüfung der Kuhmilch. Bern, 1858.

Souillier, Des substances alimentaires, de leur qualité, de leur falsification, de leur manutention, et de leur conservation. Amiens, 1858.

Monier, Mémoires sur l'analyse du lait et des farines. Paris, 1858.

Nägeli, Die Stärkemehlkörner. Zurich, 1858.

Friederich, Die Verfälschung der Speisen und Getränke. Münster, 1859.

Adriene, Recherches sur le lait au point de vue de sa composition, de son analyse, etc. Paris, 1859.

Gellée, Précis d'analyse pour la recherche des altérations et falsifications des produits chimiques et pharmaceutiques. Paris, 1860.

Gerhardt, Précis d'analyse pour la recherche des altérations, etc. Paris, 1860.

Vogel, Eine neue Milchprobe. Stuttgart, 1860.

Roussen, Falsifications des vins par l'alun. Paris, 1861.

Brinton, On Food. London, 1861.

Quarigues, Chemische künstliche Bereitung der moussirenden Weine. Weimar, 1861.

Selmi, Chimica applicata all' igiene alla economica domestica. Milan, 1861.

Wenke, Das Bier und seine Verfälschung. Weimar, 1861.

Henderson, Geschichte des Weines. 1861.

Hoskins, What we eat, and an account of the most common Adulterations of Food and Drink, with simple tests by which many of them may be detected. Boston, 1861.

Muller, A., La composition chimique d'aliments, représenté en tableaux coloriés. Brux., 1862.

Haraszthy, Grape Culture, Wines, and Wine-making. New York, 1862.

Pohl, Beihilfe zum Gallisiren der Weine. Wien, 1863.

Moir, Das Bier und dessen Untersuchungen. München, 1864.

Balling, Die Bereitung des Weines. Prag, 1865.

Ladray, L'art de faire le vin. Paris, 1865.

Pasteur, Précis théorique et pratique des substances alimentaires. Paris, 1865.

Druitt, On Wines. London, 1866.

Huber und Becker, Die pathologisch-histiologischen und bacteriologischen Untersuchungsmethoden, mit einer Darstellung der wichtigsten Bacterien. Leipzig, 1866.

Robinet, Manuel pratique et élémentaire d'analyse chimique des vins. Paris, 1866.

Gerstenbergk, Geheimnisse und Winke für Braumeister. Weimar, 1866.

Vogel, Die Bieruntersuchung. Berlin, 1866.

Feser, Der Werth der bestehenden Milchproben für die Milchpolizei. München, 1866.

Brun, Guide pratique pour reconnaitre et corriger les fraudes et maladies du vin. Paris, 1866.

Lancaster, Good Food, what it is and how to get it. London, 1867.

Feuchtwanger, Fermented Liquors, etc. New York, 1867.

Wiesner, Einleitung in die technisch Mikroscopie. Wien, 1867.

Gall, Das Gallisiren. Trier, 1867.

Monier, Guide pratique d'essai et l'analyse des sucres. Paris, 1867.

Cameron, Chemistry of Food. London, 1868.

Cammerson, Guide pour l'analyse des matières sucrées. Paris, 1868.

Pasteur, Étude sur le Vinaigre. Paris, 1868.

Dubusque, Pratique du Saccharimètre Soleil modifiée. Paris, 1868.

Wanklyn, Water Analysis. London, 1868.

Sonnenschein, Handbuch der gerichtlichen Chemie. Berlin, 1869.

Letheby, On Food, its varieties, chemical composition, etc. London, 1870.

Rion, Sämmtliche Geheimnisse der Bierbrauerei. New York, 1870.

Neubauer, Chemie des Weines. Wiesbaden, 1870.

Foellix, Gründliche Belehrung über richtiges Gallisiren oder Veredeln der Trauben-most in nicht guten Weinjahren durch Zucker- und Wasserzusatz. Mainz, 1870.

Martigny, Die Milch, ihre Wesen und ihre Verwerthung. 1871.

Huseman, Die Pflanzenstoffen. Berlin, 1871.

Hager, Untersuchungen. Leipzig, 1871.

Facen, Chimica bromatologica ossia guida per riconoscere la bonta, le alterazioni e la falsificazione delle sostanze alimentari. Compilation. Firenze, 1872.

Griffin, The Chemical Testing of Wines and Spirits. London, 1872.

Wiesner, Mikroskopische Untersuchungen. Stuttgardt, 1872.

Thudichum and Dupré, A Treatise on the Origin, Nature, and Varieties of Wine. London, 1872.

Dobell, On Diet. London, 1872.

Vogel, Nahrungs- und Genussmittel aus dem Pflanzenreiche. Wien, 1872.

Dragendorff, Untersuchungen aus dem pharmaceutischen Institut in Dorpat. St. Petersburg, 1872.

Thein, Die Weinveredelung und Künstfabrication. Prag, 1873.

Dochnahl, Die künstliche Weinbereitung. Frankfurt, 1873.

Bersch, Die Vermehrung und Verbesserung des Weines. Wien, 1873.

Smith, Ed., Handbook for Inspectors of Nuisances. London, 1873.

——, Foods. London, 1873.

Hager, Untersuchungen. Leipzig, 1873.

Atcherly, Adulterations of Food. London, 1874.

Baltzer, Die Nahrungs- und Genussmittel der Menschen. Nordhausen, 1874.

Lunel, Guide pratique pour reconnaître les falsifications des substances alimentaires. Paris, 1874.
Walchner, Die Nahrungsmittel des Menschen, ihre Verfälschungen und Verunreinigung. Berlin, 1874.
Marvaud, Les aliments d'épargne. Paris, 1874.
Smith, Ed., Manual for Medical Officers of Health. London, 1874.
Hamm, Das Weinbuch. Leipzig, 1874.
Nägeli, Stärkegruppe. Leipzig, 1874.
Schmidt, Ein Beitrag zur Kenntniss der Milch. Dorpat, 1874.
Squibb, Proper Legislation on Adulteration of Food. New York, 1874.
Wanklyn, Milk Analysis. London, 1874.
——— Tea, Coffee, and Cocoa. London, 1874.
Sharples, Food, and its Adulteration. Preston, 1874.
Passoz, Notice sur la saccharométrie chimique. Paris, 1874.
Angell and Hehner, Butter, its Analysis and Adulteration. London, 1874.
Cotter, Adulterations of Liquors. New York, 1874.
Jones, Chemistry of Wines. London, 1874.
Bowman and Bloxam, Medical Chemistry. London, 1874.
Springer, Ein Handbuch der Untersuchung, Prüfung und Werthbestimmung aller Handswaaren, Natur- und Kunsterzeugnisse, Gifte, Lebensmittel, Geheimmittel, etc. Berlin, 1874.
Attfield, General, Medicinal, and Pharmaceutical Chemistry. London, 1874.
Thiel, Nahrungs- und Genussmittel als Erzeugnisse der Industrie. Braunschweig, 1874.
Black, A Practical Treatise on Brewing. London, 1875.
Dammer, Kurzes chemische Handwörterbuch. 1875.
Blankenhorn, Bibliotheca œnologica, etc. Heidelberg, 1875.
Müller, Chemische Zusammensetzung der wichtigsten Nahrungsmittel. 1875.
Terrell, Notions pratiques sur l'analyse chimique des substances sacchariféres. Paris, 1878.
Prescott, Chemical Examination of Alcoholic Liquors. New York, 1875.
Pavy, A Treatise on Food and Dietetics. London, 1875.
Hoppe - Seyler, Handbuch der physiologisch- und pathologisch-chemische Analyse. Berlin, 1875.
Bartling, Die Englische Spiritus- fabrication und der Spiritus auf dem Englischen Markte. London, 1876.
Bastide, Vins sophistiqués. Beriés, 1876.
Blyth, Dictionary of Hygiene and Public Health. London, 1876.
Bresgen, Der Handel mit verdorbenen Getränke. Ahrenweiler, 1876.
Bolley, Handbuch der technisch-chemischen Untersuchungen. Leipzig, 1876.

Pasteur, Étude sur la bière. Paris, 1876.
————— Recherches des substances amères dans la bière. Paris, 1876.
Ritter, Des vins coloriés par la fuchsine. Paris, 1876.
Schutzenberger, On Fermentation. New York, 1876.
Bauer, Die Verfälschung der Nahrungsmittel in grossen Städten, speciell Berlin, etc. Berlin, 1877.
Grandeau, Traité d'analyse des matières agricoles. Paris, 1877.
Church, Food. New York, 1877.
Dennehl, Die Verfälschung des Bieres. Berlin, 1877.
Feltz, Etude expérimentale de l'action de la fuchsine sur l'organisme. Nancy, 1877.
Gaultier, La sophistication des vins. Paris, 1877.
Duplais, Traité de la fabrication des liqueurs et de la distillation des alcools. Paris, 1877.
Goppelsroeder, Sur l'analyse des vins. Mulhouse, 1877.
Hilger, Die wichtigen Nahrungsmittel. Erlangen, 1877.
Lieberman, Anleitung zur chemischen Untersuchung auf der Gebiete der Medicinal-polizei. Stuttgardt, 1877.
Birnbaum, Einfache Methoden zur Prüfung wichtiger Lebensmittel auf Verfälschungen. Karlsruhe, 1877.
Focke, Massregeln gegen Verfälschung der Nahrungsmittel. Chemnitz, 1877.
Hausner, Die Fabrikation der Conserven und Conditen. Leipzig, 1877.
Lobner, Massregeln gegen Verfälschung der Nahrungsmittel. Chemnitz, 1877.
Mierzinski, Die Conservirung der Thier- und Pflanzenstoffe. Berlin, 1877.
Wittstein, Taschenbuch des Nahrungs- und Genussmittel-Lehre. Nordlingen, 1877.
Lintner, Lehrbuch der Bierbraurei. 1877.
Loebner, Massregeln gegen Verfälschung der Nahrungsmittel. Chemnitz, 1877.
Reitleitner, Die Analyse des Weines. Wien, 1877.
Schnarke, Wörterbuch der Verfälschung. Jena, 1877.
Husson, Du Vin. Paris, 1877.
Bauer, Die Verfälschung des Nahrungsmittel. Berlin, 1877.
Stierlin, Ueber Weinverfälschung und Weinfarbung. Bern, 1877.
————— Das Bier und seine Verfälschung. Bern, 1877.
Pfeiffer, Analyse der Milch. Wiesbaden, 1877.
Koenig, Chemische Zusammensetzung der menschlichen Nahrungsmittel. Leipzig, 1878.
Lang, Die Fabrikation der Künstbutter, Spärbutter, und Butterin. Leipzig, 1878.
Auerbeck, Die Verfälschung der Nahrungs- und Genussmittel. Bremen, 1878.

Fox, Sanitary Examination of Water, Air, and Food. 1878.

Klencke, Illustrirtes Lexicon der Verfälschungen der Nahrungsmittel und Getränke. Leipzig, 1878.

Schmidt, Anleitung zu sanitärisch- und polizeilich-chemischen Untersuchungen. Zurich, 1878.

Birnbaum, Das Brodtbacken. Braunschweig, 1878.

Bronner and Scoffern, The Chemistry of Food and Diet. London, 1878.

Kollmann, Anhaltspunkte zur Benutzung bei Bieruntersuchung. Leipzig, 1878.

Nessler, Die Behandlung des Weines. Stuttgart, 1878.

Parkes, A Manual of Practical Hygiene. London, 1878.

Roth, Die Chemie des Rothweines. Heidelberg, 1878.

Reischauer, Die Chemie des Bieres. München, 1879.

Caldwell, Agricultural Qualitative and Quantitative Chemical Analysis. New York, 1879.

Adams, Étude sur les principales méthodes d'essai et d'analyse du lait. Paris, 1879.

Blas, De la présence de l'acide salicylique dans les bières. Paris, 1879.

Dietzsch, Die wichtigsten Nahrungs- und Genussmittel. Zurich, 1879.

Kensington, Analysis of Foods. London, 1879.

Fleischman, Das Molkerwesen. 1879.

Bourchadat et Quervenne, Instruction sur l'essai et l'analyse du lait. Paris, 1879.

Robinet, Manuel pratique d'analyse des vins, etc. Paris, 1879.

Stahlschmidt, Bolley's Handbuch der technisch-chemischen Untersuchungen. Leipzig, 1879.

Mott, Brief History of the Mégé Discovery. New York, 1880.

Elsner, Die Praxis des Nahrungs-mittel Chemikers, etc. Leipzig, 1880.

Hoppe-Seyler, Physiologische Chemie. Berlin. 1880.

Guckeisen, Die modernen Principien der Ernährung. Köln, 1880.

Griessmayer, Die Verfälschung der wichtigsten Nahrungs- und Genussmittel. 1880.

Meyer und Finkelnburg, Gesetze der Verkehr mit Nahrungsmittel, Genussmittel, etc. Berlin, 1880.

Pick, Die Untersuchung der im Handel und Gewerbe gebräuchlichsten Stoffe. Wien, 1880.

Märcker, Handbuch der Spiritusfabrikation. 1880.

Johnson, Chemistry of Common Life. New York, 1880.

Pratt, Food Adulteration. Chicago, 1880.

Muter, An Introduction to Pharmaceutical and Medical Chemistry. Philadelphia, 1880.

Flügge, Lehrbuch der hygienischen Untersuchungsmethoden. Leipzig, 1881.

Hehner, Alkoholtafeln. Wiesbaden, 1881.
Medicus, Gerichtlich-chemische Prüfung von Nahrungs- und Genuss-
    mittel. Würzburg, 1881.
Nowak, Lehrbuch der Hygiene. Wien, 1881.
Post, Handbuch der analytischen Untersuchungen zur Beaufsichti-
    gung der chemische Grossbetriber. Braunschweig, 1881.
Tucker, Manual of Sugar Analysis. New York, 1881.
Blyth, Foods, Composition and Analysis. London, 1882.
Blochman, Ueber Verfälschung der Nahrungsmittel. Köln, 1882.
Flick, Die Chemie im Dienst der öffentlichen Gesundheitspflege.
    Dresden, 1882.
Landolt, Handbook of the Polariscope (trans.). London, 1882.
Palm, Die wichtigsten und gebräuchlichsten Nahrungsmittel. St.
    Petersburg, 1882.
Prescott, Proximate Organic Analysis. New York, 1882.
Bell, James, Chemistry of Food. London, 1883.
Frankland, Agricultural Chemical Analysis. London, 1883.
Tracy, Handbook of Sanitary Information. New York, 1884.
Naquet, Legal Chemistry (trans., 2nd edition). New York, 1884.
Cornwall, Adulteration of Beer. 1885.
Husband-Audry, Aids to the Analysis of Food and Drugs. 1884.
Smee, Milk in Health and Disease. London, 1885.
Wauters, Prospect d'organisation d'un service de surveillance des
    Denrées alimentaires et Boissons. Paris, 1885.
Brieger, Untersuchung über Ptomaine. Berlin, 1886.
Cazeneuve, La coloration des vins par les couleurs de houille.
    Paris, 1886.
Jago, The Chemistry of Wheat, Flour, and Bread. London, 1886.
Merat et Delens, Dictionnaire Universelle. Paris, 1886.
Schimper, Anleitung zur mikroskopisch-chemischen Untersuchung
    der Nahrungs- und Genussmittel. Jena, 1886.
Thomann, Alleged Adulteration of Malt Liquors. New York, 1886.
Wanklyn, Bread Analysis. London, 1886.
Benedikt, Analyse der Fette, etc. Berlin, 1886.
Allen, Commercial Organic Analysis. Philadelphia, 1887.
Damner, Illustrirtes Lexikon der Verfälschungen und Verunreini-
    gungen der Nahrungs- und Genussmittel. Leipzig, 1887.
Bickerdyke, The Curiosities of Ale and Beer. New York, 1887.
Moeller, Mikroskopie der Nahrungs- und Genussmittel. Berlin, 1887.
Offinger, Die Ptomaïne oder Cadaver-Alkaloïde. Wiesbaden, 1887.

LEGISLATION.

THE following are the more important and recent laws relating to Food Adulteration, which have been enacted by American State Legislatures, and by the United States Government.

The New York State General Law, of 1881, for the prevention of the adulteration of food and drugs, is as follows :—

SECTION 1. No person shall, within this State, manufacture, have, offer for sale, or sell any article of food or drugs which is adulterated within the meaning of this Act, and any person violating this provision shall be deemed guilty of a misdemeanour, and upon conviction thereof, shall be punished by fine not exceeding fifty dollars for the first offence, and not exceeding one hundred dollars for each subsequent offence.

2. The term "food," as used in this Act, shall include every article used for food or drink by man. The term "drug," as used in this Act, shall include all medicines for internal and external use.

3. An article shall be deemed to be adulterated within the meaning of this Act :—

a.—In the case of drugs.

1. If, when sold under or by a name recognised in the United States Pharmacopœia, it differs from the standard of strength, quality, or purity laid down therein.

2. If, when sold under or by a name not recognised in the United States Pharmacopœia, but which is found in some other pharmacopœia or other standard work on Materia Medica, it differs materially from the standard of strength, quality, or purity laid down in such work.

3. If its strength or purity fall below the professed standard under which it is sold.

b.—In the case of food or drink.

1. If any substance or substances has or have been mixed with it so as to reduce or lower or injuriously affect its quality or strength.

2. If any inferior or cheaper substance or substances have been substituted wholly or in part for the article.

3. If any valuable constituent of the article has been wholly or in part abstracted.

4. If it be an imitation of, or be sold under the name of, another article.

5. If it consists wholly or in part of a diseased or decomposed, or putrid or rotten, animal or vegetable substance, whether manufactured or not, or, in the case of milk, if it is the produce of a diseased animal.

6. If it be coloured, or coated, or polished, or powdered, whereby damage is concealed, or it is made to appear better than it really is, or of greater value.

7. If it contain any added poisonous ingredient, or any ingredient which may render such article injurious to the health of the person consuming it : Provided, that the State Board of Health may, with the approval of the Governor, from time to time declare certain articles or preparations to be exempt from the provisions of this Act : And provided further, that the provisions of this Act shall not apply to mixtures or compounds recognised as ordinary articles of food, provided that the same are not injurious to health and that the articles are distinctly labelled as a mixture, stating the components of the mixture.

4. It shall be the duty of the State Board of Health to prepare and publish from time to time lists of the articles, mixtures, or compounds declared to be exempt from the provisions of this Act in accordance with the preceding section. The State Board of Health shall also from time to time fix the limits of variability permissible in any article of food or drug, or compound, the standard of which is not established by any national pharmacopœia.

5. The State Board of Health shall take cognisance of the interests of the public health as it relates to the sale of food and drugs and the adulteration of the same, and make all necessary investigations and inquiries relating thereto. It shall also have the supervision of the appointment of public analysts and chemists, and upon its recommendation whenever it shall deem any such officers incompetent, the appointment of any and every such officer shall be revoked and be held to be void and of no effect. Within thirty days after the passage of this Act, the State Board of Health shall meet and adopt such measures as may seem necessary to facilitate the enforcement of this Act, and prepare rules and regulations with regard to the proper methods of collecting and examining articles of food or drugs, and for the appointment of the necessary inspectors and analysts; and the State Board of Health shall be authorised to expend, in addition to all

sums already appropriated for said Board, an amount not exceeding ten thousand dollars for the purpose of carrying out the provisions of this Act. And the sum of ten thousand dollars is hereby appropriated out of any moneys in the treasury, not otherwise appropriated, for the purposes in this section provided.

6. Every person selling or offering or exposing any article of food or drugs for sale, or delivering any article to purchasers, shall be bound to serve or supply any public analyst or other agent of the State or Local Board of Health appointed under this Act, who shall apply to him for that purpose, and on his tendering the value of the same, with a sample sufficient for the purpose of analysis of any article which is included in this Act, and which is in the possession of the person selling, under a penalty not exceeding fifty dollars for a first offence, and one hundred dollars for a second and subsequent offences.

7. Any violation of the provisions of this Act shall be treated and punished as a misdemeanour ; and whoever shall impede, obstruct, hinder, or otherwise prevent any analyst, inspector, or prosecuting officer in the performance of his duty shall be guilty of a misdemeanour, and shall be liable to indictment and punishment therefor.

8. Any Acts or parts of Acts inconsistent with the provisions of this Act are hereby repealed.

9. All the regulations and declarations of the State Board of Health made under this Act from time to time, and promulgated, shall be printed in the statutes at large.

10. This Act shall take effect at the expiration of ninety days after it shall become a law.

AMENDMENT of April 29th, 1885.

SECTION 1. The title of chapter four hundred and seven of the laws of eighteen hundred and eighty-one, entitled " An Act to prevent the adulteration of food and drugs," is hereby amended to read as follows : " An Act to prevent the adulteration of food, drugs and spirituous, fermented or malt liquors in the State of New York."

2. Section one of chapter four hundred and seven of the laws of eighteen hundred and eighty-one is amended to read as follows :—

1. No person shall within this State manufacture, brew, distil, have, offer for sale or sell any articles of food, drugs, spirituous, fermented or malt liquors which are adulterated within the meaning of this Act, and any person violating this provision shall be deemed guilty of a misdemeanour, and upon conviction thereof, shall be punished by fine not exceeding fifty dollars for the first offence, and not exceeding one hundred dollars or imprisonment for one year, or both, for each subsequent offence, and shall in addition thereto be liable to a penalty of

one hundred dollars for each and every offence, to be sued for and recovered in the name of the people of the State of New York on complaint of any citizen, one-half of such recovery to be paid to the prosecutor of the action and the balance shall be paid to the county where such recovery shall be obtained for the support of the poor.

3. Section two is hereby amended to read as follows:—

2. The term food as used in this Act shall include every article of food or drink by man, including teas, coffees, and spirituous, fermented and malt liquors. The term drug as used in this Act shall include all medicines for internal or external use.

4. Section three is hereby amended by adding after subdivision seven the following: C. In the case of spirituous, fermented and malt liquors, if it contain any substance or ingredient not normal or healthful to exist in spirituous, fermented or malt liquors, or which may be deleterious or detrimental to health when such liquors are used as a beverage.

5. Section five is hereby amended to read as follows:—

5. The State Board of Health shall take cognisance of the interests of the public health as it relates to the sale of food, drugs, spirituous, fermented and malt liquors, and the adulteration thereof, and make all necessary inquiries relating thereto. It shall have the supervision of the appointment of public analysts and chemists, and upon its recommendation, whenever it shall deem any such officers incompetent, the appointment of any and every such officer shall be revoked and be held to be void and of no effect. Within thirty days after the passage of this Act, and from time to time thereafter as it may deem expedient, the said Board of Health shall meet and adopt such measures, not provided for by this Act, as may seem necessary to facilitate the enforcement of this Act, and for the purpose of making an examination or analysis of spirituous, fermented or malt liquors sold or exposed for sale in any store or place of business not herein otherwise provided for, and prepare rules and regulations with regard to the proper methods of collecting and examining articles of food, drugs, spirituous, fermented or malt liquors, and for the appointment of the necessary inspectors and analysts. The said Board shall at least once in the calendar year cause samples to be procured in public market or otherwise, of the spirituous, fermented or malt liquors distilled, brewed, manufactured or offered for sale in each and every brewery or distillery located in this State, and a test, sample or analysis thereof to be made by a chemist or analyst duly appointed by said Board of Health. The samples shall be kept in vessels and in a condition necessary and adequate to obtain a proper test and analysis of the liquors contained therein. The vessels containing such samples shall be properly labelled and numbered by the secretary of said Board of Health, who shall also prepare and keep an accurate and proper list of the names of the dis-

tillers, brewers or vendors, and opposite each name shall appear the number which is written or printed upon the label attached to the vessel containing the sample of the liquor manufactured, brewed, distilled or sold. Such lists, numbers and labels shall be exclusively for the information of the said Board of Health, and shall not be disclosed or published unless upon discovery of some deleterious substance prior to the completion of the analysis, except when required in evidence in a court of justice. The samples when listed and numbered shall be delivered to the chemist, analyst or other officer of said Board of Health, and shall be designated and known to such chemist, analyst or officer only by its number, and by no other mark or designation. The result of the analysis or investigation shall thereupon, and within a convenient time, be reported by the officer conducting the same to the secretary of said State Board of Health, setting forth explicitly the nature of any deleterious substance, compound or adulteration which may be detrimental to public health and which has been found upon analysis in such samples, and stating the number of the samples in which said substance was found. Upon such examination or analysis the brewer, distiller or vendor in whose sample of spirituous, fermented or malt liquor such deleterious substances, compounds or adulterations shall be found, shall be deemed to have violated the provisions of this Act, and shall be punishable as prescribed in section seven of this Act.

6. Section six of said chapter four hundred and seven of the laws of eighteen hundred and eighty-one is hereby amended to read as follows : —

6. Every person selling, offering, exposing for sale or manufacturing, brewing or distilling any article of food, spirituous, malt or fermented liquors, or delivering any such articles to purchasers, shall be bound to serve or supply any public analyst or other agent of the State or local Board of Health appointed under this Act, who shall apply to him for that purpose, and upon his tendering the value of the same, with a sample sufficient for the purpose of analysis of any article which is included in this Act, and which is in possession of the person selling, manufacturing, brewing or distilling the same, and any person who shall refuse to serve or supply such sample of any article as prescribed herein, or any person who shall impede, obstruct, hinder or otherwise prevent any analyst, inspector or prosecuting officer in the performance of his duty shall be deemed to have violated the provisions of this Act, and shall be punishable as prescribed by section seven of this Act.

7. Section seven of said chapter four hundred and seven of the laws of eighteen hundred and eighty-one is hereby amended to read as follows : —

7. Upon discovering that any person has violated any of the provisions of this Act, the State Board of Health shall immediately communicate the facts to the district attorney of the county in which the

person accused of such violation resides or carries on business, and the said district attorney, upon receiving such communication or notification, shall forthwith commence proceeding for indictment and trial of the accused as prescribed by law in cases of misdemeanour.

8. The State Board of Health shall be authorised to expend, in addition to the sums already appropriated for said board, an amount not exceeding three thousand dollars, for the purpose of carrying out the provisions of this Act, in relation to spirituous, fermented or malt liquors. And the sum of three thousand dollars is hereby appropriated out of any moneys in the treasury not otherwise appropriated and expended for the purposes of this Act.

9. This Act shall take effect immediately.

SPECIAL ACT to prevent deception in the sale of dairy products, and to preserve the public health, being supplementary to and in aid of chapter two hundred and two of the laws of eighteen hundred and eighty-four, entitled "An act to prevent deception in sales of dairy products."

(PASSED April 30, 1885).

The People of the State of New York, represented in Senate and Assembly, do enact as follows :—

SECTION 1. No person or persons shall sell or exchange, or expose for sale or exchange, any unclean, impure, unhealthy, adulterated or unwholesome milk, or shall offer for sale any article of food made from the same, or of cream from the same. The provisions of this section shall not apply to skim milk sold to bakers or housewives for their own use or manufacture, upon written orders for the same, nor to skim milk sold for use in the county in which it is produced. This provision shall not apply to pure skim cheese made from milk which is clean, pure, healthy, wholesome and unadulterated, except by skimming. Whoever violates the provisions of this section is guilty of a misdemeanour, and shall be punished by a fine of not less than twenty-five dollars, nor more than two hundred dollars, or by imprisonment of not less than one month or more than six months, or both such fine and imprisonment for the first offence, and by six months' imprisonment for each subsequent offence.

2. No person shall keep cows for the production of milk for market, or for sale or exchange, or for manufacturing the same, or cream from the same, into articles of food, in a crowded or unhealthy, condition, or feed the cows on food that is unhealthy, or that produces impure, unhealthy, diseased or unwholesome milk. No person shall manufacture from impure, unhealthy, diseased or unwholesome milk, or of cream from the same, any article of food. Whoever violates the pro-

T

visions of this section is guilty of a misdemeanour and shall be punished by a fine of not less than twenty-five dollars, nor more than two hundred dollars, or by imprisonment of not less than one month or more than four months, or by both such fine and imprisonment for the first offence, and by four months' imprisonment for each subsequent offence.

3. No person or persons shall sell, supply or bring to be manufactured to any butter or cheese manufactory, any milk diluted with water or any unclean, impure, unhealthy, adulterated or unwholesome milk, or milk from which any cream has been taken (except pure skim milk to skim cheese factories), or shall keep back any part of the milk commonly known as " strippings," or shall bring or supply milk to any butter or cheese manufactory that is sour (except pure skim milk to skim cheese factories). No butter or cheese manufactories, except those who buy all the milk they use, shall use for their own benefit, or allow any of their employés or any other person to use for their own benefit, any milk, or cream from the milk, or the product thereof, brought to said manufactories without the consent of the owners thereof. Every butter or cheese manufacturer, except those who buy all the milk they use, shall keep a correct account of all the milk daily received, and of the number of packages of butter and cheese made each day, and the number of packages and aggregate weight of cheese and butter disposed of each day, which account shall be open to inspection to any person who delivers milk to such manufacturer. Whoever violates the provisions of this section shall be guilty of a misdemeanour, and shall be punished for each offence by a fine of not less than twenty-five dollars, or more than two hundred dollars, or not less than one month or more than six months' imprisonment, or both such fine and imprisonment.

4. No manufacturer of vessels for the package of butter shall sell or dispose of any such vessels without branding his name and the true weight of the vessel or vessels on the same, with legible letters or figures not less than one-fourth of an inch in length. Whoever violates the provisions of this section is guilty of a misdemeanour, and shall be punished for each offence by a fine of not less than fifty dollars, nor more than one hundred dollars, or by imprisonment of not less than thirty days or more than sixty days, or by both such fine and imprisonment.

5. No person shall sell, or offer or expose for sale, any milk except in the county from which the same is produced, unless each can, vessel or package containing such milk shall be distinctly and durably branded with letters not less than one inch in length, on the outside, above the center, on every can, vessel or package containing such milk, the name of the county from which the same is produced ; and the same marks shall be branded or painted in a conspicuous place on

the carriage or vehicle in which the milk is drawn to be sold ; and such milk can only be sold in, or retailed out of a can, vessel, package or carriage so marked. Whoever violates the provisions of this section shall be guilty of a misdemeanour, and shall be punished by a fine of not less than twenty-five dollars nor more than two hundred dollars, or not less than two months' or more than four months' imprisonment, or both such fine and imprisonment, for the first offence, and by four months' imprisonment for each subsequent offence.

6. No person shall manufacture out of any oleaginous substance or substances, or any compound of the same, other than that produced from unadulterated milk, or of cream from the same, any article designed to take the place of butter or cheese produced from pure un-adulterated milk or cream of the same, or shall sell, or offer for sale, the same as an article of food. This provision shall not apply to pure skim-milk cheese made from pure skim milk. Whoever violates the provisions of this section shall be guilty of a misdemeanour, and be punished by a fine of not less than two hundred dollars nor more than five hundred dollars, or not less than six months or more than one year's imprisonment, or both such fine and imprisonment for the first offence, and by imprisonment for one year for each subsequent offence.

7. No person by himself or his agents or servants shall render or manufacture out of any animal fat or animal or vegetable oils not pro-duced from unadulterated milk or cream from the same, any article or product in imitation or semblance of or designed to take the place of natural butter or cheese produced from pure unadulterated milk or cream of the same, nor shall he or they mix, compound with, or add to milk, cream or butter any acids or other deleterious substance or any animal fats or animal or vegetable oils not produced from milk or cream, with design or intent to render, make or produce any article or substance or any human food in imitation or semblance of natural butter or cheese, nor shall he sell, keep for sale, or offer for sale any article, substance or compound made, manufactured or produced in violation of the provisions of this section, whether such article, sub-stance or compound shall be made or produced in this State or in any other State or country. Whoever violates the provisions of this section shall be guilty of a misdemeanour and be punished by a fine of not less than two hundred dollars nor more than five hundred dollars or not less than six months' or more than one years' imprisonment for the first offence, and by imprisonment for one year for each subsequent offence. Nothing in this section shall impair the provisions of section six of this Act.

8. No person shall manufacture, mix or compound with or add to natural milk, cream or butter any animal fats or animal or vegetable oils, nor shall he make or manufacture any oleaginous substance not produced from milk or cream, with intent to sell the same for butter or

cheese made from unadulterated milk or cream, or have the same in his possession, or offer the same for sale with such intent, nor shall any article or substance or compound so made or produced, be sold for butter or cheese, the product of the dairy. If any person shall coat, powder or colour with annatto or any colouring matter whatever, butterine or oleomargarine, or any compounds of the same, or any product or manufacture made in whole or in part from animal fats or animal or vegetable oils not produced from unadulterated milk or cream, whereby the said product, manufacture or compound shall be made to resemble butter or cheese, the product of the dairy, or shall have the same in his possession, or shall sell or offer for sale or have in his possession any of the said products which shall be coloured or coated in semblance of or to resemble butter or cheese, it shall be conclusive evidence of an intent to sell the same for butter or cheese, the product of the dairy. Whoever violates any of the provisions of this section shall be guilty of a misdemeanour, and be punished by a fine of not less than two hundred dollars nor more than one thousand dollars. This section shall not be construed to impair or affect the prohibitions of sections six and seven of this Act.

9. Every manufacturer of full-milk cheese may put a brand upon each cheese indicating "full-milk cheese," and the date of the month and year when made ; and any person using this brand upon any cheese made from which any cream whatever has been taken shall be guilty of a misdemeanour, and shall be punished for each offence by a fine of not less than one hundred dollars nor more than five hundred dollars.

10. No person shall offer, sell or expose for sale in full packages, butter or cheese branded or labelled with a false brand or label as to county or state in which the article is made. Whoever violates the provisions of this section is guilty of a misdemeanour, and shall be punished by a fine of not less than twenty-five dollars or more than fifty dollars, or imprisonment of not less than fifteen days or more than thirty days for the first offence, and fifty dollars or thirty days' imprisonment for each subsequent offence.

11. No person shall manufacture, sell or offer for sale any condensed milk, unless the same shall be put up in packages upon which shall be distinctly labelled or stamped the name, or brand, by whom or under which the same is made. No condensed milk shall be made or offered for sale unless the same is manufactured from pure, clean, healthy, fresh, unadulterated and wholesome milk, from which the cream has not been removed, or unless the proportion of milk solids contained in the condensed milk shall be in amount the equivalent of twelve per centum of milk solids in crude milk, and of such solids twenty-five per centum shall be fat. When condensed milk shall be sold from cans, or packages not hermetically sealed, the vendor shall brand or label such cans or packages with the name of the county or

counties from which the same was produced, and the name of the vendor. Whoever violates the provisions of this section shall be guilty of a misdemeanour, and be punished by a fine of not less than fifty dollars or more than five hundred dollars, or by imprisonment of not more than six months, or by both such fine and imprisonment for the first offence, and by six months' imprisonment for each subsequent offence.

12. Upon the expiration of the term of office of the present commissioner, the Governor, by and with the advice and consent of the Senate, shall appoint a commissioner, who shall be known as the New York State Dairy Commissioner, who shall be a citizen of this State, and who shall hold his office for the term of two years, or until his successor is appointed, and shall receive a salary of three thousand dollars per annum, and his necessary expenses incurred in the discharge of his official duties under this Act. Said commissioner shall be charged, under the direction of the Governor, with the enforcement of the various provisions thereof, and with all laws prohibiting or regulating the adulteration of butter, cheese, or milk. The said commissioner is hereby authorised and empowered to appoint such assistant commissioners and to employ such experts, chemists, agents, and such counsel as may be deemed by him necessary for the proper enforcement of this law, their compensation to be fixed by the commissioner. The said commissioner is also authorised to employ a clerk at an annual salary not to exceed twelve hundred dollars. The sum of fifty thousand dollars is hereby appropriated, to be paid for such purpose out of any moneys in the Treasury not otherwise appropriated. All charges, accounts and expenses authorised by this Act shall be paid by the Treasurer of the State upon the warrant of the comptroller, after such expenses have been audited and allowed by the comptroller. The entire expenses of said commissioner shall not exceed the sum appropriated for the purposes of this Act. The said commissioner shall make annual reports to the legislature, on or before the fifteenth day of January of each year, of his work and proceedings, and shall report in detail the number of assistant commissioners, experts, chemists, agents, and counsel he has employed, with their expenses and disbursements. The said commissioner shall have a room in the new capitol, to be set apart for his use by the capitol commissioner. The said commissioner and assistant commissioners and such experts, chemists, agents, and counsel as they shall duly authorise for the purpose, shall have full access, egress, and ingress to all places of business, factories, farms, buildings, carriages, vessels, and cans used in the manufacture and sale of any dairy products or any imitation thereof. They shall also have power and authority to open any package, can, or vessel containing such articles which may be manufactured, sold, or exposed for sale, in violation of the provisions of this Act, and may inspect the contents therein and may take

therefrom samples for analysis. This section shall not affect the
tenure of the office of the present commissioner.

13. Upon the application for a warrant under this Act, the certificate of the analyst or chemist of any analysis made by him shall be
sufficient evidence of the facts therein stated. Every such certificate
shall be duly signed and acknowledged by such analyst or chemist
before an officer authorised to take acknowledgments of conveyances
of real estate.

14. Courts of special sessions shall have jurisdiction of all cases
arising under this Act, and their jurisdiction is hereby extended so as
to enable them to enforce the penalties imposed by any or all sections
thereof.

15. In all prosecutions under this Act, one-half of the money shall
be paid by the court or clerk thereof to the city or county where the
recovery shall be had, for the support of the poor, except in the city
and county of New York shall be equally divided between the pension
funds of the police and fire departments, and the residue shall be paid
to the Dairy Commissioner, who shall account therefor to the Treasury
of the State, and be added to any appropriation made to carry out the
provisions of this Act. All sums of money expended by the Dairy
Commissioner under the provisions of this Act shall be audited and
allowed by the Comptroller of the State. Any bond given by any
officer shall be subject to the provisions of this section.

16. In all prosecutions under this Act relating to the sale and
manufacture of unclean, impure, unhealthy, adulterated, or unwholesome milk, if the milk be shown to contain more than eighty-eight
per centum of water or fluids, or less than twelve per centum of milk
solids, which shall contain not less than three per centum of fat, it
shall be declared adulterated, and milk drawn from cows within fifteen
days before, and five days after, parturition, or from animals fed on
distillery waste, or any substance in the state of putrefaction or fermentation, or upon any unhealthy food whatever, shall be declared
unclean, unhealthy, impure and unwholesome milk. This section
shall not prevent the feeding of ensilage from silos.

17. The doing of any thing prohibited being done, and the not
doing of any thing directed to be done in this Act, shall be presumptive evidence of a wilful intent to violate the different sections and
provisions thereof. If any person shall suffer any violation of the
provisions of this Act by his agent, servant, or in any room or building
occupied or controlled by him, he shall be deemed a principal in such
violation and punished accordingly.

18. Chapters four hundred and sixty-seven of the laws of eighteen
hundred and sixty-two, five hundred and forty-four, and five hundred
and eighteen of the laws of eighteen hundred and sixty-four, five
hundred and fifty-nine of the laws of eighteen hundred and sixty-five,

four hundred and fifteen of the laws of eighteen hundred and seventy-seven, two hundred and twenty, and two hundred and thirty-seven of the laws of eighteen hundred and seventy-eight, four hundred and thirty-nine of the laws of eighteen hundred and eighty, and two hundred and fourteen of the laws of eighteen hundred and eighty-two, are hereby repealed.

19. If any person shall, by himself or other, violate any of the provisions of sections one, two, three, four or five of this Act, or knowingly suffer a violation thereof by his agent, or in any building or room occupied by him, he shall, in addition to the fines and punishments therein described for each offence, forfeit and pay a fixed penalty of one hundred dollars. If any person, by himself or another, shall violate any of the provisions of sections six, seven, or eight of this Act, he shall, in addition to the fines and penalties herein prescribed for each offence, forfeit and pay a fixed penalty of five hundred dollars. Such penalties shall be recovered with costs in any court of this State having jurisdiction thereof in an action to be prosecuted by the Dairy Commissioner, or any of his assistants in the name of the people of the State of New York.

20. This Act and each section thereof is declared to be enacted to prevent deception in the sale of dairy products, and to preserve the public health which is endangered by the manufacture, sale or use of the articles or substances herein regulated or prohibited.

21. This Act shall take effect immediately. Sections six and seven shall not apply to any product manufactured, or in process of manufacture at the time of the passage of this Act; but neither this exemption nor this Act shall impair the power to prosecute any violations heretofore committed of section six of the Act of which this Act is supplemental.

AN ACT to amend chapter two hundred and two of the laws of eighteen hundred and eighty-four, entitled "An Act to prevent deception in sales of dairy products."

(PASSED April 30, 1885).

The people of the State of New York, represented in Senate and Assembly, do enact as follows :—

SECTION I. Section seven of chapter two hundred and two of the laws of eighteen hundred and eighty-four, entitled "An Act to prevent deception in sales of dairy products," is hereby amended to read as follows :—

7. No person shall offer, sell, or expose for sale butter or cheese branded or labelled with a false brand or label as to the quality of the article, or the county or State in which the article is made. The New

York State Dairy Commissioner is hereby authorised and directed to procure and issue to the cheese manufactories of the State, upon proper application therefor and under such regulations as to the custody and use thereof as he may prescribe, a uniform stencil brand bearing a suitable device or motto, and the words " New York State Full Cream Cheese." Every brand issued shall be used upon the outside of the cheese and also upon the package containing the same, and shall bear a different number for each separate manufactory, and the commissioner shall keep a book in which shall be registered the name, location and number of each manufactory using the said brand, and the name or names of the persons at each manufactory authorised to use the same. It shall be unlawful to use or permit such stencil brand to be used upon any other than full cream cheese or packages containing the same. Whoever violates the provisions of this section is guilty of a misdemeanour, and for each and every cheese or package so falsely branded shall be punished by a fine of not less than twenty-five dollars or more than fifty dollars, or imprisonment of not less than fifteen or more than thirty days.

2. This Act shall take effect immediately.

AN ACT to protect butter and cheese manufacturers.

(PASSED June 8, 1885, three-fifths being present.)

The people of the State of New York, represented in Senate and Assembly, do enact as follows :—

SECTION 1. Whoever shall with intent to defraud, sell, supply, or bring to be manufactured to any butter or cheese manufactory in this State, any milk diluted with water, or in any way adulterated, unclean or impure, or milk from which any cream has been taken, or milk commonly known as skimmed milk, or whoever shall keep back any part of the milk as strippings, or whoever shall knowingly bring or supply milk to any butter or cheese manufactory that is tainted or sour, or whoever shall knowingly bring or supply to any butter or cheese manufactory, milk drawn from cows within fifteen days before parturition, or within three days after parturition, or any butter or cheese manufacturers who shall knowingly use or allow any of his or her employés or any other person to use for his or her benefit, or for their own individual benefit, any milk or cream from the milk brought to said butter or cheese manufacturer, without the consent of all the owners thereof, or any butter or cheese manufacturer who shall refuse or neglect to keep or cause to be kept a correct account, open to the inspection of any one furnishing milk to such manufacturer, of the amount of milk daily received, or of the number of pounds of butter and the number of cheeses made each day, or of the number cut or otherwise disposed of, and the weight of each, shall for each and every offence forfeit and pay a sum not less than twenty-five dollars nor more than one hundred dollars, with costs of suit, to be sued for in any court of competent jurisdiction for the benefit of the person or persons, firm or association, or corporation or their assigns upon whom such fraud or neglect shall be committed. But nothing in this Act shall affect, impair, or repeal any of the provisions of chapter two hundred and two of the laws of eighteen hundred and eighty-four, or of the acts amendatory thereof or supplementary thereto.

2. This Act shall take effect immediately.

SPECIAL ACT in relation to the manufacture and sale of vinegar.

(PASSED June 9, 1886.)

The People of the State of New York, represented in Senate and Assembly, do enact as follows :—

SECTION 1. Every person who manufactures for sale, or offers or exposes for sale as cider vinegar, any vinegar not the legitimate product of pure apple juice, known as apple cider, or vinegar not made exclusively of said apple cider, or vinegar into which foreign substances, drugs or acids have been introduced, as may appear by proper test, shall for each offence be punishable by a fine of not less than fifty, nor more than one hundred dollars.

2. Every person who manufactures for sale, or offers for sale, any vinegar found upon proper tests to contain any preparation of lead, copper, sulphuric acid, or other ingredient injurious to health, shall for each such offence be punishable by fine of not less than one hundred dollars.

3. The mayor of cities shall, and the supervisor of towns may, annually, appoint one or more persons to be inspectors of vinegar, who shall be sworn before entering upon their duties, and who shall have power and authority to inspect and examine all vinegar offered for sale.

4. No person shall by himself, his servant or agent, or as the servant or agent of any other person, sell, exchange, deliver, or have in his custody or possession, with intent to sell or exchange, or expose or offer for sale or exchange any adulterated vinegar, or label, brand or sell as cider vinegar, or as apple vinegar, any vinegar not the legitimate product of pure apple juice, or not made exclusively from apple cider.

5. All vinegars shall be without artificial colouring matter, and shall

have an acidity equivalent to the presence of not less than four and one-half per cent., by weight, of absolute acetic acid, and in the case of cider vinegar, shall contain in addition not less than two per cent. by weight of cider vinegar solids upon full evaporation over boiling water ; and if any vinegar contains any artificial colouring matter or less than the above amount of acidity, or in the case of cider vinegar, if it contains less than the above amount of acidity or of cider vinegar solids, it shall be deemed to be adulterated within the meaning of this Act.

6. Every person making or manufacturing cider vinegar shall brand on each head of the cask, barrel or keg containing such vinegar the name and residence of the manufacturer, the date when same was manufactured, and the words cider vinegar.

7. Whoever violates any of the provisions of this Act shall be punished by a fine not exceeding one hundred dollars. Any person who may have suffered any injury or damage by reason of the violation of any of the provisions of this Act, may maintain an action in his own name against any person violating any of the provisions of this Act, to recover the penalties provided for such violation, and one-half of the sum recovered shall be retained by him for his own use and the other half shall be paid into the city or county treasury where such offence was committed for the benefit of such city or county.

8. This Act shall take effect immediately.

The following are the Statutes of the State of Massachusetts relating to the adulteration of food and drugs :—

GENERAL LAWS RELATING TO ADULTERATION.

FOOD AND DRUGS.

Adulteration prohibited.
1882, 263, § 1.

SECTION 1. No person shall, within this commonwealth, manufacture for sale, offer for sale, or sell any drug or article of food which is adulterated within the meaning of this Act.

Definition of terms " drug " and " food."
1882, 263, § 2.

2. The term "drug" as used in this Act shall include all medicines for internal or external use, antiseptics, disinfectants, and cosmetics. The term "food" as used herein shall include all articles used for food or drink by man.

Drugs, how adulterated.
1882, 263, § 3.
Specifications.

3. An article shall be deemed to be adulterated within the meaning of this Act—

(a.) In the case of drugs,—(1.) If, when sold under or by a name recognised in the United States Pharmacopœia, it differs from the standard of strength, quality, or purity laid down therein, unless the order calls for an article inferior to such standard, or unless such

Officinal drugs may be sold as called for, or as variation is difference is made known or so appears to the purchaser at the time of such sale; (2.) If, when sold under or by a name not recognised in the United States Pharmacopœia, but which is found in some other pharmacopœia, or other standard work on *materia medica*, it differs materially from the standard of strength, quality, or purity laid down in such work; (3.) If its strength or purity falls below the professed standard under which it is sold: made known to the purchaser. 1884, 289, § 7.

(*b.*) In the case of food—(1.) If any substance or substances have been mixed with it so as to reduce, or lower, or injuriously affect its quality or strength; (2.) If any inferior or cheaper substance or substances have been substituted wholly or in part for it; (3.) If any valuable constituent has been wholly or in part abstracted from it; (4.) If it is an imitation of, or is sold under the name of another article; (5.) If it consists wholly or in part of a diseased, decomposed, putrid, or rotten animal or vegetable substance, whether manufactured or not, or in the case of milk, if it is the produce of a diseased animal; (6.) If it is coloured, coated, polished, or powdered, whereby damage is concealed, or if it is made to appear better or of greater value than it really is; (7.) If it contains any added or poisonous ingredient, or any ingredient which may render it injurious to the health of a person consuming it. Food, how adulterated. Specifications.

4. The provisions of this Act shall not apply to mixtures or compounds recognised as ordinary articles of food or drinks, provided that the same are not injurious to health, and are distinctly labelled as mixtures or compounds. And no prosecutions shall at any time be maintained under the said Act concerning any drug the standard of strength or purity whereof has been raised since the issue of the last edition of the United States Pharmacopœia, unless and until such change of standard has been published throughout the commonwealth. Provisions of Act not to apply to labelled compounds or mixtures when not injurious to health. No prosecution to be made relative to drugs, if standard of same has been raised since the issue of the last edition of the Pharmacopœia until such change has been published. 1884, 289, § 5.

5. The State Board of Health, Lunacy, and Charity, shall take cognisance of the interests of the public health relating to the sale of drugs and food and the adulteration of the same, and shall make all necessary investigations and inquiries in reference thereto, and for these purposes may appoint inspectors, analysts, and chemists, who shall be subject to its supervision and removal. State Board shall make investigations and may appoint inspectors, analysts and chemists. 1882, 263, § 5.

Within thirty days after the passage of this Act the said Board shall adopt such measures as it may deem necessary to facilitate the enforcement hereof, and shall prepare rules and regulations with regard to the proper methods of collecting and examining drugs and articles of food. Said Board may expend annually an amount not exceeding ten thousand dollars for the purpose of carrying out the provisions of The Board shall make regulations as to collecting and examining of food and drugs, and may expend ten thousand dollars in carrying out

the provisions of
this Act.
1882, 263, § 5.
1884, 289, § 2.
Three-fifths to
be expended in
relation to milk
and its products.
1884, 289, § 1.

this Act : provided, however, that not less than three-fifths of the said
amount shall be annually expended for the enforcement of the laws
against the adulteration of milk and milk products.

Samples to be
furnished to offi-
cers or agents.
1882, 263, § 6.

6. Every person offering or exposing for sale, or delivering to a
purchaser, any drug or article of food included in the provisions of
this Act, shall furnish to any analyst or other officer or agent appointed hereunder, who shall apply to him for the purpose and shall
tender him the value of the same, a sample sufficient for the purpose
of the analysis of any such drug or article of food which is in his
possession.

Obstruction and
its penalty.
1882, 263, § 7.

7. Whoever hinders, obstructs, or in any way interferes with any
inspector, analyst, or other officer appointed hereunder, in the performance of his duty, and whoever violates any of the provisions of
this Act, shall be punished by a fine not exceeding fifty dollars for the
first offence, and not exceeding one hundred dollars for each subsequent offence.

State Board to
report prosecu-
tions and money
expended.
1883, 263, § 2.
1884, 289, § 2.
Powers of in-
spectors.
1884, 289, § 3.

8. The State Board of Health, Lunacy, and Charity shall report
annually to the Legislature the number of prosecutions made under
said chapter, and an itemised account of all money expended in
carrying out the provisions thereof.

9. An inspector appointed under the provisions of said chapter two
hundred and sixty-three of the Acts of the year eighteen hundred and
eighty-two shall have the same powers and authority conferred upon
a city or town inspector by section two of chapter fifty-seven of the
Public Statutes.

Act of 1882 does
not affect chap-
ter 57 of the
Public Statutes.
1884, 289, § 4.

10. Nothing contained in chapter two hundred and sixty-three of
the Acts of the year eighteen hundred and eighty-two shall be in any
way construed as repealing or amending anything contained in chapter
fifty-seven of the Public Statutes.

Samples to be
sealed for bene-
fit of defendant.
1884, 289, § 8.

11. Before commencing the analysis of any sample the person
making the same shall reserve a portion which shall be sealed ; and
in case of a complaint against any person the reserved portion of the
sample alleged to be adulterated shall upon application be delivered
to the defendant or his attorney.

Selling corrupt
or unwholesome
provisions with-
out notice.
Public Statutes,
chap. 208, § 1.
12 Cush. 499.

12. Whoever knowingly sells any kind of diseased, corrupted, or
unwholesome provisions, whether for meat or drink, without making
the same fully known to the buyer, shall be punished by imprisonment
in the jail not exceeding six months, or by fine not exceeding two
hundred dollars.

Adulterating
food.
Public Statutes,
chap. 208, § 3.

13. Whoever fraudulently adulterates, for the purpose of sale, bread
or any other substance intended for food, with any substance injurious to health, or knowingly barters, gives away, sells, or has in

possession with intent to sell, any substance intended for food, which has been adulterated with any substance injurious to health, shall be punished by imprisonment in the jail not exceeding one year, or by fine not exceeding three hundred dollars ; and the articles so adulterated shall be forfeited, and destroyed under the direction of the court.

14. Whoever adulterates, for the purpose of sale, any liquor used or intended for drink, with Indian cockle, vitriol, grains of paradise, opium, alum, capsicum, copperas, laurel-water, logwood, Brazil wood, cochineal, sugar of lead, or any other substance which is poisonous or injurious to health, and whoever knowingly sells any such liquor so adulterated, shall be punished by imprisonment in the State prison not exceeding three years ; and the articles so adulterated shall be forfeited. *Adulterating liquor used for drink, with Indian cockle, etc. Public Statutes, chap. 208, § 4.*

15. Whoever fraudulently adulterates, for the purpose of sale, any drug or medicine, or sells any fraudulently adulterated drug or medicine, knowing the same to be adulterated, shall be punished by imprisonment in the jail not exceeding one year, or by fine not exceeding four hundred dollars ; and such adulterated drugs and medicines shall be forfeited, and destroyed under the direction of the court. *Adulteration of drugs or medicines. Public Statutes, chap. 208, § 5.*

16. Whoever sells arsenic, strychnine, corrosive sublimate, or prussic acid, without the written prescription of a physician, shall keep a record of the date of such sale, the name of the article, the amount thereof sold, and the name of the person or persons to whom delivered ; and for each neglect shall forfeit a sum not exceeding fifty dollars. Whoever purchases deadly poisons as aforesaid, and gives a false or fictitious name to the vendor, shall be punished by fine not exceeding fifty dollars. *Persons selling certain poisons to keep record, etc.* *Purchasers who give false name, etc. Public Statutes, chap. 208, § 6.*

LAWS RELATIVE TO SPECIAL ARTICLES OF FOOD.

OF THE INSPECTION AND SALE OF MILK AND MILK PRODUCTS.

1. The mayor and aldermen of cities shall, and the selectmen of towns may, annually appoint one or more persons to be inspectors of milk for their respective places, who shall be sworn before entering upon the duties of their office. Each inspector shall publish a notice of his appointment for two weeks in a newspaper published in his city or town, or if no newspaper is published therein, he shall post up such notice in two or more public places in such city or town. *Appointment of inspectors of milk. Public Statutes, chap. 57, § 1.*

2. Such inspectors shall keep an office, and shall record in books kept for the purpose the names and place of business of all persons engaged in the sale of milk within their city or town. Said inspectors may enter all places where milk is stored or kept for sale, and all *Their duties and powers. 1884, 310, § 3. 11 Allen, 264.*

persons engaged in the sale of milk shall, on the request in writing of an inspector, deliver to the person having the request a sample or specimen sufficient for the purpose of analysis of the milk then in his possession from such can or receptacle as shall be designated by the inspector or the person bearing the request. Said inspector shall cause the sample or specimen of milk so delivered to be analysed or otherwise satisfactorily tested, the results of which analysis or test they shall record and preserve as evidence. The inspectors shall receive such compensation as the mayor and alderman or selectmen may determine.

Persons selling milk from carriages to be licensed. Public Statutes, chap. 57, § 3.

3. In all cities, and in all towns in which there is an inspector of milk, every person who conveys milk in carriages or otherwise for the purpose of selling the same in such city or town shall annually, on the first day of May, or within thirty days thereafter, be licensed by the inspector or inspectors of milk of such city or town to sell milk within the limits thereof, and shall pay to such inspector or inspectors fifty cents each to the use of the city or town. The inspector or inspectors shall pay over monthly to the treasurer of such city or town all sums collected by him or them. Licenses shall be issued only in the names of the owners of carriages or other vehicles, and shall for the purposes of this chapter be conclusive evidence of ownership. No license shall be sold, assigned, or transferred. Each license shall record the name, residence, place of business, number of carriages or other vehicles used, name and residence of every driver or other person engaged in carrying or selling said milk, and the number of the license. Each licensee shall before engaging in the sale of milk, cause his name, the number of his license, and his place of business, to be legibly placed on each outer side of all carriages or vehicles used by him in the conveyance and sale of milk, and he shall report to the inspector or inspectors any change of driver or other person employed by him which may occur during the term of his license. Whoever, without being first licensed under the provisions of this section, sells milk or exposes it for sale from carriages or other vehicles, or has it in his custody or possession with intent so to sell, and whoever violates any of the provisions of this section, shall for a first offence be punished by fine of not less than thirty nor more than one hundred dollars ; for a second offence by fine of not less than fifty nor more than three hundred dollars ; and for a subsequent offence by fine of fifty dollars and by imprisonment in the house of correction for not less than thirty nor more than sixty days.

Persons selling milk in stores, etc., to be registered. Public Statutes, chap. 57, § 4. 1 Allen, 593. 2 Allen, 157.

4. Every person before selling milk or offering it for sale in a store, booth, stand, or market-place in a city or in a town in which an inspector or inspectors of milk are appointed, shall register in the books of such inspector or inspectors, and shall pay to him or them fifty cents to the use of such city or town ; and whoever neglects so

to register shall be punished for each offence by fine not exceeding twenty dollars.

5. Whoever by himself or by his servant or agent, or as the servant or agent of any other person, sells, exchanges, or delivers, or has in his custody or possession with intent to sell or exchange, or exposes or offers for sale or exchange, adulterated milk, or milk to which water or any foreign substance has been added, or milk produced from cows fed on the refuse of distilleries or from sick or diseased cows, shall for a first offence be punished by fine of not less than fifty nor more than two hundred dollars; for a second offence by fine of not less than one hundred nor more than three hundred dollars, or by imprisonment in the house of correction for not less than thirty nor more than sixty days; and for a subsequent offence by fine of fifty dollars and by imprisonment in the house of correction for not less than sixty nor more than ninety days.

Penalty for selling, etc., adulterated milk, etc. Public Statutes, chap. 57, § 5. 9 Allen, 499. 10 Allen, 199. 11 Allen, 264. 107 Mass., 194.

6. Whoever by himself or by his servant or as the servant or agent of any other person, sells, exchanges, or delivers, or has in his custody or possession with intent to sell or exchange, or exposes or offers for sale as pure milk, any milk from which the cream or a part thereof has been removed, shall be punished by the penalties provided in the preceding section.

Penalty for selling milk from which cream has been removed. Public Statutes, chap. 57, § 6.

7. No dealer in milk, and no servant or agent of such a dealer, shall sell, exchange, or deliver, or have in his custody or possession, with intent to sell, exchange, or deliver, milk from which the cream or any part thereof has been removed, unless in a conspicuous place above the centre upon the outside of every vessel, can, or package from or in which such milk is sold, the words "skimmed milk" are distinctly marked in letters not less than one inch in length. Whoever violates the provisions of this section shall be punished by the penalties provided by section 5.

Vessels containing milk from which cream has been removed to be marked "skimmed milk." Public Statutes, chap. 57, § 7.

8. Any inspector of milk, and any servant or agent of an inspector who wilfully connives at or assists in a violation of the provisions of this chapter, and whoever hinders, obstructs, or in any way interferes with any inspector of milk, or any servant or agent of an inspector in the performance of his duty, shall be punished by fine of not less than one hundred nor more than three hundred dollars, or by imprisonment for not less than thirty nor more than sixty days.

Penalty on inspectors, etc., for conniving, etc. Public Statutes, chap. 57, § 8. 1884, 310, § 5.

9. In all prosecutions under this chapter, if the milk is shown upon analysis to contain more than eighty-seven per cent. of watery fluid, or to contain less than thirteen per cent. of milk solids, it shall be deemed for the purposes of this chapter to be adulterated.

What milk to be deemed adulterated. Public Statutes, chap. 57, § 9.

10. It shall be the duty of every inspector to institute a complaint for a violation of any of the provisions of this chapter on the information of any person who lays before him satisfactory evidence by which to sustain such complaint.

Inspectors to institute complaints. Public Statutes, chap. 57, § 10.

Names, etc., of persons convicted to be published.
Public Statutes, chap. 57, § 11.

11. Each inspector shall cause the name and place of business of every person convicted of selling adulterated milk, or of having the same in his possession with intent to sell, to be published in two newspapers in the county in which the offence was committed.

Milk cans to hold eight quarts when, etc.
Public Statutes, chap. 57, § 12.

12. When milk is sold by the can, such can shall hold eight quarts, and no more.

Spurious butter sold in boxes, tubs and firkins to be plainly marked as such.
1884, 310, § 1.

13. Whoever, by himself or his agents, sells, exposes for sale, or has in his possession with intent to sell, any article, substance or compound, made in imitation or semblance of butter, or as a substitute for butter, and not made exclusively and wholly of milk or cream, or containing any fats, oils or grease not produced from milk or cream, shall have the words "imitation butter," or " oleomargarine," stamped, labelled or marked, in printed letters of plain Roman type, not less than one inch in length, so that said word cannot be easily defaced, upon the top and side of every tub, firkin, box or package containing

Retail packages to be marked on outside of wrapper.

any of said article, substance, or compound. And in cases of retail sales of any of said article, substance or compound, not in the original packages, the seller shall, by himself or his agents, attach to each package so sold, and shall deliver therewith to the purchaser, a label or wrapper bearing in a conspicuous place upon the outside of the package the words " imitation butter " or " oleomargarine " in printed letters of plain Roman type, not less than one half inch in length.

Spurious cheese to be plainly marked as such.
Public Statutes, chap. 56, § 18.

14. Whoever, by himself or his agents, sells, exposes for sale, or has in his possession with intent to sell, any article, substance, or compound, made in imitation or semblance of cheese, or as a substitute for cheese, and not made exclusively and wholly of milk or cream, or containing any fats, oils or grease not produced from milk or cream, shall have the words "imitation cheese" stamped, labelled, or marked in printed letters of plain Roman type not less than one inch in length, so that said words cannot be easily defaced, upon the side of every cheese cloth or band around the same, and upon the top and side of every tub, firkin, box, or package containing any of said article, sub-

Wrappers to be marked.

stance or compound. And in case of retail sales of any of said article, substance or compound not in the original packages, the seller shall, by himself or his agents, attach to each package so sold at retail, and shall deliver therewith to the purchaser a label or wrapper bearing in a conspicuous place upon the outside of the package the words "imitation cheese," in printed letters of plain Roman type not less than one half inch in length.

Penalty for fraudulent sales.
Public Statutes, chap. 56, § 19.

15. Whoever sells, exposes for sale, or has in his possession with intent to sell, any article, substance, or compound made in imitation or semblance of butter, or as a substitute for butter, except as provided in section one ; whoever sells, exposes for sale, or has in his possession with intent to sell, any article, substance, or compound

made in imitation or semblance of cheese, or as a substitute for cheese, except as provided in section two, and whoever shall deface, erase, cancel, or remove any mark, stamp, brand, label, or wrapper provided for by this Act, or change the contents of any box, tub, article, and package marked, stamped, or labelled as aforesaid, with intent to deceive as to the contents of said box, tub, article, or package, shall for every such offence forfeit and pay a fine of one hundred dollars, and for a second and each subsequent offence a fine of two hundred dollars, to be recovered with costs in any court of this commonwealth of competent jurisdiction ; and any fine paid shall go to the city or town where the offence was committed.

16. Inspectors of milk shall institute complaints for violations of the provisions of the three preceding sections when they have reasonable cause to believe that such provisions have been violated, and on the information of any person who lays before them satisfactory evidence by which to sustain such complaint. Said inspectors may enter all places where butter or cheese is stored or kept for sale, and said inspectors shall also take specimens of suspected butter and cheese and cause them to be analysed or otherwise satisfactorily tested, the result of which analysis or test they shall record and preserve as evidence ; and a certificate of such result, sworn to by the analyser, shall be admitted in evidence in all prosecutions under this and the three preceding sections. The expense of such analysis or test, not exceeding twenty dollars in any one case, may be included in the costs of such prosecutions. Whoever hinders, obstructs, or in any way interferes with any inspector, or any agent of an inspector, in the performance of his duty, shall be punished by a fine of fifty dollars for the first offence, and of one hundred dollars for each subsequent offence.

Complaints for violations to be instituted by inspectors of milk. 1884, 310, § 2.

17. For the purposes of the four preceding sections the terms " butter " and " cheese " shall mean the products which are usually known by these names, and are manufactured exclusively from milk or cream, with salt and rennet, and with or without colouring matter.

Terms "butter" and "cheese" defined. Public Statutes, chap. 56, § 21.

18. Before commencing the analysis of any sample the person making the same shall reserve a portion which shall be sealed ; and in case of a complaint against any person the reserved portion of the sample alleged to be adulterated shall upon application be delivered to the defendant or his attorney.

Portion of sample to be reserved for defendant. 1884, 310, § 4.

      *   *   *   *   *   *

OF THE SALE OF CHOCOLATE.

28. No manufacturer of chocolate shall make any cake of chocolate except in pans in which are stamped the first letter of his christian name, the whole of his surname, the name of the town where he

Chocolate, how to be stamped. Public Statutes, chap. 60, § 8.

U

APPENDIX.

resides, and the quality of the chocolate in figures, No. 1, No. 2, No. 3, as the case may be, and the letters MASS.

Ingredients of.

29. Number one shall be made of cocoa of the first quality, and number two of cocoa of the second quality, and both shall be free from adulteration ; number three may be made of the inferior kinds and qualities of cocoa. Each box containing chocolate shall be branded on the end thereof with the word chocolate, the name of the manufacturer, the name of the town where it was manufactured, and the quality, as described and directed in the preceding section for the pans.

**Boxes, how branded.
Public Statutes, chap. 60, § 9.**

30. If chocolate manufactured in this commonwealth is offered for sale or found within the same, not being of one of the qualities described in the two preceding sections and marked as therein directed, the same may be seized and libelled.

**Boxes, when may be seized, etc.
Public Statutes, chap. 60, § 10.**

OF THE ADULTERATION OF VINEGAR.

**Sale of adulterated vinegar.
Penalty.
Public Statutes, chap. 60, § 69.
1883, 257, § 1.**

31. Every person who manufactures for sale or offers or exposes for sale as cider vinegar, any vinegar not the legitimate product of pure apple juice, known as apple cider or vinegar, not made exclusively of said apple cider or vinegar, into which any foreign substances, ingredients, drugs or acids have been introduced, as may appear by proper tests, shall for each such offence be punished by fine of not less than fifty nor more than one hundred dollars.

**Sale of vinegar containing ingredients injurious to health.
Penalty.
Public Statutes, chap. 60, § 70.**

32. Every person who manufactures for sale, or offers or exposes for sale, any vinegar found upon proper tests to contain any preparation of lead, copper, sulphuric acid, or other ingredients injurious to health, shall for each such offence be punished by fine of not less than one hundred dollars.

**Appointment of inspectors.
Public Statutes, chap. 60, § 71.**

33. The mayor and aldermen of cities shall, and the selectmen of towns may, annually appoint one or more persons to be inspectors of vinegar for their respective places, who shall be sworn before entering upon their duties.

**Compensation of inspectors.
1883, chap. 257, § 2.**

34. Any city or town in which an inspector shall be appointed under the preceding section, may provide compensation for such inspector from the time of such appointment, and in default of such provision shall be liable in an action at law for reasonable compensation for services performed under such appointment.

(CHAP. 307, ACTS OF 1884.)

AN ACT to prevent the adulteration of vinegar.

Be it enacted &c., as follows :—

SECTION 1. No person shall by himself, his servant or agent or as the servant or agent of any other person, sell, exchange, deliver or have in his custody or possession with intent to sell or exchange, or expose or offer for sale or exchange any adulterated vinegar, or label, brand or sell as cider vinegar, or as apple vinegar, any vinegar not the legitimate product of pure apple juice, or not made exclusively from apple cider. *Sale of adulterated vinegar.*

2. All vinegar shall have an acidity equivalent to the presence of not less than five per cent. by weight of absolute acetic acid, and in the case of cider vinegar shall contain in addition not less than one and one-half per cent. by weight of cider vinegar solids upon full evaporation over boiling water, and if any vinegar contains less than the above amount of acidity, or if any cider vinegar contains less than the above amount of cider vinegar solids, such vinegar shall be deemed to be adulterated within the meaning of this Act. *Standard of vinegar prescribed.*

3. It shall be the duty of the inspectors of milk who may be appointed by any city or town to enforce the provisions of this Act. *Milk inspectors to enforce Act.*

4. Whoever violates any of the provisions of this Act shall be punished by fine not exceeding one hundred dollars. *Penalty for violation.*

5. All Acts or parts of Acts inconsistent with this Act are hereby repealed.

Approved June 2, 1884.

The method of testing vinegar, used by Dr. B. F. Davenport, late Vinegar Inspector of Boston, is as follows :—

The following detailed practical method of determining whether a sample of "cider vinegar or apple vinegar" conforms to the requirements of the Statute of April 1885, relating thereto, which requires that it should be not only the legitimate and exclusive product of pure apple juice or cider, but also that it should not fall below the quality of possessing an acidity equivalent to the presence of not less than $4\frac{1}{2}$ per cent. by weight of absolute—that is, monohydrated—acetic acid, and should yield upon full evaporation at the temperature of boiling water not less than 2 per cent. by weight of cider vinegar solids, may prove of interest to those dealing in the article. As the limits set by the Statute are in per cents. by weight, the portion of vinegar taken for the tests should, for perfect accuracy, be also taken by weight—that is, the quantities of 6 and of 10 grammes are to be taken for the tests of strength and of residue ; but as taking it by measure, if of about the ordinary atmospheric temperature of 60 to 70 degrees F. will make the apparent percentage at most only 1 to 2 per cent. of itself greater than the true—that is, will make a true 5 per cent. vinegar appear to be, say, from 5·05 to 5·10 per cent.—measuring proves in practice to be accurate enough for all common commercial purposes, and therefore the quantities of 6 and of 10 cubic centimetres by measure may be taken in place of as many grammes.

All the measuring apparatus necessary for making the legal tests is one of the measuring tubes called burettes. It is most convenient to have this of a size to contain 25 to 50 c.c.—that is, cubic centimetres —and have these divided into tenths. The best form of burette is the Mohr's, which is closed by a glass stop-cock. Besides this, only a dropping-tube, called a pipette, graduated to deliver 6 and 10 c.c., will be needed. These tubes are to be obtained of any philosophical or chemical apparatus dealer, being articles generally kept in stock by them for common use, like yard-sticks.

The only two chemicals needed in determining the strength of a vinegar are such as can be obtained of any competent apothecary in any city of the State. They are simply a small vial of a 1 per cent. solution of Phenol-phthalein in diluted alcohol, and a sufficient quantity of a solution of caustic soda, prepared as directed for "Volumetric Solution of Soda" upon page 399 of the last 'U. S. Pharmacopœia,' a book which is in the hands of every competent apothecary, as it contains the formulæ according to which he is required by the law of the State to prepare all such medicinal preparations as are mentioned therein.

Having these, the procedure for making the test will be as follows : —Fill the pipette by suction, and then quickly close the top of it with the forefinger. Raise the tube out of the sample of vinegar, and let it empty out by drops exactly down to the top graduation-mark, this bearing the mark of o· c.c. Then holding it over a white mug or cup, let it run out exactly down to the 6 c.c. mark. Dilute the 6 c.c. of vinegar thus measured out into the mug with sufficient clean water to make it look about white, and then add to it about three drops of the Phenol-phthalein solution. Then having prepared the burette by filling it up to the top, zero, or any other noted mark of the graduation, with the volumetric solution of soda, let the soda solution run out cautiously into the diluted vinegar, which should be constantly stirred about. As soon as the vinegar in the mug begins to darken, the soda should then only be allowed to run into it by drops. This dropping is thus continued until at last a final drop of soda turns the vinegar suddenly to a permanent pink or cherry colour, which will not disappear upon further stirring. By now reading off from the graduations of the

burette the number of full c.c. divisions and of tenths which have been
emptied out to bring about this change of colour in the vinegar is known
the per cents. and tenths of acidity equivalent to true acetic acid contained in the vinegar being examined. This, if it is a pure cider
vinegar, and well made, will be upon the average about 6 per cent.,
but never under 5 per cent. If, in like manner, 10 c.c. of the vinegar
is exactly measured off by the pipette into a small light porcelain dish,
and then evaporated fully to dryness over boiling water, the number of
grammes weight gained by the dish, when multiplied by ten, gives the
percentage of solid residue contained in the vinegar.

There are certain characteristics peculiar to the residue of a pure
cider vinegar, the principal of which are the following :—It will be
about 3 per cent. in weight, and never less than 2 per cent. It is
always soft, viscid, of apple flavour, somewhat acid and astringent in
taste. A drop of it taken up in a clean loop of platinum or of iron
wire, and ignited in a colourless Bunsen gas-lamp flame, imparts to it
the pale lilac colour of a pure potash salt, without any yellow, due to
sodium, being visible. The ignited residue left in the loop of wire will
be a fusible bead of quite a good size, and it will have a strong alkaline
reaction upon moistened test-paper, effervescing briskly when immersed
in an acid. The presence in a vinegar of the *slightest* trace of any
free mineral acid will prevent the ignited residue having any alkaline
reaction, or effervescing with acids. The presence of any practical
amount of commercial acetic acid added to " tone up " the strength of
the vinegar will cause the igniting residue to impart another colour to
the Bunsen flame, and the residue itself will have a smoky pyroligneous
taste or odour. Any corn glucose used in the vinegar will cause its
residue when ignited to emit the characteristic odour of burning corn,
and, as the last spark glows through the carbonised mass, to usually
emit the familiar garlic odour of arsenic, for the common oil of vitriol
usually used in the production of glucose is now mostly derived from
pyrites, which almost always contain arsenic. A glucose vinegar which
has been made without vaporising the alcohol after the fermentation
of the glucose will also have a strong reducing action upon a copper
salt in an alkaline solution, and also will give a heavy precipitation of
lime with ammonium oxalate. A true malt vinegar always contains
phosphates, and a wine vinegar cream of tartar. The presence of any
acrid vegetable substance in a vinegar is known by the residue having
a pungent taste, especially if before the evaporation the vinegar has
been exactly neutralised with soda.

In a pure apple cider vinegar hydrogen sulphide gas will not cause
any discoloration, nor will the addition of a solution of either barium
nitrate, silver nitrate, or ammonium oxalate cause anything more than
the *very slightest* perceptible turbidity. But the addition of some
solution of lead acetate—that is, of sugar of lead—will cause an im-

mediate voluminous and flocculent precipitation, which will all settle out in about ten minutes, leaving a clear fluid above. In most of the so-called "apple vinegars," made with second pressings of the fermenting pumice, the addition of some of this lead solution will cause but a slight turbidity, without any precipitate settling out for several hours, and even then the precipitate will not be of the same appearance as in apple cider vinegar.

Sophistications of cider vinegar that will not be detected by some one or more of the above given tests are not likely to be met with, for the simple reason that they are not profitable. To translate percentages of acid strength into the old commercial terms of grains of soda bicarbonate per troy ounce, the per cent. may be multiplied by 6·72, or, *vice versâ*, divide the grains by the same factor. To reduce it into grains of potash bicarbonate 8 would be the factor to be used in like manner.

The general Adulteration of Food Law of the State of New Jersey is the same as that of New York. The following is a copy of a special Act in relation to the sale of adulterated milk :—

AN ACT to prevent the adulteration of milk and to regulate the sale of milk.

Persons selling or offering for sale skimmed milk, to solder a label or tag upon can or package.

1. Be it enacted by the Senate and General Assembly of the State of New Jersey, that every person who shall sell, or who shall offer or expose for sale, or who shall transport or carry, or who shall have in possession with intent to sell, or offer for sale, any milk from which the cream, or any part thereof has been removed, shall distinctly, durably and permanently solder a label, tag or mark of metal in a conspicuous place upon the outside and not more than six inches from the top of every can, vessel or package containing such milk, and said metal label, tag or mark shall have the words "skimmed milk" stamped, engraved or indented thereon in letters not less than one inch in height, and such milk shall only be sold or shipped in or retailed

Penalty for violating this section.

out of a can, vessel or package so marked, and every person who shall violate the provisions of this section shall be deemed guilty of a misdemeanour, and on conviction thereof shall be subject to the penalties prescribed in section eight of this Act.

Penalty for selling or offering for sale impure or adulterated milk.

2. And be it enacted, that every person who shall sell, or who shall offer for sale, or who shall transport or carry, for the purposes of sale, or who shall have in possession with intent to sell or offer for sale, any impure, adulterated or unwholesome milk, shall be deemed guilty of a

misdemeanour, and on conviction thereof shall be subject to the penalties prescribed in section eight of this Act.

3. And be it enacted, that every person who shall adulterate milk or who shall keep cows for the production of milk, in a crowded or unhealthful condition, or feed the same on food that produces impure, diseased or unwholesome milk, shall be deemed guilty of a misdemeanour, and on conviction thereof, shall be subject to the penalties prescribed in section eight of this Act.

Penalty for adulterating milk and keeping cows in an unhealthy condition, etc.

4. And be it enacted, that the addition of water or any substance or thing is hereby declared an adulteration; and milk that is obtained from animals that are fed on distillery waste, usually called " swill," or upon any substance in a state of putrefaction or rottenness, or upon any substance of an unhealthful nature, is hereby declared to be impure and unwholesome, and any person offending as aforesaid shall be deemed guilty of a misdemeanour, and on conviction thereof shall be subject to the penalties prescribed in section eight of this Act.

Addition of water or other substance declared an adulteration.

5. And be it enacted, that every person who shall feed cows on distillery waste, usually called " swill," or upon any substance in a state of putrefaction, or rottenness or upon any substance of an unwholesome nature, shall be deemed guilty of a misdemeanour, and on conviction thereof shall be subject to the penalties prescribed in section eight of this Act.

Penalty for feeding cows on unwholesome substances.

6. And be it enacted, that every person who shall sell, or who shall offer for sale any milk that has been exposed to, or contaminated by the emanations, discharge or exhalations from persons sick with scarlet fever, measles, diphtheria, small pox, typhoid fever, or any contagious disease by which the health or life of any person may be endangered or compromised, shall be guilty of a misdemeanour, and on conviction thereof shall be subject to the penalties prescribed in section eight of this Act.

Penalty for selling or offering for sale milk exposed to certain diseases.

7. And be it enacted, that in all prosecutions under this Act, if the milk shall be shown, upon analysis, to contain more than eighty-seven per centum of watery fluids, or to contain less than thirteen per centum of milk solids, it shall be deemed, for the purposes of this Act, to be adulterated.

When milk is deemed to be adulterated.

8. And be it enacted, that every person who shall violate any of the provisions of this Act shall be deemed guilty of a misdemeanour, and, upon conviction thereof, shall be punished by a fine of not less than fifty dollars, nor more than two hundred dollars, or imprisonment in the county jail for not less than thirty days, nor more than ninety days, or both, at the discretion of the court, and if the fine is not immediately paid, shall be imprisoned for not less than thirty days, or until said fine shall be paid, and for a second offence by a fine of not less than one hundred dollars, nor more than three hundred dollars, or by imprisonment in the county jail for not less than sixty days, nor

Penalty for violating the provisions of this Act.

more than ninety days, or both, at the discretion of the court, and for any subsequent offence by a fine of fifty dollars and imprisonment in the county jail not less than sixty nor more than ninety days; and on trial for such misdemeanour or penalty, the sale, or offer for sale, or exposure for sale, of milk or articles contrary to the provisions of this Act, shall be presumptive evidence of knowledge by the accused of the character of the milk or article so sold, or offered, or exposed for sale, and that the can, vessel or package was not marked as required by this Act.

Penalties—how recovered.

9. And be it enacted, that all penalties imposed under the provisions of this Act may be sued for in any court having competent jurisdiction, one-half the fine to go to the person making the complaint, and the other half to be paid to the county collector for the benefit of the county; any court of competent jurisdiction in this state shall have jurisdiction to try and dispose of all and any of the offences arising in the same county against the provisions of this Act, and every justice of the peace shall have jurisdiction within his county of actions to recover any penalty hereby given or created.

State Board of Health empowered to appoint an inspector of milk. Compensation and expenses—how paid.

Duties of inspector.

10. And be it enacted, that the State Board of Health is hereby empowered and directed to appoint, each year, a competent person, who shall act as State inspector of milk, at a salary of eight hundred dollars per annum, payable by the treasurer of this State, by warrant of the comptroller, in quarterly payments, for the purposes of this Act, and in addition thereto, said inspector shall be paid his actual travelling expenses while in the performance of his duties, and actual expenses of suits brought by him under this Act, payable by the treasurer of this State by warrant of the comptroller; said inspector shall act until removed by said board, or until his successor is appointed, and shall make such reports to said board, at such time as it may direct; said inspector, having reason to believe the provisions of this Act are being violated, shall have power to open any can, vessel, or package containing milk and not marked as directed by the first section of this Act, whether sealed, locked or otherwise, or whether in transit or otherwise; and if, upon inspection, he shall find such can, vessel or package to contain any milk which has been adulterated, or from which the cream, or any part thereof, has been removed, or which is sold, offered or exposed for sale, or held in possession with intent to sell or offer for sale, in violation of any section of this Act, said inspector is empowered to condemn the same and pour the contents of such can, vessel or package upon the ground, and bring suit against

Inspector to advertise name and place of business of persons convicted of violating this Act.

the person or party so violating the law, and the penalty, when so collected by such suit, shall be paid into the treasury of this State, and said inspector is directed to cause the name and place of business of all persons convicted of violating any section of this Act to be published once in two newspapers in the county in which the offence is committed; and said inspector is empowered to appoint one or more deputies, who shall have power to inspect milk, as provided by this Act, and who shall be empowered to act as complainant, as provided by section nine of this Act; provided, that no expense be incurred to the State by action or appointment in lieu thereof of said deputies. Proviso.

11. And be it enacted, that said State inspector of milk shall also be a public analyst, and shall make analyses and investigations of food, drugs, and other substances, as he may be directed so to do by the State Board of Health. Inspector to be a public analyst.

12. And be it enacted, that an Act entitled "An Act to prevent the adulteration of milk, and to prevent traffic in impure and unwholesome milk," approved April seventh, one thousand eight hundred and seventy-five, and an Act, entitled "An Act to regulate the sale of milk," approved April fifth, one thousand eight hundred and seventy-eight, and an Act entitled "A supplement to an Act to regulate the sale of milk, approved April fifth, one thousand eight hundred and seventy-eight," approved March twelfth, one thousand eight hundred and eighty," are hereby repealed. Certain Acts repealed.

13. And be it enacted, that this Act shall take place immediately.

Approved March 22, 1881.

The New Jersey State Board of Health has adopted the following rules for the government of its inspectors and analysts :—

Duties of Inspectors.

1. The inspector is to buy samples of food or drugs, and to seal each sample in the presence of a witness.

2. The inspector must affix to each sample a label bearing a number, his initials, and the date of purchase.

3. Under no circumstance is the inspector to inform the analyst as to the source of the sample before the analysis shall have been completed and formally reported to the President or Secretary of the State Board of Health.

4. Inspectors are to keep a record of each sample as follows :—

    (1). Number of sample.
    (2). Date and time of purchase.
    (3). Name of witness to sealing.
    (4). Name and address of seller.

(5) Name and address of producer, manufacturer or wholesaler, when known, with marks on original package.

(6) Name of analyst and date of sending.

(7) How sent to analyst.

5. If the seller desires a portion of the sample, the inspector is to deliver it under seal. The duplicate sample left with seller should have a label containing the same marks as are affixed to the portion taken by the inspector.

6. The inspector is to deliver the sample to the analyst, taking his receipt for the same, or he may send it by registered mail, express or special messenger.

DUTIES OF THE ANALYSTS.

1. The analyst is to analyse the samples immediately upon receipt thereof.

2. Samples, with the exception of milk and similar perishable articles, are to be divided by the analyst and a portion sealed up, and a copy of the original label affixed. These duplicates are to be sent to the Secretary of the State Board of Health at the end of each month, and to be retained by him until demanded for another analysis, as provided for in section 3 of these Rules.

3. Should the result obtained by any analyst be disputed in any case, an appeal may be made to the State Board of Health, through its secretary, by the defendant or person selling the sample, or his attorney, and said secretary shall then require another member of the Committee of Public Analysts to repeat the analysis, using the duplicate sample for such purpose. But when an appeal shall be made, a sum of money sufficient to cover the expenses of the second analysis shall be deposited with the President of the State Board of Health, which sum shall be paid over to the analyst designated by the President and Secretary of the Board to perform the second analysis, in case the analysis shall be found to agree with the first in all essential particulars.

4. In the case of all articles having a standard of purity fixed by any of the laws of the State, the certificate of the analyst should show the relation of the article in question to that standard.

5. Where standards of strength, purity or quality are not fixed by law, the Committee of Analysts shall present to the State Board of Health such standard as in their judgment should be fixed.

6. Each analyst should keep a record book, in which should be entered notes, as follows:—

(1) From whom the sample is received.

(2) Date, time and manner in which the sample was received.

(3) Marks on package, sealed or not.

(4) Results of analysis in detail.

This record should be produced at each meeting of the committee.

7. At the completion of the analysis a certificate in the form given below should be forwarded to the person from whom the sample was received, and a duplicate copy sent to the State Board of Health.

CERTIFICATE.

To whom it may concern.

I, _____, a member of the Committee of Public Analysts, appointed by the State Board of Health of New Jersey under the provisions of an Act entitled " An Act to prevent the adulteration of food and drugs," approved March 25th, 1881, do hereby certify that I received from _____, on the _____ day of _____, 188 ___, a sample of _____, sealed as require by the rules of said Board, and bearing the following marks, to wit :_____

I carefully mixed said samples and have analysed the same, and hereby certify and declare the results of my analysis to be as follows :_____

_____ [*Signature.*]

EXCEPTIONS.

The following exceptions are adopted :—

Mustard.—Compounds of mustard, with rice flour, starch, or flour, may be sold if each package is marked " Compound Mustard," and if not more than 25 per cent. of such substance is added to the mustard.

Coffee.—Compounds of coffee with chicory, rye, wheat, or other cereals, may be sold if the package is marked " A Mixture," and if the label states the per cent. of coffee contained in said mixture.

Oleomargarine and other imitation dairy products may be sold if each package is marked with the name of the substance, and in all respects fulfils the terms of the special law as to these.

Syrups.—When mixed with glucose, syrup may be sold if the package is marked " A Mixture."

The following is a summary of the laws of various States and Territories relative to Oleomargarine :*—

STATES.

California.

" An Act to prevent the sale of oleomargarine, under the name and pretence that the said commodity is butter."

This law is restrictive, requires the word " oleomargarine " to be branded on the package.

* Second Report of the New York State Dairy Commissioner.

The penalty is from fifty dollars to two hundred dollars, or imprisonment from fifty to two hundred days, or both.

"An Act to prevent fraud and deception in the sale of butter and cheese."

This law is restrictive, requiring the article to be manufactured and sold under its appropriate name.

Penalty is from ten dollars to five hundred dollars or imprisonment from ten to ninety days, or both.

Approved, March 2, 1881.

"An Act to prevent the sale or disposition as butter of the substance known as 'oleomargarine,' or 'oleomargarine butter,' and when 'oleomargarine' or 'oleomargarine butter' is sold or disposed of requiring notice thereof to be given."

This law is restrictive, requiring branding, also requiring hotel-keepers, etc., to keep posted up in their places of business in three places, the words "oleomargarine sold here."

Penalty from five dollars to five hundred dollars, or imprisonment for not more than three months, or both such fine and imprisonment.

Approved, March 1, 1883.

"An Act to protect and encourage the production and sale of pure and wholesome milk, and to prohibit and punish the production and sale of unwholesome or adulterated milk."

This law makes it a misdemeanour to sell or expose for sale adulterated or unwholesome milk, or to keep cows for producing the same in an unhealthy condition, or feeding them on feed that will produce impure milk, etc.

Penalty is one hundred dollars for the first offence, and double that amount for each subsequent offence.

Approved, March 12, 1870.

Colorado.

"An Act to encourage the sale of milk, and to provide penalties for the adulteration thereof."

This law makes it a misdemeanour to sell adulterated milk or milk from which the cream has been taken, or for withholding the strippings without the purchasers being aware of the fact.

Penalty is from twenty-five dollars to one hundred dollars, or imprisonment for six months, or by both such fine and imprisonment.

In force, May 20, 1881.

"An Act to regulate the manufacture and sale of oleomargarine, butterine, suine or other substances made in imitation of, or having the semblance of butter, and to provide penalties for the violation of the provisions hereof."

This law requires that a license shall be necessary to manufacture, import, or sell oleomargarine or kindred products within the State. License to manufacture or import not less than one thousand ; license to sell not less than five hundred.

Penalty from fifty dollars to five hundred dollars, or imprisonment not to exceed one year or both.

Approved, April 6, 1885.

Connecticut.

" An Act concerning the sale of oleomargarine and other articles."

This law requires that the article shall be properly branded, and that the seller shall keep a sign posted up in his place of business that such commodity is sold there.

Penalty seven dollars, or imprisonment from ten to thirty days or both.

Approved, April 4, 1883.

Delaware.

"An Act to regulate the manufacture and sale of oleomargarine."
This law is restrictive in its nature.
Penalty fifty dollars, commitment until the fine is paid.
Approved, February 10, 1879.

"An Act to amend chapter 154, volume 16, Laws of Delaware."
This amendment has reference to the fact that the substance manufactured is " artificial butter."

Passed, March 21, 1883.

Florida.

Chapter 80, sections 34-35, McClellans' Digest, 1881.

Section 34 makes it a misdemeanour to sell spurious preparations as butter; section 35 has reference to hotels and boarding-houses.

Penalty, not to exceed one hundred, or imprisonment not to exceed thirty days, or both.

Illinois.

" An Act to prevent and punish the adulteration of articles of food, drink and medicine, and the sale thereof when adulterated."

Section 3 of this law has reference to colouring matter in food, drink or medicine.

Section 4 of this law has reference to mixing oleomargarine with butter, cheese, etc., requiring the seller to inform the buyer of the fact and the proportion of the mixture.

Penalty, first offence, twenty-five dollars to two hundred dollars; second offence, one hundred dollars to two hundred dollars, or imprisonment from one to six months or both; third offence, from five hundred dollars to two thousand dollars and imprisonment not less than one year nor more than five years.

Approved, June 1, 1881.

"An Act to require operators of butter and cheese factories on the co-operative plan to give bonds, and to prescribe penalties for the violation thereof."

This law requires the filing of a bond in the penal sum of six thousand dollars that certain reports will be made on the first of each month and a copy filed with the town clerk, etc.

Penalty, from two hundred dollars to five hundred dollars, or imprisonment from thirty days to six months, or both.

Approved, June 18, 1883.

Indiana.

Section 2071, Revised Statutes. "Selling unwholesome milk."

This section provides against the sale of unwholesome milk, whether from adulteration or from the feed given the cows; also against the use of poisonous or deleterious material in the manufacture of butter and cheese.

Penalty, from fifty dollars to five hundred dollars.

"An Act to prevent the sale of impure butter, and the keeping on any table at any hotel or boarding-house of impure butter, providing penalties declaring an emergency."

This law requires the branding with the word "oleomargarine."

Penalty from ten dollars to fifty dollars.

Approved, March 3, 1883.

Iowa.

Section 4042, Code.

This section provides against the adulteration of milk in any way.

Penalty, twenty-five dollars to one hundred dollars, and makes the offender liable in double that amount to the party injured.

"An Act to protect the dairy interests and for the punishment of fraud connected therewith."

This law requires that "oleo" and kindred products shall be branded with the word "oleomargarine."

Penalty, from twenty dollars to one hundred dollars or imprisonment from ten to ninety days.

"An Act to prevent and punish the adulteration of articles of food, drink, and medicine, and the sale thereof when adulterated."

This law provides that skimmed milk cheese shall be so branded, and when oleomargarine is mixed with any other substance for sale it shall be distinctly branded with the true and appropriate name.

Penalty, first offence, from ten dollars to fifty dollars ; second, from twenty-five dollars to one hundred dollars, or confined in the county jail not more than thirty days ; third, from five hundred dollars to one thousand dollars and imprisonment not less than one year nor more than five years.

Maryland.

"An Act to repeal the Act of 1883, chapter 493, entitled 'An Act for the protection of dairymen, and to prevent deception in the sale of butter and cheese, and to re-enact new sections in lieu thereof.'"

This law requires that substances made in semblance of butter and cheese not the true product of the dairy shall be branded with the word "oleomargarine" so as to be conspicuous, and that the buyer shall be apprised of the nature of the article that he has bought.

Penalty, one hundred dollars, or imprisonment not less than thirty or more than ninety days for the second offence, and not less than three months nor more than one year for the third offence.

Approved, April 8, 1884.

Maine.

"An Act to amend chapter 128 of the Revised Statutes, relating to the sale of unwholesome food."

This law is prohibitive as to oleomargarine and kindred products.

Penalty, for the first offence one hundred dollars, and for each subsequent offence two hundred dollars, to be recovered with costs.

Massachusetts.

This State has a law against selling adulterated milk.

Penalty, for first offence, fifty dollars to one hundred dollars ; for the second offence, one hundred dollars to three hundred dollars, or by imprisonment for thirty to sixty days ; and for each subsequent offence, fifty dollars and imprisonment from sixty to ninety days.

Michigan.

"An Act to prevent deception in the manufacture and sale of dairy products and to preserve the public health."

This law prohibits the manufacture and sale of oleomargarine and kindred products.

Penalty, two hundred dollars to five hundred dollars or not less than six months' nor more than one year's imprisonment, or both, for the first offence, and by imprisonment for one year for each subsequent offence.

Approved, June 12, 1885.

Minnesota.

"An Act to prohibit and prevent the sale or manufacture of unhealthy or adulterated dairy products."

This law prohibits the sale of impure or adulterated milk.

Penalty, twenty-five dollars to two hundred dollars, or imprisonment from one to six months, or both for the first offence, and six months' imprisonment for each subsequent offence.

This law also prohibits the manufacture and sale of oleaginous substances or compounds of the same.

Penalty, from one hundred dollars to five hundred dollars, or from six months' to one year's imprisonment, or both, such fine and imprisonment for the first offence, and by imprisonment one year for each subsequent offence.

Approved, March 5, 1885.

Missouri.

This State passed the first prohibitory law.

Penalty, confinement in the county jail not to exceed one year, or fine not to exceed one thousand dollars, or both.

Nebraska.

Section 2345, "Skimmed milk or adulterated milk."

This section provides against the sale of adulterated milk, and makes a penalty of from twenty-five dollars to one hundred dollars and be liable to double the amount to the person or persons upon whom the fraud is perpetrated.

New Hampshire.

"An Act relating to the sale of imitation butter."

This law provides that no artificial butter shall be sold unless it is coloured pink.

Penalty, for the first offence, fifty dollars, and for a second offence a fine of one hundred dollars. "A certificate of the analysis sworn to by the analyser shall be admitted in evidence in all prosecutions."

"The expense of the analysis, not exceeding twenty dollars, included in the costs."

New Jersey.

Law similar to the New York law.

Ohio.

This State has a law that is prohibitory except as to oleomargarine made of beef suet and milk.

Penalty, one hundred dollars to five hundred dollars, or from three to six months' imprisonment, or both, for the first offence ; and by such fine and imprisonment for one year for each subsequent offence.

Passed, April 27, 1885.

Oregon.

The law in this State provides against adulterated and unwholesome milk, against keeping cows in an unhealthy condition, and against feeding them upon unhealthful food.

It also provides that oleaginous substances sold upon the market shall be so branded as to distinguish them from the true dairy product ; and that in hotels, boarding-houses, restaurants, etc., where such substances are used as an article of food, the bill of fare shall state the fact, and that the name of the said substance shall be posted up in the dining-room in a conspicuous place.

Passed, February 20, 1885.

Pennsylvania.

" An Act to protect dairymen, and to prevent deception in sales of butter and cheese."

This act requires the branding of imitation butter and cheese.

Penalty, one hundred dollars. Violations of this Act by exportation to a foreign country are punished by a fine of from five dollars to two hundred dollars, or by imprisonment from ten to thirty days, or by both such fine and imprisonment.

Approved, May 24, 1883.

" An Act for the protection of the public health and to prevent adulteration of dairy products and fraud in the sale thereof."

This law prohibits the sale of oleomargarine and kindred products.

Penalty, one hundred dollars to three hundred dollars, or by imprisonment from ten to thirty days for the first offence, and by imprisonment for one year for each subsequent offence.

Approved, May 21, 1885.

Rhode Island.

" Of the sale of butter, potatoes, onions, berries, nuts, and shelled beans."

This law provides that artificial butter shall be stamped " Oleomar-

X

garine," and that the retailer shall deliver to the purchaser a label upon which shall be the word " Oleomargarine."

Penalty, one hundred dollars.

Tennessee.

Code of 1884, chapter 14, sections 2682, 2683, 2684.

This law requires that the substance shall be manufactured under its true and appropriate name, and that it shall be distinctly branded with the true and appropriate name.

Penalty, from ten dollars to three hundred dollars, or imprisonment from ten to ninety days.

Vermont.

"An Act to prevent fraud in the sale of oleomargarine and other substances as butter."

This law provides that oleomargarine and kindred products shall not be sold as butter.

Penalty, five hundred dollars.

Approved, November 1884.

Chapters 192, Laws of 1874, 76 of 1870, 51 of 1855, provide against the adulteration of milk.

Virginia.

Code of Virginia, 1873, chapter 865, title 26, section 56.

" Provision against adulterating milk intended for the manufacture of cheese."

This law provides against the adulteration of milk carried to cheese manufactories, etc.

Penalty, from twenty-five dollars to one hundred dollars, with costs of suit.

West Virginia.

Chapter 41, Acts of West Virginia, 1885.

" An Act to prevent the manufacture and sale of mixed and impure butter and cheese and imitations thereof."

This law requires that the true and appropriate name of the substance shall be printed thereon, etc.

Penalty, from ten dollars to one hundred dollars, or imprisonment.

Wisconsin.

Section 1494, chapter 61, Revised Statutes.

This Act provides that no cream shall be taken from the manufactory where it is being worked up, also that the persons manufacturing cheese at factories shall keep certain records.

Chapter 361, R. S.

"An Act to prevent the manufacture and sale of oleaginous substances or compounds of the same in imitation of the pure dairy products, and to repeal sections 1 and 3 of chapter 49 of the laws of 1881."

This law prohibits the manufacture and sale of oleomargarine and kindred products.

Penalty, not to exceed one thousand dollars, or imprisonment not to exceed one year, or by both such fine and imprisonment.

Published, April 13, 1885.

TERRITORIES.

Arizona.

"An Act to regulate the sale and manufacture of oleomargarine or other substitutes for butter in the Territory of Arizona."

This law requires that oleomargarine and kindred substances sold in the territory shall be appropriately branded with the word "oleomargarine." And that the seller shall deliver to the purchaser a printed label on which is the word "oleomargarine." Also that dealers shall keep posted up in their places of business this sign, "Oleomargarine sold here."

Penalty for the first offence not less than five dollars, for the second offence not less than one hundred dollars or imprisonment for sixty days, and for each succeeding offence five hundred dollars and imprisonment for ninety days.

Approved, March 8, 1883.

Dakota.

"An Act to secure the public health and safety against unwholesome provisions."

This law requires that all oleaginous substances shall be branded with their true and proper names. Costs of analyses, not exceeding twenty dollars, shall or may be included in the costs of prosecutions.

Penalty, first offence, one hundred dollars, and every subsequent offence, two hundred dollars.

Passed at the session of 1883.

The following States and Territories have no law on the subject :—

STATES.—Alabama, Arkansas, Georgia, Kansas, Kentucky, Louisiana, Mississippi, Nevada, North Carolina, South Carolina, Texas.

TERRITORIES.—Alaska, Idaho, Montana, New Mexico, Utah, Washington, Wyoming.

X 2

The complete text of the United States Oleomargarine
Tax Law is as follows :—

SECTION 1. Be it enacted by the Senate and House of Repre-
sentatives of the United States of America, in Congress assembled.
That for the purposes of this Act the word "butter" shall be understood to mean the food product usually known as butter, and which is
made exclusively from milk or cream, or both, with or without common
salt, and with or without additional colouring matter.

2. That for the purposes of this Act certain manufactured substances
certain extracts, and certain mixtures and compounds, including such
mixtures and compounds with butter, shall be known and designated
as "oleomargarine," namely : All substances heretofore known as
oleomargarine, oleo, oleomargarine oil, butterine, lardine, suine, and
neutral ; all mixtures and compounds of oleomargarine, oleo, oleomargarine oil, butterine, lardine, suine, and neutral ; all lard extracts
and tallow extracts ; and all mixtures and compounds of tallow, beef
fat, suet, lard, lard oil, vegetable oil, annatto and other colouring matter,
intestinal fat, and offal fat made in imitation or semblance of butter, or
when so made, calculated or intended to be sold as butter or for butter.

3. That special taxes are imposed as follows :—Manufacturers of
oleomargarine shall pay six hundred dollars. Every person who
manufactures oleomargarine for sale shall be deemed a manufacturer
of oleomargarine.

4. Wholesale dealers in oleomargarine shall pay four hundred and
eighty dollars. Every person who sells or offers for sale oleomargarine
in the original manufacturer's packages shall be deemed a wholesale
dealer in oleomargarine. But any manufacturer of oleomargarine who
has given the required bond and paid the required special tax, and
who sells only oleomargarine of his own production, at the place of
manufacture, in the original packages to which the tax-paid stamps
are affixed, shall not be required to pay the special tax of a wholesale
dealer in oleomargarine on account of such sale.

Retail dealers in oleomargarine shall pay forty-eight dollars. Every
person who sells oleomargarine in less quantities than ten pounds at
one time shall be regarded as a retail dealer in oleomargarine. And
Sections 3232, 3233, 3234, 3235, 3236, 3237, 3238, 3239, 3240, 3241,
and 3243 of the Revised Statutes of the United States are, so far as
applicable, made to extend to and include and apply to the special
taxes imposed by this section, and to the persons upon whom they are
imposed. (See page 10 for Revised Statutes.) Provided, That in case
any manufacturer of oleomargarine commences business subsequent to
the thirtieth day of June in any year, the special tax shall be reckoned
from the first day of July in that year, and shall be five hundred dollars.

4. That every person who carries on the business of a manufacturer

of oleomargarine without having paid the special tax therefor, as required by law, shall, besides being liable to the payment of the tax, be fined not less than one thousand dollars and not more than five thousand dollars ; and every person who carries on the business of a wholesale dealer in oleomargarine without having paid the special tax therefor, as required by law, shall, besides being liable to the payment of the tax, be fined not less than five hundred dollars nor more than two thousand dollars, and every person who carries on the business of a retail dealer in oleomargarine without having paid the special tax therefor, as required by law, shall, besides being liable to the payment of the tax, be fined not less than fifty dollars nor more than five hundred dollars for each and every offence.

5. That every manufacturer of oleomargarine shall file with the Collector of Internal Revenue of the district in which his manufactory is located, such notices, inventories, and bonds, shall keep such books and render such returns of materials and products, shall put up such signs and affix such number to his factory, and conduct his business under such surveillance of officers and agents as the Commissioner of Internal Revenue, with the approval of the Secretary of the Treasury may, by regulation, require. But the bond required of such manufacturer shall be with sureties satisfactory to the Collector of Internal Revenue, and in a penalȝ sum of not less than five thousand dollars, and the sum of said bond may be increased from time to time, and additional sureties required at the discretion of the Collector, or under instructions of the Commissioner of Internal Revenue.

6. That all oleomargarine shall be packed by the manufacturer thereof in firkins, tubs, or other wooden packages not before used for that purpose, each containing not less than ten pounds, and marked, stamped and branded as the Commissioner of Internal Revenue, with the approval of the Secretary of the Treasury, shall prescribe ; and all sales made by manufacturers of oleomargarine and wholesale dealers in oleomargarine shall be in original stamped packages. Retail dealers in oleomargarine must sell only from original stamped packages, in quantities not exceeding ten pounds, and shall pack the oleomargarine sold by them in suitable wooden or paper packages, which shall be marked and branded as the Commissioner of Internal Revenue with the approval of the Secretary of the Treasury, shall prescribe. Every person who knowingly sells or offers for sale, or delivers or offers to deliver, any oleomargarine in any other form than in new wooden or paper packages as above described, or who packs in any package any oleomargarine in any manner contrary to law, or who falsely brands any package or affixes a stamp on any package denoting a less amount of tax than that required by law, shall be fined for each offence not more than one thousand dollars, and be imprisoned not less than six months nor more than two years.

7. That every manufacturer of oleomargarine shall securely affix, by pasting, on each package containing oleomargarine manufactured by him, a label on which shall be printed, besides the number of the manufactory and the district and State in which it is situated, these words :—" Notice.—The manufacturer of the oleomargarine herein contained has complied with all the requirements of law. Every person is cautioned not to use this package again or the stamp thereon again nor to remove the contents of this package without destroying said stamp, under the penalty provided by law in such cases." Every manufacturer of oleomargarine who neglects to affix such label to any package containing oleomargarine made by him, or sold or offered for sale by or for him, and every person who removes any such label so affixed from any such package, shall be fined fifty dollars for each package in respect to which such offence is committed.

8. That upon oleomargarine which shall be manufactured and sold, or removed for consumption or use, there shall be assessed and collected a tax of two cents per pound, to be paid by the manufacturer thereof; and any fractional part of a pound in a package shall be taxed as a pound. The tax levied by this section shall be represented by coupon stamps ; and the provisions of existing laws governing the engraving, issue, sale, accountability, effacement and destruction of stamps relating to tobacco and snuff, as far as applicable, are hereby made to apply to stamps provided for by this section.

9. That whenever any manufacturer of oleomargarine sells, or removes for sale or consumption, any oleomargarine upon which the tax is required to be paid by stamps, without the use of the proper stamps, it shall be the duty of the Commissioner of Internal Revenue, within a period of not more than two years after such sale or removal, upon satisfactory proof, to estimate the amount of tax which has been omitted to be paid, and to make an assessment therefor and certify the same to the collector. The tax so assessed shall be in addition to the penalties imposed by law for such sale or removal.

10. That all oleomargarine imported from foreign countries shall, in addition to any import duty imposed on the same, pay an internal revenue tax of 15 cents per pound, such tax to be represented by coupon stamps as in the case of oleomargarine manufactured in the United States. The stamps shall be affixed and cancelled by the owner or importer of the oleomargarine while it is in the custody of the proper custom-house officers ; and the oleomargarine shall not pass out of the custody of said officers until the stamps have been so affixed and cancelled, but shall be put up in wooden packages, each containing not less than ten pounds ; as prescribed in this Act for oleomargarine manufactured in the United States, before the stamps are affixed ; and the owner or importer of such oleomargarine shall be liable to all the penal provisions of this Act prescribed for manu-

facturers of oleomargarine manufactured in the United States. Whenever it is necessary to take any oleomargarine so imported to any place other than the public stores of the United States for the purpose of affixing and cancelling such stamps, the Collector of Customs of the port where such oleomargarine is entered, shall designate a bonded warehouse to which it shall be taken, under the control of such customs officer as such collector shall direct; and every officer of customs who permits such oleomargarine to pass out of his custody or control without compliance by the owner or importer thereof with the provisions of this section relating thereto, shall be guilty of a misdemeanour, and shall be fined not less than one thousand dollars nor more than five thousand dollars, and imprisoned not less than six months nor more than three years. Every person who sells or offers for sale any imported oleomargarine, or oleomargarine purporting or claimed to have been imported, not put up in packages and stamped as provided by this Act, shall be fined not less than five hundred dollars nor more than five thousand dollars, and be imprisoned not less than six months nor more than two years.

11. That every person who knowingly purchases or receives for sale any oleomargarine which has not been branded or stamped according to law, shall be liable to a penalty of fifty dollars for each such offence.

12. That every person who knowingly purchases or receives for sale any oleomargarine from any manufacturer who has not paid the special tax shall be liable for each offence to a penalty of one hundred dollars, and to forfeiture of all articles so purchased or received, or of the full value thereof.

13. That whenever any stamped package containing oleomargarine is emptied, it shall be the duty of the person in whose hands the same is to destroy utterly the stamps thereon, and any person who wilfully neglects or refuses so to do shall for each such offence be fined not exceeding fifty dollars, and imprisoned not less than ten days nor more than six months. And any person who fraudulently gives away or accepts from another, or who sells, buys, or uses for packing oleomargarine, any such stamped package, shall for each such offence be fined not exceeding one hundred dollars and be imprisoned not more than one year. Any revenue officer may destroy any emptied oleomargarine package upon which the tax-paid stamp is found.

14. That there shall be in the office of the Commissioner of Internal Revenue an analytical chemist and a microscopist, who shall each be appointed by the Secretary of the Treasury, and shall each receive a salary of two thousand five hundred dollars per annum; and the Commissioner of Internal Revenue may, whenever in his judgment the necessities of the service so require, employ chemists and microscopists, to be paid such compensation as he may deem proper, not exceeding in the aggregate any appropriation made for that purpose.

And such commissioner is authorised to decide what substances, extracts, mixtures or compounds which may be submitted for his inspection in contested cases are to be taxed under this Act ; and his decision in matters of taxation under this Act shall be final. The commissioner may also decide whether any substances made in imitation or semblance of butter, and intended for human consumption, contains ingredients deleterious to the public health ; but in case of doubt or contest his decisions in this class of cases may be appealed from to a board hereby constituted for the purpose, and composed of the Surgeon-General of the Army, the Surgeon-General of the Navy, and the Commissioner of Agriculture, and the decisions of this body shall be final in the premises.

15. That all packages of oleomargarine subject to tax under this Act that shall be found without stamps or marks as herein provided, and all oleomargarine intended for human consumption which contains ingredients adjudged, as hereinbefore provided, to be deleterious to the public health, shall be forfeited to the United States. Any person who shall wilfully remove or deface the stamps, marks or brands on the package containing oleomargarine taxed as provided herein shall be guilty of a misdemeanour, and shall be punished by a fine of not less than one hundred dollars nor more than two thousand dollars, and by imprisonment for not less than thirty days nor more than six months.

16. That oleomargarine may be removed from the place of manufacture for export to a foreign country without payment of tax or affixing stamps thereto, under such regulations and the filing of such bonds and other security as the Commissioner of Internal Revenue, with the approval of the Secretary of the Treasury, may prescribe. Every person who shall export oleomargarine shall brand upon every tub, firkin, or other package containing such article the word " oleomargarine" in plain Roman letters not less than one-half inch square.

17. That whenever any person engaged in carrying on the business of manufacturing oleomargarine defrauds, or attempts to defraud, the United States of the tax on the oleomargarine produced by him, or any part thereof, he shall forfeit the factory and manufacturing apparatus used by him, and all oleomargarine and all raw material for the production of oleomargarine found in the factory and on the factory premises, and shall be fined not less than five hundred dollars nor more than five thousand dollars, and be imprisoned not less than six months nor more than three years.

18. That if any manufacturer of oleomargarine, any dealer therein, or any importer or exporter thereof shall knowingly or wilfully omit, neglect, or refuse to do, or cause to be done, any of the things required by law in the carrying on or conducting of his business, or shall do anything by this Act prohibited, if there be no specific penalty or

punishment imposed by any other section of this Act for the neglect-
ing, omitting, or refusing to do, or for the doing or causing to be done,
the thing required or prohibited, he shall pay a penalty of one thousand
dollars; and if the person so offending be the manufacturer of or a
wholesale dealer in oleomargarine, all the oleomargarine owned by
him, or in which he has any interest as owner, shall be forfeited to the
United States.

19. That all fines, penalties and forfeitures imposed by this Act may
be recovered in any court of competent jurisdiction.

20. That the Commissioner of Internal Revenue with the approval
of the Secretary of the Treasury, may make all needful regulations for
the carrying into effect of this Act.

21. That this Act shall go into effect on the ninetieth day after its
passage ; and all wooden packages containing ten or more pounds of
oleomargarine found on the premises of any dealer on or after the
ninetieth day succeeding the date of the passage of this Act shall be
deemed to be taxable under section eight of this Act, and shall be
taxed, and shall have affixed thereto the stamps, marks, and brands
required by this Act or by regulations made pursuant to this Act ; and
for the purposes of securing the affixing of the stamps, marks and
brands required by this Act, the oleomargarine shall be regarded as
having been manufactured and sold, or removed from the manufactory
for consumption or use, on or after the day this Act takes effect; and
such stock on hand at the time of the taking effect of this Act may be
stamped, marked and branded under special regulations of the Commissioner of Internal Revenue, approved by the Secretary of the
Treasury; and the Commissioner of Internal Revenue may authorise
the holder of such packages to mark and brand the same and to affix
thereto the proper tax-paid stamps.

The following is the United States' Tea Adulteration Law :—

SECTION 1. Be it enacted by the Senate and House of Represen-
tatives of the United States of America in Congress assembled, That
from and after the passage of this Act it shall be unlawful for any
person or persons or corporation to import or bring into the United
States any merchandise for sale as tea, adulterated with spurious leaf
or with exhausted leaves, or which contains so great an admixture of
chemicals or other deleterious substances as to make it unfit for use;
and the importation of all such merchandise is hereby prohibited.

2. That on making entry at the custom house of all tea or merchandise described as tea imported into the United States, the importer or consignee shall give a bond to the collector of the port that
such merchandise shall not be removed from warehouse until released

by the custom house authorities, who shall examine it with reference
to its purity and fitness for consumption ; and that for the purpose of
such examination samples of each line in every invoice shall be submitted by the importer or consignee to the examiner, with his written
statement that such samples represent the true quality of each and
every part of the invoice, and accord with the specification therein
contained ; and in case the examiner has reason to believe that such
samples do not represent the true quality of the invoice, he shall make
such further examination of the tea represented by the invoice, or any
part thereof, as shall be necessary : Provided, That such further examination of such tea shall be made within three days after entry
thereof has been made at the custom house : And provided further,
That the bond above required shall also be conditioned for the payment of all custom house charges which may attach to such merchandise prior to being released or destroyed (as the case may be)
under the provisions of this Act.

3. That if, after an examination, as provided in section two, the tea
is found by the examiner not to come within the prohibition of this
Act, a permit shall at once be granted to the importer or consignee
declaring the tea free from the control of the custom authorities ; but
if on examination such tea, or merchandise described as tea, is found,
in the opinion of the examiner, to come within the prohibitions of this
Act, the importer or consignee shall be immediately notified, and the
tea, or merchandise described as tea, so returned shall not be released
by the custom house, unless on a re-examination called for by the
importer or consignee, the return of the examiner shall be found
erroneous : Provided, That should a portion of the invoice be passed
by the examiner, a permit shall be granted for that portion, and the
remainder held for further examination, as provided in section four.

4. That in case of any dispute between the importer or consignee
and the examiner, the matter in dispute shall be referred for arbitration
to a committee of three experts, one to be appointed by the collector,
one by the importer, and the two to choose a third, and their decision
shall be final ; and if upon such final re-examination the tea shall be
found to come within the prohibitions of this Act, the importer or
consignee shall give a bond, with securities satisfactory to the collector, to export such tea, or merchandise described as tea, out of the
limits of the United States, within a period of six months after such
final re-examination ; but if the same shall not have been exported
within the time specified, the collector, at the expiration of that time
shall cause the same to be destroyed.

5. That the examination and appraisement herein provided for shall
be made by a duly qualified appraiser of the port at which said tea is
entered, and when entered at ports where there are no appraisers,
such examination and appraisement shall be made by the revenue

officers to whom is committed the collection of duties, unless the Secretary of the Treasury shall otherwise direct.

6. That leaves to which the term "exhausted" is applied in this Act shall mean and include any tea which has been deprived of its proper quality, strength, or virtue by steeping, infusion, decoction, or other means.

7. That teas actually on shipboard for shipment to the United States at the time of the passage of this Act shall not be subject to the prohibition thereof.

8. That the Secretary of the Treasury shall have the power to enforce the provisions of this Act by appropriate regulations.

Approved, March 2, 1883.

The following is the text of the California Wine Adulteration Law, passed Feb. 17th, 1887 :—

The People of the State of California, represented in Senate and Assembly, do enact as follows :—

SECTION 1. For the purposes of this Act, pure wine shall be defined as follows : The juice of grapes fermented, preserved, or fortified for use as a beverage, or as a medicine, by methods recognised as legitimate according to the provisions of this Act; unfermented grape juice, containing no addition of distilled spirits, may be denominated according to popular custom and demand as wine only when described as "unfermented wine," and shall be deemed pure only when preserved for use as a beverage or medicine, in accordance with the provisions of this Act. Pure grape must shall be deemed to be the juice of grapes, only, in its natural condition, whether expressed or mingled with the pure skins, seeds, or stems of grapes. Pure condensed grape must shall be deemed to be pure grape must from which water has been extracted by evaporation for purposes of preservation or increase of saccharine strength. Dry wine is that produced by complete fermentation of saccharine contained in must. Sweet wine is that which contains more or less saccharine appreciable to the taste. Fortified wine is that wine to which distilled spirits have been added to increase alcoholic strength, for purposes of preservation only, and shall be held to be pure, when the spirits so used are the product of the grape only. Pure champagne or sparkling wine is that which contains carbonic acid gas or effervescence produced only by natural fermentation of saccharine matter of musts, or partially fermented wine in bottle.

2. In the fermentation, preservation, and fortification of pure wine,

it shall be specifically understood that no materials shall be used
intended as substitutes for grapes, or any part of grapes ; no colouring
matters shall be added which are not the pure products of grapes
during fermentation, or by extraction from grapes with the aid of pure
grape spirits ; no foreign fruit juices, and no spirits imported from
foreign countries, whether pure or compounded with fruit juices, or
other material not the pure product of grapes, shall be used for any
purpose ; no aniline dyes, salicylic acid, glycerine, alum, or other
chemical antiseptics, or ingredients recognised as deleterious to the
health of consumers, or as injurious to the reputation of wine as pure,
shall be permitted ; and no distilled spirits shall be added except for
the sole purpose of preservation, and without the intention of enabling
trade to lengthen the volume of fortified dry wine by the addition of
water, or other wine weaker in alcoholic strength.

3. In the fermentation and preservation of pure wine, and during
the operations of fining or clarifying, removing defects, improving
qualities, blending and maturing, no methods shall be employed which
essentially conflict with the provisions of the preceding sections of this
Act, and no materials shall be used for the promotion of fermentation,
or the assistance of any of the operations of wine treatment which are
injurious to the consumer or the reputation of wine as pure ; *provided*,
that it shall be expressly understood that the practices of using pure
tannin in small quantities, leaven to excite fermentation only, and not
to increase the material for the production of alcohol ; water before or
during, but not after fermentation, for the purpose of decreasing the
saccharine strength of musts to enable perfect fermentation ; and the
natural products of grapes in the pure forms as they exist in pure
grape musts, skins, and seeds ; sulphur fumes, to disinfect cooperage
and prevent disease in wine ; and pure gelatinous and albuminous
substances, for the sole purpose of assisting fining or clarification, shall
be specifically permitted in the operations hereinbefore mentioned, in
accordance with recognised legitimate custom.

4. It shall be unlawful to sell, or expose, or offer to sell under the
name of wine, or grape musts, or condensed musts, or under any names
designating pure wines, or pure musts as hereinbefore classified and
defined, or branded, labelled, or designated in any way as wine or
musts, or by any name popularly and commercially used as a designation of wine produced from grapes, such as claret, burgundy, hock,
sauterne, port, sherry, madeira, and angelica, any substance, or compound, except pure wine, or pure grape must, or pure grape condensed
must, as defined by this Act, and produced in accordance with and
subject to restrictions herein set forth ; *provided*, that this Act shall
not apply to liquors imported from any foreign country, which are
taxed upon entry by custom laws in accordance with a specific duty
and contained in original packages or vessels and prominently

branded, labelled, or marked so as to be known to all persons as foreign products, excepting, however, when such liquors shall contain adulterations of artificial colouring matters, antiseptic chemicals, or other ingredients known to be deleterious to the health of consumers; *and provided further*, that this Act shall not apply to currant wine, gooseberry wine, or wines made from other fruits than the grape, which are labelled or branded and designated and sold, or offered or exposed for sale under names, including the word wine, but also expressing distinctly the fruit from which they are made, as gooseberry wine, elderberry wine, or the like. Any violation of any of the provisions of any of the preceding sections shall be a misdemeanour.

5. Exceptions from the provisions of this Act shall be made in the case of pure champagne, or sparkling wine, so far as to permit the use of crystallised sugar in sweetening the same according to usual custom, but in no other respect.

6. In all sales and contracts for sale, production, or delivery of products defined in this Act, such products, in the absence of a written agreement to the contrary, shall be presumed to be pure as herein defined, and such sale or contracts shall, in the absence of such an agreement, be void, if it be established that the products so sold or contracted for were not pure as herein defined. And in such case the concealment of the true character of such products shall constitute actual fraud for which damages may be recovered, and in a judgment for damages, reasonable attorney fees to be fixed by the Court, shall be taxed as costs.

7. The Controller of the State shall cause to have engraved plates, from which shall be printed labels which shall set forth that the wine covered by such labels is pure California wine in accordance with this Act, and leaving blanks for the name of the particular kind of wine, and the name or names of the seller of the wine and place of business. These labels shall be of two forms or shapes, one a narrow strip to cap over the corks of bottles, the other, round or square, and sufficiently large, say three inches square, to cover the bungs of packages in which wine is sold. Such labels shall be furnished upon proper application to actual residents, and to be used in this State only, and only to those who are known to be growers, manufacturers, traders, or handlers, or bottlers of California wine, and such parties will be required to file a sworn statement with said Controller, setting forth that his or their written application for such labels is and will be for his or their sole use and benefit, and that he or they will not give, sell, or loan such label to any other person or persons whomsoever. Such labels shall be paid for at the same rate and price as shall be found to be the actual cost price to the State, and shall be supplied from time to time as needed upon the written application of such parties as are before mentioned. Such label when affixed to bottle or wine package

shall be so affixed, that by drawing the cork from bottle or opening the bung of package, such label shall be destroyed by such opening; and before affixing such labels all blanks shall be filled out by stating the variety or kind of wine that is contained in such bottle or package, and also by the name or names and Post Office address of such grower, manufacturer, trader, handler, or bottler of such wine.

8. It is desired and required that all and every grower, manufacturer, trader, handler, or bottler of California wine, when selling or putting up for sale any California wine, or when shipping California wine to parties to whom sold, shall plainly stencil, brand, or have printed where it will be easily seen, first, " Pure California Wine," and secondly his name, or the firm's name, as the case may be, both on label of bottle or package in which wine is sold and sent, or he may, in lieu thereof, if he so prefers and elects, affix the label which has been provided for in section seven. It shall be unlawful to affix any such stamp or label as above provided to any vessel containing any substance other than pure wine, as herein defined, or to prepare or use on any vessel containing any liquid any imitation or counterfeit of such stamp, or any paper in the similitude or resemblance thereof, or any paper of such form and appearance as to be calculated to mislead or deceive any unwary person, or cause him to suppose the contents of such vessel to be pure wine. It shall be unlawful for any person or persons, other than the ones for whom such stamps were procured, to in any way use such stamps, or to have possession of the same. A violation of any of the provisions of this section shall be a misdemeanour, and punishable by fine of not less than fifty dollars and not more than five hundred dollars, or by imprisonment in the county jail for a term of not exceeding ninety days, or by both such fine and imprisonment. All moneys collected by virtue of prosecutions had against persons violating any provisions of this or any preceding sections shall go one half to the informer and one half to the District Attorney prosecuting the same.

9. It shall be the duty of the Controller to keep an account, in a book to be kept for that purpose, of all stamps, the number, design, time when, and to whom furnished. The parties procuring the same are hereby required to return to the Controller semi-annual statements under oath, setting forth the number used, and how many remain on hand. Any violation of this section, by the person receiving such stamps, is a misdemeanour.

10. It shall be the duty of any and all persons receiving such stamps to use the same only in their business, in no manner or in nowise to allow the same to be disposed of except in the manner authorised by this Act; to not allow the same to be used by any other person or persons. It shall be their duty to become satisfied that the wine contained in the barrels or bottles is all that said label imports as

defined by this Act. That they will use the said stamps only in this State, and shall not permit the same to part from their possession, except with the barrels, packages, or bottles upon which they are placed as provided by this Act. A violation of any of the provisions of this section is hereby made a felony.

12. This Act shall take effect and be in force ninety days after its passage.

INDEX.

A.

Acetous fermentation, 225
Acids, acetic, 146
—— butyric, 63
—— malic, 173
—— nitrous, 210
—— phosphoric, 147
—— picric, 153
—— salicylic, 149, 177
—— succinic, 174
—— sulphuric, 176, 227
—— tannic, 22, 174
—— tartaric, 102, 173
—— in beer, 146
—— —— butter, 63, 71
—— —— wine, 172
Adams' test for milk, 59
Adulteration, excuses for, 1
—— extent of, 5, 7
—— varieties of, 9, 10
Albuminoid ammonia, 207
Albuminoids in beer, 145
—— —— flour, 89
—— —— water, 207
Alcohol in beer, 143
—— —— bread, 94
—— —— liquors, 195
Alcoholometric tables, 144, 196
Alkaloids in beer, 150
—— —— flour, 91
—— —— milk, 62
Allspice, 253
Aloes, 152

Alum in baking powders, 102
—— —— bread, 98
—— —— flour, 92
American adulteration, 8
—— cheese, 85
—— wine, 158
Ammonia in water, 207
Amylic alcohol, 197
Annato in butter, 77
—— —— cheese, 86
Aniline dyes in wine, 178–183
Artesian wells in New York, 257
Artificial bitters in beer, 141
—— butter, 66
—— cheese, 85
—— coffee, 31–40
—— honey, 122
—— jelly, 256
—— liquors, 193
—— spices, 245
—— sugar, 105
—— tea, 19, 28
—— wine, 167
Ash of beer, 136
—— —— bread, 96
—— —— chicory, 35
—— —— cocoa, 44
—— —— coffee, 31, 35
—— —— flour, 89
—— —— milk, 52
—— —— mustard, 242
—— —— pepper, 244
—— —— pickles, 232
—— —— sugar, 110

Ash of tea, 16, 22
——— —— wine, 175
Asparagus, 254

B.

Bacteria in water, 220
Bakers' chemicals, 101
Baking powders, 102
Banana essence, 129
Barley malt, 132
Beans in coffee, 31
Beech leaves in tea, 18
Beer, 132
—— adulteration of, 137
—— acids in, 146
—— alcohol in, 142
—— albuminoids in, 145
—— alkaloids in, 150
—— American, 134
—— analysis of, 142
—— ash of, 136, 147
—— bitters in, 137, 141
—— carbonic acid in, 143
—— composition of, 135
—— extract of, 134, 144
—— flavourings for, 137
—— glucose in, 138
—— glycerine in, 150
—— lager, 134
—— malt substitutes in, 138
—— manufacture of, 133
—— phosphates in, 147
—— picric acid in, 153
—— picrotoxine in, 153
—— production of, 134
—— salicylic acid in, 149
—— salt in, 147
—— soda in, 140
—— standards for, 148
—— sugar in, 144
—— sulphites in, 156
—— Wittstein's test for, 151
—— varieties of, 133
Bees' wax, 128
Bibliography, 258

Biological examination of water, 216
Bitters in beer, 141
Bleaching of flour, 90
——— —— sugar, 108
Blending of beer, 140
——— liquors, 185
——— wine, 164
Blue pigments, 14, 107
Boards of Health, 6
Borax in milk, 61
Bouquet of liquors, 187
——— —— wine, 164
Brandy, 186
Bread, 94
—— aerated, 95
—— alcohol in, 94
—— alum in, 98
—— analysis of, 97
—— ash of, 96
—— composition of, 96
—— salt in, 96
—— soda in, 95
—— starch in, 96
—— water in, 96
Brewing in the United States, 134
Butter, 63
—— acids in, 71
—— adulteration of, 66
—— analysis of, 65
—— Angell & Hehner's test, 72
—— annato in, 77
—— artificial, 66
—— ash of, 65
—— carrotin in, 77
—— colouring of, 77
—— composition of, 63
—— examination of, 65, 68
—— fat crystals in, 79
—— fusing point of, 63, 69
—— gelatine in, 76
—— Hübl's process for, 75
—— Koettstorfer's process for, 71
—— microscopic appearance of, 78
—— oleomargarine in, 66
—— photomicrographs of 78

322 INDEX.

Butter, Reichert's process for, 73
—— saffron in, 77
—— salt in, 65
—— soluble acids in, 71
—— specific gravity of, 67
—— tests for purity of, 70
—— volatile acids in, 71
—— water in, 65
Butterine, 66, 67
Butter fat, melting point, 69
—— —— specific gravity, 68
Butyric acid, 63
—— alcohol, 188
—— ether, 187

C.

Caffeine, 21, 39
California wine, 158, 160
Cane sugar, 104
Canned vegetables, 254
Capsicum, 229
Carbohydrates, 99
Carbonic acid, 95, 143
Carotine, 77
Caseine, 50, 85
Cassia, 252
Cayenne pepper, 247
Cereals in coffee, 31, 34
Cheese, 83
—— adulteration of, 85
—— American, 84
—— analysis, 86
—— artificial, 85
—— composition of, 83
—— fats in, 84
—— lard, 85
—— varieties of, 83, 84
Chicory, 31
—— ash, 35
—— colouring power of, 34
—— extract, 38
—— in coffee, 32, 34
—— sugar in, 37
—— tests for, 32
Chlorine in water, 206

Chocolate, 42
—— ash of, 45
—— fats in, 45
—— flavourings for, 42
—— flour in, 42
—— sugar in, 45
Chrome yellow in coffee, 40
—— —— —— candy, 131
Cider vinegar, 230
Cinnamon, 253
Cloves, 252
Coal-tar colours in candy, 130
—— —— —— mustard, 240
—— —— —— wine, 178, 183
Cocoa, 42
—— adulteration of, 42, 45
—— analysis of, 45
—— composition of, 43
—— starch in, 42
—— theobromine in, 44
Cocoanut oil in butter, 73
Coffee, 29
—— adulteration of, 31
—— analysis of, 30
—— artificial, 31, 40
—— ash of, 31, 35
—— caffeine in, 39
—— cereals in, 31, 34
—— chicory in, 31, 32
—— colouring of, 40
—— composition of, 30
—— density of infusion, 33
—— examination of, 32
—— extract of, 31
—— facing of, 40
—— fat in, 30
—— sugar in, 37, 38
—— tests for purity of, 32, 33
Cognac essence, 193
—— oil, 193
Colouring agents, 15, 77, 130
—— —— aniline, 130
—— —— annato, 77
—— —— carrotin, 77
—— —— gypsum, 14

Colouring agents, indigo, 14
—— —— lead, 131
—— —— logwood, 178
—— —— Martius' yellow, 77
—— —— mineral, 15
—— —— Prussian blue, 15
—— —— saffron, 77
—— —— turmeric, 15, 77
—— —— vegetable, 130
—— —— Venetian red, 40
Cocculus indicus, 153
Condensed milk, 53
Confectionery, 129
Copper in grains, 255
—— —— pickles, 232

D.

Dairy Commissioner, 50
Darnel in flour, 90
Dextrine, 24, 146
Dextrose, 105
Dialysis, 180, 183
Diastase, 132
Digestion of alumed bread, 98
—— —— butter, 82
—— —— oleomargarine, 82

E.

Elaidin test, 234
Elm leaves, 18
Ergot in flour, 90
Essences, artificial, 129
Ethers, 129, 174

F.

Facing of coffee, 40
—— —— tea, 15
Fats in butter, 63, 71
—— —— chocolate, 46
—— —— crystals, 79
—— fixed, 73
—— insoluble, 71
—— milk, 57
—— soluble, 71, 73

Fats, volatile, 73
Fehling's test, 37, 111
Feser's lactoscope, 57
Flavourings for beer, 137
—— —— candy, 129
—— —— chocolate, 42
—— —— liquors, 194
—— —— wine, 165
Flour, 88
—— adulteration of, 90
—— albuminoids in, 89
—— alkaloids in, 91
—— alum in, 90, 92
—— analysis of, 89
—— ash of, 89
—— composition of, 87
—— fungi in, 91
—— gluten in, 89
—— phosphates in, starch in, 89
—— tests for, 92
—— water in, 89
Forchammer's test, 203
Frankland's method, 211
Fruit, canned, 254
—— essences, 129
—— wine, 168
Fusel oil in candy, 129
—— —— liquors, 197

G.

Gall's method for wine, 162
Gelatine in butter, 76
Gentian in beer, 150
Gin, 191
Ginger, 253
Glucose, commercial, 105
—— estimation of, 111
—— in beer, 138
—— in honey, 124
—— in wine, 171
—— manufacture of, 105
—— tests for, 110, 124
Gluten in flour, 89
Glycerine in beer, 150
—— —— wine, 171

Granules of starch, 100
Gypsum in sugar, 110
——— —— tea, 14
—— —— wine, 163, 176

H.
Honey, 121
—— adulteration of, 122
—— analysis of, 124
—— artificial, 122
—— ash of, 123
—— comb, 122, 128
—— glucose in, 123
—— sugar in, 123
—— water in, 123
Hop-substitutes, 137, 150
Hordeine, 133
Hawthorn leaves, 18
Hubl's test, 75

I.
Ice, impure, 224
Indigo, 14, 19, 40, 129
Iodine test, 99

J.
Jellies, 256

K.
Kœttstorfer's test, 71

L.
Lactometer, 53, 54
Lactoscope, 57
Levulose, 107
Lard cheese, 85
Leaves in tea, 17, 18
Legislation, 268
Liquors, 186
—— adulteration of, 192
Logwood test, 92

M.
Mace, 253
Malic acid, 173
Malt, 132, 137

Maltose, 107
Malt substitutes in beer, 137, 148
Maple sugar, 109
Marble dust, 131
Marc of wines, 157
Martius' yellow, 77, 240
Meat extracts, 255
Micro-organisms in water, 214
Microscopic examination of butter, 78
—— —— coffee, 40
—— —— fats, 78, 79
—— —— milk, 61
—— —— spices, 246
—— —— starches, 100
—— —— tea, 17
—— —— water, 216
Milk, 49
—— Adam's method for, 59
—— adulteration of, 49
—— analysis of, 53
—— ash of, 52
—— caseine in, 59
—— composition of, 51
—— condensed, 53
—— cream in, 57
—— fats in, 57
—— globules, 61
—— nitrites in, 62
—— photo-micrographs of, 61
—— ptomaines in, 62
—— skimmed, 50
—— specific gravity of, 53, 55
—— standards for, 59–60
—— sugar of, 59
—— total solids, 58
—— water in, 56
Miscellaneous adulteration, 254
Molasses, 105
Moore's test for carotine, 77
Mustard, 239
—— adulteration of, 240
—— analysis of, 241
—— ash of, 242
—— colouring of, 240

Mustard, composition of, 239
—— flour in, 240
—— oil of, 241
—— sulphur in, 241

N.

Nessler's solution, 208
Nitrates in water, 210
Nitrites in milk, 62
—— —— vinegar, 231
—— —— water, 210
Nitrogen in flour, 89
—— —— tea, 21
—— —— water, 210

O.

Oenanthic ether, 158
Oils, bitter almond, 129
—— cocoanut, 73
—— cognac, 193
—— cotton seed, 234, 236
—— fusel, 197
—— lard, 68
—— mustard, 241
—— nut, 235
—— olive, 233
—— poppy, 235
—— rape seed, 236
—— sesamé, 236
—— turpentine, 191
Oleic acid, 63
Oleomargarine, 66
—— composition of, 67
—— digestion of, 82
—— effects of, 80, 81
—— exportation of, 66
—— manufacture of, 66
—— photo-micrographs of, 79
—— tests for, 70
Olive oil, 233
—— —— adulteration of, 233
—— —— American, 233
—— —— cotton seed oil in, 236
—— —— examination of, 234

Olive oil, specific gravity of, 234
—— —— standard for, 237
Organisms in ice, 219
—— —— water, 217

P.

Pepper, 243
—— adulteration of, 244
—— analysis of, 245
—— ash of, 244
—— cayenne, 247
—— composition of, 243
—— starch in, 246
Pepperette, 248
Phosphates in beer, 147
—— —— bread, 89
—— —— wine, 176
Photogravures of leaves, 18
—— —— water, 217
—— —— polariscope, 112
—— —— tea, 17
—— —— tea plant, *Frontispiece.*
Photo-micrographs of butter, 79
—— —— cream, 61
—— —— digestion of fats, 82
—— —— fats, 79
—— —— milk, 61
—— —— oleomargarine, 79
—— —— spices, 252
—— —— starches, 100
Pickles, 232
Picric acid, 153
Polariscope, 112
Polarisation of beer, 148
—— —— honey, 123
—— —— glucose, 118
—— —— lactose, 59
—— —— sugar, 112
—— —— wine, 171
Poplar leaves, 18
Preservatives in beer, 149, 156
—— —— butter, 77
—— —— milk, 61
—— —— wine, 177

Preserved milk, 53
Prussian blue in candy, 131
—— —— coffee, 40
—— —— tea, 14
Ptomaines in ice cream, 62
—— —— milk, 62

Q.

Quassia in beer, 152

R.

Raisin wine, 168
Reichert's test, 73
"Rock and rye" drops, 129
Rose leaves, 18
Rum, 190

S.

St. Andrew's cross in fats, 79
Sal aeratus, 101
Salicine in beer, 137
Salt in beer, 147
—— —— butter, 65
Salicylic acid in beer, 149
—— —— wine, 175
Sand in tea, 14
Soda water syrups, 257
Specific gravity of beer, 142
—— —— butter, 63, 68
—— —— fats, 68
—— —— milk, 50, 53
—— —— oils, 232
—— —— spirits, 185–189
—— —— tables, 55, 144, 145, 196
—— —— vinegar, 226
—— —— wine, 159
Spices, 249
—— microscopic examination of, 249
Standards for beer, 148
—— —— butter, 72, 74, 75
—— —— cocoa, 46
—— —— milk, 59, 60
—— —— tea, 25
—— —— water, 213, 214

Standards for wine, 184
Starch, 99
—— estimation of, 99
—— granules, 100
—— in mustard, 240
—— in pepper, 246
—— photo-micrographs of, 100
—— in spices, 252
Strychnine in beer, 151
Sugar, 104
—— adulteration of, 107
—— analysis of, 109
—— ash of, 110
—— cane, 104
—— fruit, 105
—— grape, 105, 119
—— invert, 104
—— malt, 107
—— maple, 109
—— milk, 59, 107
—— tin salts in, 107
Sulphates in wine, 176
Sulphuric acid in vinegar, 228
—— —— wine, 176
Syrups, adulteration of, 108
—— glucose, 108

T.

Tables, of adulteration, 10
—— alcoholometric, 144
—— coffee infusion, 33
—— lactometric, 55
—— malt extract, 145
—— specific gravity, 55, 143, 196
Tannic acid in tea, 22
—— —— in wine, 174
Tartar, cream of, 101
—— —— in wine, 173
Tartaric acid in baking powder, 103
—— —— in wine, 173
Tea, 12
—— adulteration of, 14
—— analysis of, 21, 26, 27
—— ash of, 16, 17, 22

Tea, Ching Suey, 28
—— colouring of, 14
—— composition of, 15
—— dust, 16
—— examination of, 21
—— extract of, 23
—— facing of, 15
—— factitious, 19, 28
—— foreign leaves in, 14, 18
—— gypsum in, 14
—— gum in, 24
—— indigo in, 19
—— insoluble ash in, 23
—— —— leaf in, 28
—— leaves, 7, 17, 18
—— lie, 19
—— microscopic examination of, 18
—— Ping Suey, 8
—— sand in, 14
—— soapstone in, 19
—— soluble ash, 23
—— South American, 26
—— spent, 15
—— standards for, 25
—— tannin in, 22
—— theine in, 21
—— volatile oil in, 22
Te-mo-ki leaves, 18
Theine in tea, 21
Tin in canned fruits, 254
Tin salts in sugar, 107

U.

Ultramarine in sugar, 107

V.

Vanilla in chocolate, 42
Vegetables, canned, 254
Vinegar, 225
—— adulteration of, 229
—— analysis of, 227
—— cider, 230
—— extract of, 227
—— malt, 226

Vinegar, standards for, 227
—— sulphuric acid in, 228
—— whisky, 230
—— wine, 226
Volatile acids in butter, 73
—— ethers in wine, 174

W.

Water, 200
—— albuminoid ammonia in, 207
—— American supply, 220
—— bacteria in, 216
—— biological examination of, 216
—— carbon in, 212
—— chlorine in, 206
—— croton, 219
—— examination of, 201
—— Forchammer's process, 203
—— Frankland's process, 211
—— free ammonia in, 207
—— Hudson river, 222
—— microscopic examination of, 216
—— nitrates in, 210
—— nitrites in, 210
—— nitrogen in, 210
—— organic matter in, 203
—— organisms in, 219
—— sewage in, 207, 210
—— standards for, 213
—— total solids in, 202
—— urea in, 207
—— Wanklyn's process, 207
Wheat, 87
Wheaten flour, 87
—— starch, 88, 100
Whey, 50
Whisky, 188
—— vinegar, 230
Willow leaves, 18
Wine, 157
—— acids in, 172
—— adulteration of, 163
—— alcohol in, 169
—— American, 158

Wine, ash of, 175
—— blending of, 164
—— California, 160
—— colouring of, 166, 178
—— ethers in, 174
—— examination of, 169
—— extract of, 170
—— fruit, 168
—— glycerine in, 170
—— imitation, 167
—— improving, 161
—— malic acid in, 173
—— natural, 160
—— Pasteuring, 161
—— Petiot's process, 161
—— phosphoric acid in, 176
—— plastering of, 163

Wine, polarisation of, 171
—— raisin, 168
—— salicylic acid in, 177
—— Scheele's process for, 162
—— standards for, 184
—— succinic acid in, 174
—— sulphates in, 176
—— sulphurous acid in, 177
—— sugar in, 170
—— table of, 159
—— tannin in, 174
—— tartrates in, 178
—— tartaric acid in, 173
—— varieties of, 159
Willow leaves, 18
Wisteria —— 18

PRINTED BY E. AND F. N. SPON, NEW YORK AND LONDON.

www.ingramcontent.com/pod-product-compliance
Lightning Source LLC
Chambersburg PA
CBHW021107270326
41929CB00009B/768